Headache Medicine

Headache Medicine

Edited by Roy Harrington

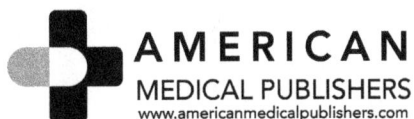

AMERICAN
MEDICAL PUBLISHERS
www.americanmedicalpublishers.com

American Medical Publishers,
41 Flatbush Avenue,
1st Floor, New York,
NY 11217, USA

Visit us on the World Wide Web at:
www.americanmedicalpublishers.com

ISBN: 978-1-63927-299-0

Cataloging-in-Publication Data

Headache medicine / edited by Roy Harrington.
    p. cm.
Includes bibliographical references and index.
ISBN 978-1-63927-299-0
1. Headache. 2. Head--Diseases. 3. Head--Diseases--Treatment. 4. Pain. I. Harrington, Roy.
RC392 .H43 2022
616.849 1--dc23

Table of Contents

Preface

Every book is initially just a concept; it takes months of research and hard work to give it the final shape in which the readers receive it. In its early stages, this book also went through rigorous reviewing. The notable contributions made by experts from across the globe were first molded into patterned chapters and then arranged in a sensibly sequential manner to bring out the best results.

Headache is the pain in the face, head or neck. It can occur as a migraine, tension-type headache or cluster headache. There are various causes of headache. These include dehydration, fatigue, sleep deprivation, stress, the effects of medications, the effects of recreational drugs, viral infections, loud noises, common colds, head injury, etc. In severe headaches, there is a high risk of depression. Its treatment depends on the underlying cause. Oral medications such as non-steroidal anti-inflammatory drugs are commonly used for the treatment of headaches. Complementary strategies such as cognitive behavioral therapy, relaxation training, electromyographic feedback, etc. may also be used for the management of headache. The topics included in this book on headache medicine are of utmost significance and bound to provide incredible insights to readers. The topics included in this book on headache medicine are of utmost significance and bound to provide incredible insights to readers. It is compiled in such a manner, that it will provide an in-depth knowledge about the incidence of headaches, their diagnosis and treatment. This book is a resource guide for experts as well as students.

It has been my immense pleasure to be a part of this project and to contribute my years of learning in such a meaningful form. I would like to take this opportunity to thank all the people who have been associated with the completion of this book at any step.

Editor

Paroxysmal hemicrania: a retrospective study of a consecutive series of 22 patients and a critical analysis of the diagnostic criteria

Sanjay Prakash[1*], Pooja Belani[2], Ashish Susvirkar[2], Aditi Trivedi[2], Sunil Ahuja[3] and Animesh Patel[3]

Abstract

Background: Paroxysmal hemicrania (PH) is a probably underreported primary headache disorder. It is characterized by repeated attacks of severe, strictly unilateral pain lasting 2 to 30 minutes localized to orbital, supraorbital, and temporal areas accompanied by ipsilateral autonomic features. The hallmark of PH is the absolute cessation of the headache with indomethacin. However, these all features may not be present in all cases and a few cases may remain unclassified according to the 2nd Edition of The International classification of Headache Disorders (ICHD-II) criteria for PH.

Methods: Twenty-two patients were included in this retrospective observation.

Results: We describe 17 patients, observed over six years, who fulfilled the ICHD-II criteria for PH. In parallel, we identified five more patients in whom one of the features of the diagnostic criteria for PH was missing. Two patients did not show any evidence of cranial autonomic feature during the attacks of headache. Another two patients did not fulfill the criteria for PH as the maximum attack frequency was less than five. One patient had an incomplete response to indomethacin.

Conclusion: A subset of patients may not have all the defined features of PH and there is a need for refinement of the existing diagnostic criteria.

Keywords: Chronic daily headache, Paroxysmal hemicrania, Hemicrania continua, Cluster headache

Background

Paroxysmal hemicrania (PH) is a rare primary headache disorder. It is classified in group 3 of the 2nd Edition of The International classification of Headache Disorders (ICHD-II) along with other trigeminal autonomic cephalalgias (TACs). The characteristic features of PH are: (a) repeated attacks of severe unilateral, orbital, supraorbital or temporal pain lasting for 2–30 min; (b) at least one ipsilateral cranial autonomic feature; (c) attacks frequency > 5 per day for more than half of the time, (d) complete response to therapeutic doses of indomethacin. All four characteristic features are essential to satisfy the ICHD-II criteria for PH [1]. However, a few patients may have atypical presentation [2,3].

Herein, in a retrospective study, we report 17 patients who fulfilled the ICHD-II criteria for PH. In parallel, we identified a group of patients (5 patients) who met all criteria minus one (either absence of cranial autonomic features or headache frequency < 5 per day or complete response to indomethacin).

Methods

We performed a retrospective chart review of all patients with a putative diagnosis of PH, seen in the neurology department at our institute from February 2006 to July 2012. The patients having a diagnosis of PH or PH like headache and with a minimum follow-up of 3 months duration were included in the study. We reviewed the charts of each individual. A few patients were interviewed by telephone to complete the follow-up. Exclusion criteria were: (a) a possible secondary PH; (b) patients who were never subjected for neuroimaging, as we did not rule out the possibility of

* Correspondence: drprakashs@yahoo.co.in
[1]Department of Neurology, Medical College, O-19, doctor's quarter, jail road, Baroda, Gujarat 390001, India
Full list of author information is available at the end of the article

secondary PH in these patients; and (c) a follow-up of < 3 months duration. The study did not require approval by the local ethics committee as per the local regulations for retrospective observation. The majority of patients were seen and examined by a neurologist (SP). The patients fulfilling the ICHD-II criteria for PH were tabulated. Data are presented as percentages or as arithmetic mean with SD. Student's t-test was used to compare the continuous data between the subgroups. The chi-square test with Yates's correction was used for categorical data. A p-value < 0.05 was defined as statistically significant. Patients with atypical features were tabulated separately.

Results

A total of 28 patients were identified with a putative diagnosis of PH or PH-like headache. One patient was excluded because of the possibility of secondary PH (pituitary adenoma). One patient was never subjected to neuroimaging and was excluded from the final analyses. Two other patients were excluded because of the incomplete follow-up (< 3 months). Two patients were excluded because of the incomplete data entry. Finally, twenty-two patients were identified. Seventeen patients (77%) fulfilled the ICHD-II criteria for PH. Two patients (9%) did not show any evidence of cranial autonomic features. Two patients (9%) did not fulfill the criteria for PH as the maximum attack frequency was less than five. One patient (5%) did not show a complete response to indomethacin.

Epidemiological profiles, and clinical features of patients fulfilling the criteria for PH (17 patients) are noted in Table 1. Patients with atypical features (with no cranial autonomic features or headache frequency < 5 per day or incomplete response to indomethacin) were summarized separately in Table 2.

Epidemiological and clinical features of patients fulfilling the ICHD-II criteria for PH

The mean age of participants was 38 years, 53% were female. The mean illness duration was 38.2 ± 38.1 months. All patients had strictly unilateral pain. None of the patients reported bilateral or side-shifting pain. All patients reported pain in the distribution defined in the ICHD-II diagnostic criteria for PH. Orbital/retro orbital was the most common site of pain (88%). Temporal and frontal regions were two other common sites of pain. Two patients (12%) reported pain even in the neck. All patients had at least one autonomic feature as defined in the diagnostic criteria for PH. However, autonomic features were not consistent in each attack in every patient. Only six patients (35%) reported autonomic features in each or most of the attacks. In five patients (29%), cranial autonomic features were noted in less than half of the attacks.

Table 1 Epidemiological and clinical features of patients with parosysmal hemicrania

Parameters	(n-17)
Age (years)(mean, range)	38 ± 12.3, 21–60
Sex (M:F)	1:1.1 (8:9)
Duration of illness	
Mean (SD)	38.2 ± 38.1 months
Range	3 months-10 yrs
Median	18 months
Laterality, n (%)	
Rt	8 (47)
Lt	9 (53)
Course, n (%)	
Chronic	15 (88)
Episodic	2 (12)
Site of headache, n (%)	
Orbital\retroorbital	15(88)
Temporal	10 (59)
Frontal	10 (59)
Parieto-occipital	7 (41)
Infra- orbital /maxillary	4 (24)
Peri auricular	2 (12)
Neck	2 (12)
Character of pain	
Throbbing	9 (53)
Non throbbing	12 (71)
Both throbbing and non throbbing	4 (24)
Severe or very severe	15 (88)
Interictal pain	
Present	8 (47)
Intermittent	7 (41)
Continuous	1 (6)
Restlessness / agitation	13 (76)
Autonomic symptoms, n (%)	
Tearing	13 (76)
Conjunctival injection	11 (65)
Feeling of sand / itching in eye	8 (47)
Nasal stuffiness	7 (41)
Rhinorrhea	7 (41)
Ptosis	5 (29)
Lid edema	3 (18)
Miosis	1 (06)
Migrainous symptoms, n (%)	
At least one migrainous symptom	9 (53)
Nausea	5 (29)
Vomiting	1 (6)

Table 1 Epidemiological and clinical features of patients with parosysmal hemicrania (Continued)

Photophobia	4 (24)
Phonophobia	4 (24)
Co morbid conditions	
Hypertension	4(24)
Diabetes Mellitus	3(18)
Restless Leg Syndrome	1(6)
Follow up duration (months)	
(mean,SD, range)	12.5 ± 6.7, 3–24

Lacrimation (76%) and conjunctival injection (65%) were the two most common cranial autonomic features. Other common cranial autonomic features were feeling of sand/itching in the eye (47%), nasal stuffiness (41%), rhinorrhea (41%), and ptosis (29%).

Most patients (88%) reported their pain as severe or very severe. Only two patients (12%) reported their pain as moderately severe. Seventy-six percent patients used the word "excruciating" to define their pains. Fifty-three percent patients reported their pain as throbbing. Interictal pain was noted in eight (47%) patients. The ipsilateral interictal pain was mild in comparison to attack pain in all

patients. Most patients (7 out of 8 patients) had intermittent interictal pain. The diagnosis of hemicrania continua (HC) was not considered in these patients because of the mild and intermittent interictal pain. The frequency and duration of the attacks were in accordance with the diagnostic criteria for PH. Moreover, these all patients denied the presence of interictal pain during early periods of illness. In the subgroup analyses, we compared patients having interictal pain to the patients not having such background headache. There were statistically significant differences in two parameters (Table 3). The patients having interictal pain have a more chronic course (69.0 vs 10.7 months, p = 0.0006). The indomethacin dose requirement was also higher in patients with interictal pain (187.5 vs 113.9, p = 0.0018). There were no other differences between the groups (data not shown).

The usual duration of the attacks was between 2–30 minutes (in accordance to the ICHD-II criteria for PH) (Table 4). However, the duration of attacks varied between a few seconds to 3 hours. The longest attack duration was more than 30 min in four patients (24%). Two patients reported longest headache duration of 3 hours. The possibility of cluster headache (CH) was less likely in these patients as the overall duration of attacks (and frequency of attacks) were more compatible with the

Table 2 Atypical Cases of parosysmal hemicrania

	Case 1	Case 2	Case 3	Case 4	Case 5
Age	34	36	24	40	42
Sex	M	F	F	M	F
Duration of illness (months)	9	14	9	6	24
Course	Chronic	Chronic	Chronic	Chronic	Chronic
Laterality	Right	Left	Left	Right	Right
Site of pain	Orb, tem,	Orb, tem, front	Orb, tem	Orb, tem, front	Orb, tem,
Character of pain	Severe, throb, nonthrob	Severe non throb	Severe throb	Severe nonthrob	Severe throb,
Interictal pain	Yes	–	–	–	–
Autonomic features	–	–	lacri, conj	conj, rhin	Conj, lacri,
Migrainous features	nau, phot,	nau,	–	nau, phot, phon	–
Restlessness	yes	yes	yes	yes	yes
Nocturnal attacks	yes	yes	–	yes	yes
Frequency of attacks (range /day)	4–10	4–15	0–5	1–4	5–15
Duration of attacks	5–20 min	Few sec- 20 min	5–20 min	5–30 min	5–20 min
Response to indomethacin					
	Complete	Complete	Complete	Complete	Incomplete
Doses (mg/day)	150	75	150	75	225[*]
Days taken to show complete response	4	2	4	3	–
Side effects of indomethacin	pain abd,	–	Nau, vom	–	–

* = maximum tried dose.

abd: abdomen; *conj*: conjunctival injection; *front*: frontal; *lacri*: lacrimation; *nau*: nausea; *nonthrob*: nonthrobbing; *orb*: orbital; *phon*: phonophobia; *phot*: photophobia; *rhin*: rhinorrhea; *tem*: temporal; *throb*: throbbing; *vom*: vomiting.

Table 3 A comparison between patients with interictal pain to patients without interictal pain

Parameters	Interictal pain (n-8)	Without interictal pain (n-9)	p value
Duration of illness (months)	69.0 ± 40.0	10.7 ± 6.2	0.0006*
Indomethacin dose (mg/day)	187.5 ± 40.1	113.9 ± 39.7	0.0018*

* p = <0.005: significant.

diagnosis of PH. None of the patients showed any circadian periodicity. Absence of circadian rhythmicity and periodicity (clustering) also favors the diagnosis of PH.

The ICHD-II criteria for the frequency of attacks in PH are > 5 attacks per day for more than half of the time. All included patients fulfilled this criterion. The maximum attack frequencies in these 17 patients were 10–20 per day. The minimum attack frequencies were 0–5 per day. Three patients never had frequency of more than 5 attacks per day. We described it separately as atypical PH (Table 2). Nocturnal attacks were noted in 6 patients (35%). However, none of the patients reported nocturnal preponderance or periodicity. Agitation or a sense of restlessness was present in 13 patients (76%).

There was at least one migrainous feature of nausea, or vomiting, photophobia, or phonophobia in 9 (53%) patients.

Periodicity and chronicity of PH

PH is classified as episodic paroxysmal hemicrania (EPH) or chronic paroxysmal hemicrania (CPH) depending on the presence of a remission period. Fifteen (88%) patients had a chronic course. Fourteen of these patients had a chronic course since onset (primary chronic CPH). The headache began as EPH and transitioned to CPH in one patient. The course of headache was like primary EPH in two patients (12%).

Table 4 Durations and frequency of attacks in PH

Parameters	PH (n-17)
Durations of attacks	
< 2 minutes	7 (41%)
2–30 minutes	17 (100%)
> 30 minutes	4 (24%)
Attacks frequency	
>5/day for more than half of the time	17 (100%)
maximum attack frequency	10–20/day
minimum attack frequency	0–5/day
Nocturnal attacks	6 (35%)

Response to indomethacin

A response to indometacin is considered as a *sine qua non* in PH [1]. All patients responded to indomethacin. The details of response to indomethacin are summarized in Table 5. The mean effective daily dose of indomethacin was 149 mg (range 50–225). As noted earlier, the indomethacin dose requirement was higher in patients with interictal pain (187.5 vs 113.9, p = 0.0018). Fifteen patients (88%) showed a complete response in a week (7 days). Another two patients (12%) took 1–2 weeks to show the complete response to indomethacin. None of the patient was subjected to "indo" test because of the non availability of injectable indomethacin. Eight patients (47%) were subjected to tapering off indomethacin. Only one patient was successfully weaned off the drug. The patient did not have recurrence of headaches in the next 6 months follow up. There was no prior history of episodic pattern of PH in this patient. Sudden withdrawal of indomethacin (because of the side effects of indomethacin or poor compliance) was noted in 7 patients. Withdrawal of the drugs led to a recurrence of headaches within 2–10 days.

Prospectively, we gave topiramate to 4 patients. Topiramate was started because of the development of side effects of indomethacin. Two patients showed a complete response to the drug. Both the patients showed complete response at the dosage of 100 mg bid.

None of the patients received a correct diagnosis before reporting to us. Migraine (65%), cluster headache (59%) and atypical facial (35%) pain were the most common diagnoses. Various drugs have been used in the past in these patients. The details were not available for each drug

Table 5 Details of indomethacin used in patients with PH

Parameters	PH (n-17)
Indomethacin dose	
Mean ± SD (mg\daily)	149 ± 54
≤ 75 mg\daily	3 (18)
> 75–150 mg/daily	10 (59)
> 150–225 mg/daily	4 (23)
> 225 mg/daily	0 (0)
Time interval between indomethacin administration and complete response	
< 24 hrs	4 (23)
1–7 days	11 (65)
> 7 days	2 (12)
Side effects by indomethacin	
Nausea/vomiting	9 (53)
Abdominal pain	4 (23)
Diarrhea	2 (12)
Dizziness/vertigo	2 (12)
somnolence	1 (6)

in each patient. However, five patients responded partly (> 50%) to either verapamil (3 patients) or lithium (2 patients). These all four patients (diagnosed previously as CH) showed a complete response to indomethacin. Frequencies, duration, pattern (without periodicity) of the attacks were also more compatible with the diagnosis of PH.

Atypical paroxysmal hemicrania

We identified 5 patients in whom one of the features of the diagnostic criteria for PH was missing. We identified 2 patients with PH-like headaches without any cranial autonomic features. These 2 patients look like CPH, with respect to the frequency and duration of attacks and response to indomethacin. They fulfilled the ICHD-II diagnostic criteria for CPH, with the exception of autonomic symptoms. There was no better alternative diagnosis for these patients. We considered these patients as atypical or probable PH. In parallel, we identified 2 additional patients with PH-like headaches except the absence of the required number of the attacks per day to fulfill the ICHD-II criteria for PH. The ICHD-II criteria for the number of attacks per day are more than five attacks for more than half of the time. The attack frequency in these two patients was ≤ 5 / day. These 2 patients resemble CPH in respect to other features of PH according to the ICHD-II criteria. There was no better alternative diagnosis for these patients. We considered even these patients as atypical or probable PH. One patient fulfilled all the features of PH except the complete response to indomethacin. This patient showed marked improvement in frequency (5–15 /day to 0–5/day). The intensity and duration of attacks also reduced markedly. The patient had never felt such type of improvement with any drug in the past.

Discussion

Prevalence and other epidemiological feature

PH is considered as a rare primary headache disorder. It is suggested that cases of PH are probably overlooked or underreported [4]. PH was first described in 1974 [5]. In the first 15 yrs (up to 1989), a total 84 cases of PH were reported in the literature [6]. However, in the next 10 years (up to 1998), only 27 cases were reported [7]. In 2002, Boes and Dodick reported 74 patients with CPH (Goadsby and Lipton's criteria) [2]. Isolated PH cases are no longer reported now days [4]. However, the literature is scarce even for larger case series. During the last 12 years, only one large case series (31 patients) has been reported [8]. These suggest that cases of PH are underreported or overlooked.

In the early years, the prevalence of PH was estimated in relation to the prevalence of CH, and it was 0.9 to 3% [6]. This estimation was done by Antonaci and Sjasstad in 1989 (within the first 15 yrs of the discovery of the first case of PH) [6]. The authors predicted "this ratio may change considerably in the foreseeable future". After 1989, we noted at least two studies where PH was compared to CH. In 2002, Faud and Jones [9] reported 11 patients with PH. In parallel, they reported 30 patients with CH over the same period. The ratio of PH to CH was 30%. In the same way, this ratio was 15% in Zidverc-Trajkovic et al. study [10]. According to these two studies, the prevalence of PH (with respect to CH) may be more than 15% of CH. This indicates that PH is probably more common than it was anticipated earlier. Seidel et al. [11] reported 63 consecutive patients with unilateral headache not resembling migraine or CH. Only twenty-four patients received a diagnosis of primary headache disorders. Six of them had PH. Blankenburg [12] reported 8 children with PH among 628 children (1.3%) with chronic daily headache and suggested that PH is under diagnosed even in children. A possibility of misdiagnosis also exists. Initially, PH was considered as a disease of the female (2.3 to 7: 1) [4]. However, in Cittadini case series (31 patients), female preponderance was not obvious. The authors suggested that it may be because of mis-diagnosis of males with PH as cluster headache, as it is the more common with a distinct male preponderance. Our all patients were never diagnosed previously before reporting to us. This suggests that a possibility of mis-diagnosis or unawareness to PH may be very high.

Taken together, PH is probably an under diagnosed and underreported primary headache disorder. We observed 17 patients with PH (and 5 probable PH) over 6 years duration. Our case series is probably the third largest case series in the literature.

The mean age of onset (38 yrs) was comparable to other studies. In Cittadini et al. series [8], it was 37 yrs and in a review of 84 patients, mean age was 34 yrs [6]. PH is classically considered as a disease with female preponderance. However, in Cittadini et al. series [8], male outnumbered female (17 vs 14). In our series male: female was 1:1.1 (8 male vs 9 female). These two observations suggest that both male and female may be equally affected.

Duration and frequency of attacks

Seventeen patients fulfilled the criteria for PH. The closet differential diagnosis of PH is CH [4]. Clinical characteristics for both PH and CH is similar. PH is usually distinguished from other TACs by the duration and frequency of attacks and by a response to indomethacin in patients with PH [1,4]. However, as there is overlap in the diagnostic criteria for PH and CH, a possibility of misdiagnosis always exist in patients with PH and vice-versa [8,13]. Presence of indomethacin responsive CH may further complicate the issue [13].

In our all 17 cases of (typical) PH, duration and frequency of attacks were more compatible with the diagnosis of PH. All patients had headache duration between 5–30 minutes (as defined in the ICHD-II criteria for PH). Only four patients (24%) had a few headache attacks of more than 30 minutes. In Cittadini et al. series [8], 55% patients had the longest attack duration of more than 30 min. In Boes and Dodick case series [2], the maximum attack duration was more than 60 minutes in 41% patients. A patient may have a few attacks of many hours. This indicates that a few attacks in a patient may be more than of 30 minutes (an upper limit defined in ICHD-II criteria for PH). This may create diagnostic confusion, and a misdiagnosis as CH or migraine exists if patient or physician focuses mainly on maximum attack duration. Therefore, mean or average duration of the attacks should be considered in making the diagnosis of PH and other TACs.

In the same way, the frequency of attacks is also an important point in making the diagnosis of PH. More than 5 attacks per day for more than half of the time is essential to make the diagnosis of PH. All 17 patients (typical PH) fulfilled this criterion. The maximum attack frequency was ≥ 10 / day in all 17 patients. However, we observed 2 more patients who never had 5 or more attacks in a day. Other clinical features, including response to indomethacin were according to the ICHD-II criteria for PH. We considered these two patients as atypical PH. Although ICHD-II acknowledges the presence of lower frequency in patients with PH, ≥ 5 / day for more than half of the time is must to fulfill the criteria. In review of the literature, we noted a number of patients with the maximum attack frequency of < 5 / day. The maximum attack frequency was between 2 and 5 in 37% patients in Boes and Dodick case series [2]. In Cittadini case series [8], at least three patients had a maximum attack frequency of less than five in a day. In Zidverc-Trajkovic et al. observations [10], two patients (out of eight patients) had attack duration shorter than proposed by ICHD-II criteria. These observations suggest that a few patients may never have attack frequency of more than 5 in a day.

Cranial autonomic features
Patients with PH are required to have at least one of the cranial autonomic features according to ICHD-II criteria. Our three patients (16%) never had autonomic features. Two (4%) patients in Boes and Dodick case series [2] had no autonomic features. One patient in Cittadini case series had not any classical autonomic features and reported only a sense of ear fullness during the attacks. Maggioni [3] reported a case of episodic PH with no cranial autonomic feature and suggested a possibility of a subgroup of PH. Similar observations have also been noted in patients with CH and HC. Three to seven percent patients with CH may never have cranial autonomic features during CH attacks [14]. Various case series suggest that a large number of patients with HC may never have autonomic feature during the exacerbation of attacks [15]. Feeling of sand or itching in eye is classically described as an autonomic feature in patients with HC [15]. Our 8 patients (47%) mentioned the feeling of sand or itching in eye during the headache episodes. These observations need to be confirmed prospectively in other case series.

It is suggested that the presence of autonomic features is related to the intensity of the headaches [14]. Autonomic features are less likely to occur in patients with moderate to severe rather than excruciating attacks of pain. As the intensity of pain attacks in PH is much less than attacks of CH, absence of autonomic feature is possible even in patients with PH. ICHD-II acknowledges the diagnosis of CH in the absence of cranial autonomic features (if patient has restlessness) [1]. The similar suggestion has been given even for making the diagnosis of HC (i.e. HC should be diagnosed even in the absence of cranial autonomic feature) [15]. Therefore, we suggest that ICHD-II should acknowledge the diagnosis of PH even in the absence of autonomic symptoms.

Restlessness/agitation
Restlessness or agitation is classically described in patients with CH and it is one of the components of the ICHD-II diagnostic criteria for CH. It provides an alternative to make the diagnosis of CH even in the absence of autonomic feature. A few authors suggest that restlessness or agitation should also be included in the diagnostic criteria for HC [15,16]. Review of the literature suggests that restlessness or agitation may be noted in 50-90% of patients with PH. Our 76% reported restlessness or agitation. We suggest that like CH, restlessness / agitation should be included in the diagnostic criteria for PH, as it would provide alternative to make the diagnosis of PH in the absence of autonomic feature.

Lack of complete indomethacin response
A response to indometacin is considered as a *sine qua non* in PH. Our one patient had an incomplete response to indomethacin. In Boes and Dodick case series [2], 25% (10/40) patients did not exhibit responses to indomethacin. A few other patients (6 patients) had only a partial response to indomethacin. In the other two patients, a complete response to indomethacin was not sustained.

HC is another indomethacin responsive primary headache disorder. However, recent observations indicate that the indomethacin resistant HC is a distinct possibility [15,17,18]. In an earlier review, we suggested a possibility of under reporting of HC unresponsive to indomethacin, as it is difficult to classify such patients according to the present ICHD-II classification [18]. The same possibility may exist for PH unresponsive to indomethacin and it may be the reason for underreporting of PH in the literature. In a review, we noted that CH may be wrongly diagnosed as PH if patients with CH show a response to indomethacin [13]. Therefore, a possibility exists that PH unresponsive to indomethacin (especially borderline cases) can be diagnosed as CH. As the prevalence of CH is very high than PH, a possibility of misdiagnosis of PH as CH is more likely (than CH diagnosed as PH). Patients with PH also show response to lithium, verapamil, and topiramate. Therefore, a patient will not receive the diagnosis of PH, if a patient shows a response to another drug before a trial to indomethacin. Our five patients (29%) showed a partial response to lithium and verapamil (before a trial of indomethacin), and were labeled as CH. Prospectively our 2 patients showed a response to topiramate.

Interictal pain
Eight of 17 patients (47%) reported interictal pain. Seven of these (88%) had intermittent pain. This interparoxysmal pain was usually mild and was mainly described as discomfort in that area. The presence of interictal pain may create diagnostic confusion with HC [15]. However, "mild" and "intermittent" nature of interparoxysmal pain favors the diagnosis of PH. Moreover, frequency and duration of attacks were more compatible with the diagnosis of PH. Frequency and duration of the exacerbations in patients with HC are highly variable and duration of attacks frequently crosses the upper defined levels of PH (and CH) [15]. The exacerbations in a patient with HC vary between a few minutes to many hours (may be upto days) [15]. One patient reported continuous inteictal pain. The interictal pain was mild, and periodic exacerbations matched with the frequency and duration described for PH. Moreover, the patient did not have interictal pain during the early years of the disease.

We compared patients with interictal pain to patients with no such pain. The mean duration of illness was significantly higher in patients with interictal pain (69.0 vs 10.7 months, p = 0.0006). In the same way, patients with interictal pain required a high dose of indomethacin (188 vs 114 mg, p = 0.0018). These observations indicate that patients with longer duration of history are more likely to have interictal pain and these patients may require higher doses of indomethacin. Such type of observations was also noted in patients with CH [19]. In Marmura et al's case series [19], patients with a long history of disease were more likely to have interictal pain. The patients with a long history of disease and interictal pain were more refractory to the therapy. Various

mechanisms have been suggested for these observations. It is said that any longstanding chronic pain may lead to cortical changes in the brain and it may be responsible for the interictal pain and refractoriness to therapy [19-21]. As these patients may require higher doses of indomethacin, an early diagnosis is very important.

Taken together, our case series and review of the literature suggest that a subgroup of patients may not fulfill the all the features of ICHD-II diagnostic criteria of PH and a possibility of a subgroup of PH exist. Therefore, we suggest the inclusion of a more accommodating alternative diagnostic criteria or probable PH in the appendix section.

There are marked overlap in clinical features and therapeutic responses among TACs. Clinical features and therapeutic responses in patients with HC also overlap with TACs. Most pathophysiological studies on TACs have been done in CH. The literature is relatively sparse on PH, SUNCT, and HC. However, it is also suggested that all three TACs and HC have common pathophysiology [22]. In the absence of clear cut biological marker, it will be difficult to differentiate borderline or atypical cases of TACs and HC. In Seidel et al. [11] case series of 63 consecutive patients with unilateral headache not resembling migraine or CH, only twenty-four patients (38%) received a diagnosis of primary headache disorders. Headaches could not be classified according to present ICHD-II criteria in 49% patients. This suggests that there is need of refinement of diagnostic criteria of PH and other unilateral headache disorders.

Migraine is the best studied primary headache disorder with well defined pathophysiology. In spite of these, ICHD-II has provided an alternative diagnostic criterion in the appendix section. In the same way, there is need of alternative diagnostic criteria of various other primary headache disorders, including PH. Therefore, till we get biological marker of PH or other TACs, it will be better to have more accommodating type of criteria in the appendix section so that we can refine rare primary headache disorders in the future.

Limitations of our observations
This is a retrospective study and a possibility of unrecognized selection bias and recall bias exists. Although we included only those patients who had normal neuroimaging, we cannot rule out secondary headaches, as full evaluation for secondary headache was not performed on each patient. In addition, we did not have the facilities to do 'indotest'. Our observation did not have large enough numbers to reveal true differences between the typical PH (ICHD-II fulfilled) and atypical PH. Despite these limitations, our observations and review of the literature suggests that a few patients may not fulfill all the ICHD-II criteria for PH and there is need for refinement of the criteria.

Conclusion

Present diagnostic criteria for PH are too restrictive and a subset of patients may not have all the defined features of PH. There is a need for refinement of the existing diagnostic criteria.

Consent

Written informed consent was taken from the patients to publish the report.

Competing interests

The authors declare that they have no competing interests.

Authors' contributions

Conception and design: SP, PB, AS, AT. Analysis and interpretation of the data: SP, PB, SA, AP. Literature search: SP. Drafting of the article: SP, PB, AS. Critical revision of the article for important intellectual content: AT, SA, AP. All authors read, revised and approved the final manuscript.

Author details

[1]Department of Neurology, Medical College, O-19, doctor's quarter, jail road, Baroda, Gujarat 390001, India. [2]Department of Medicine, Medical College, BarodaGujarat, India. [3]Department of Psychiatry, Medical College, Baroda, Gujarat 390001, India.

References

1. Headache Classification Committee of the International Headache Society (2004) Classification and diagnostic criteria for headache disorders, cranial neuralgias, and facial pain. 2nd Ed. Cephalalgia 24:1–160
2. Boes CJ, Dodick DW (2002) Refining the clinical spectrum of chronic paroxysmal hemicrania: a review of 74 patients. Headache 42:699–708
3. Maggioni F (2010) Episodic paroxysmal hemicrania without autonomic symptoms: are there possible subgroups in PH? Cephalalgia 30(4):504–506
4. Boes C, Vincent, Russel M (2006) Paroxysmal hemicrania. In: Olesen J, Goadsby PJ, Ramadan NM, Tfelt-Hansen P, Welch KMA (eds) The headaches, 3rd edn. Lippincott Williams & Wilkins, Philadelphia, PA, pp 815–822
5. Sjaastad O, Dale I (1974) Evidence for a new (?) treatable headache entity. Headache 14:105–108
6. Antonaci F, Sjaastad O (1989) Chronic paroxysmal hemicrania (CPH): a review of the clinical manifestations. Headache 29:648–656
7. Benoliel R, Sharav Y (1998) Paroxysmal hemicrania: Case studies and review of the literature. Oral Surg Oral Med Oral Path Oral Radiol Endod 85:285–292
8. Cittadini E, Matharu MS et al (2008) Paroxysmalhemicrania: a prospective clinical study of 31 cases. Brain 131(Pt 4):1142–1155
9. Fuad F, Jones NS (2002) Paroxysmal hemicrania and cluster headache: two discrete entities or is there an overlap? Clin Otolaryngol Allied Sci 27:472–479
10. Zidverc-Trajkovic J, Pavlovic A, Mijajlovic M, Jovanovic Z, Sternic N, Kostic V (2005) Cluster headache and paroxysmal hemicrania: differential diagnosis. Cephalalgia 25:244–248
11. Seidel S, Lieba-Samal D, Vigl M, Wöber C (2011) Clinical features of unilateral headaches beyond migraine and cluster headache and their response to indomethacin. Wien Klin Wochenschr 123(17–18):536–541
12. Blankenburg M, Hechler T, Dubbel G, Wamsler C, Zernikow B (2009) Paroxysmal hemicrania in children—symptoms, diagnostic criteria, therapy and outcome. Cephalalgia 29:873–882
13. Prakash S, Shah ND, Chavda BV (2010) Cluster headache responsive to indomethacin: case reports and a critical review of the literature. Cephalalgia 30:975–982
14. Martins IP, Gouveia RG, Parreira E (2005) Cluster headache without autonomic symptoms: why is it different? Headache 45:190–195
15. Prakash S, Golwala P (2012) A proposal for revision of hemicrania continua diagnostic criteria based on critical analysis of 62 patients. Cephalalgia 32:860–868
16. Cittadini E, Goadsby PJ (2010) Hemicrania continua: A clinical study of 39 patients with diagnostic implications. Brain 133:1973–1986
17. Marmura M, Silberstein S, Gupta M (2009) Hemicrania continua: who responds to indomethacin? Cephalalgia 29:300–307
18. Prakash S, Shah ND, Bhanvadia RJ (2009) Hemicrania continua unresponsive or partially responsive to indomethacin: does it exist? A diagnostic and therapeutic dilemma. J Headache Pain 10:59–63
19. Marmura MJ, Pello SJ, Young WB (2010) Interictal pain in cluster headache. Cephalalgia 30(12):1531–1534
20. Marmura MJ, Young WB (2010) Interictal pain in primary headache syndromes. Curr Pain Headache Rep 16:170–174
21. Prakash S, Golwala P (2011) Phantom headache: pain memory- emotion hypothesis for chronic daily headache? J Headache Pain 12:281–286
22. Prakash S, Hansen JM (2011) Mechanisms of cluster headache and other trigeminal autonomic cephalalgias. In: Martelletti P, Timothy J, Steiner TJ (eds) Handbook of headache: practical management, 1st edn. Springer Verlag, pp 330–340

2

Gender differences of cognitive function in migraine patients: evidence from event-related potentials using the oddball paradigm

Rongfei Wang, Zhao Dong, Xiaoyan Chen, Mingjie Zhang, Fan Yang, Xiaolan Zhang, Weiquan Jia and Shengyuan Yu[*]

Abstract

Background: Migraine shows gender-specific incidence and has a higher prevalence in females. Gender plays an important role in the prevalence of migraine, but few studies have investigated the effect of gender on the cognitive functions of migraine patients. This study investigated gender differences in the cognitive function of migraine patients without aura.

Methods: We recruited 29 migraine patients (15 females; mean age 25.4 y) during the interictal period and 28 healthy age-matched participants (14 females; mean age 24.8 y). We used an auditory oddball paradigm to analyze target processing using event-related potentials.

Results: We investigated the N2 and P3 components. The P3 amplitude was decreased in patients compared with the control, and this reduction was not modulated by gender. These results of the P3 provided a new evidence for the dysfunction of cognitive function in migraine patients. The N2 amplitude was larger for male than female migraine patients, and this gender effect was not found in the control group.

Conclusions: These results of the P3 provided a new evidence for the dysfunction of cognitive function in migraine patients. And those of N2 may explain that male patients have the super-sensitivity of cerebral function relevant to the early target-selection and response preparation. Our findings emphasize the importance of considering gender when researching the cognitive function of migraine patients.

Keywords: Migraine; ERPs; P3; N2; Gender difference

Background

Migraine is one of the most common types in primary headache. It is characterized by episodic acute and severe disruptions of the brain parenchyma and be accompanied photophobia, phonophobia and gastrointestinal disturbance. As a common disabling primary headache disorder, the migraine has been ranked as the third most prevalent disorder and seventh-highest specific cause of disability worldwide [1]. Interestingly, migraine shows gender-specific incidence and has a higher prevalence in females. The prevalence of migraine is 9.3%, and the female: male is 2.09:1 in China [2].

Previous studies about gender differences in migraineurs found that the influences of migraines on the structures and functions of brain are different for males and females [3,4]. For example, Maleki et al. found that female migraineurs had thicker posterior insula and precuneus cortices than male migraineurs [3]. To date, evidence has revealed that migraine patients showed impairment in cognitive functions such as processing speed, sustained attention [5-7], working memory [8,9], and visual-spatial processing [4,10-12]. Although gender plays an important role in the prevalence of migraine, but few studies have investigated the effect of gender on the cognitive functions of migraine patients, which will be explored in the present study by recording and analyzing the event-related potentials (ERPs).

* Correspondence: yusy1963@126.com
Department of Neurology, Chinese PLA General Hospital, Fuxing Road 28, Haidian District, Beijing 100853, China

ERPs reveal coherent stimulus-related postsynaptic activity in the cortex with millisecond temporal resolution and, hence, are ideally suited for investigating the time course of cortical activation for cognitive processing. Several ERP studies have systematically assessed the cognitive function using the P3 component in migraine patients and observed reduced P3 amplitudes [13,14]. In contrast, there was also evidence that, when compared with normal participants, the P3 amplitude was enlarged and delayed in primary headache patients [15]. In addition to the P3, Boćkowski and colleague found longer N2 latencies in migraine patients without aura in comparison with migraine patients with aura and tension-type headaches patients [16]. Importantly, recent ERP studies demonstrated gender effects on N2 and P3 components [17,18]. Because the gender influences the prevalence of migraine, it is necessary to investigate the gender differences on attentional function using ERP components.

Methods

Participants

We recruited 29 patients with migraine without aura (15 females; mean age 25.4 y, range between 20 to 30 y) from the Chinese PLA General Hospital according to the International Headache Society (ICHD) criteria. Patients were verified to receive no prophylactic therapy and had to have been drug-free for at least 72 h. Migraine attack frequency was 1–6/month. The time interval between the last attack of migraine and the recording was at least 1 week. We also recruited 28 healthy age-matched participants (14 females; mean age 24.8 y, range between 21 to 30 y) with no history of headache attacks or drug/alcohol abuse. All of the participants had normal or corrected-to-normal vision, and normal hearing capability. No participants had remarkable dysfunctions in their motor and sensory systems, or deep tendon reflexes. We excluded participants who were illiterate, or suffering from depression, stroke, or brain injuries. This study was approved by the Ethical Committee of the Chinese PLA General Hospital, in accordance with the ethical principles of the Declaration of Helsinki. All participants gave their written and informed consents prior to the experiment.

The following clinical data were included for the migraine patients: 1) the history of the migraine, 2) the frequency of headaches per month over the previous year, 3) a rating of the most severe headache experienced in the previous year using a visual analog scale (VAS), and 4) with photophobia and phonophobia during the migraine attacks. The exclusion criteria were: 1) taking prophylactic medications for migraine, 2) a history of analgesic drug overuse, 3) general neurological or psychiatric disease, 4) a history of drug abuse or dependency, including that related to alcohol consumption and cigarette smoking, 5) a history of mixed headache types, 6) a history of a neurological disorder or abnormal findings on a neurological examination. There were no significant gender differences in the durations of the migraine history ($t(1,29) = 0.08$, $p = 0.94$), the migraine frequencies ($t(1,29) = 0.30$, $p = 0.77$), and the VAS scores ($t(1,29) = 0.06$, $p = 0.96$).

Stimuli and procedures

The experiment was performed in a sound attenuated room with dim light. The stimuli included 1600-Hz (target, 20% probability) and 1,000-Hz (standard, 80% probability) pure tones, with linear rise and fall times of 5 ms and with an intensity of 65 dB. Both stimuli were presented through headphones unilaterally, with the duration of 105 ms. The interstimulus interval (ISI) varied randomly from 1000 to 1500 ms (mean, 1200 ms). There were two separate blocks of 160 stimuli for each.

Participant was instructed to focus on a fixation cross in the center of the screen and to press the button as quickly and correctly as possible when they heard the target stimuli.

EEG recording and analysis

Electroencephalogram (EEG) was continuously recorded (band pass 0.05-100Hz, sampling rate 500Hz) at Fz, Cz and Pz electrode sites according to the international 10–20 system with ASA-Lab EEG/ERPs 64 Chanel Amplifier (www.ant-neuro.com), referenced to the left mastoid (right mastoid as recording site). VEOG and HEOG were recorded with two pairs of electrodes, one placed above and below the right eye, and the other 10 mm from the lateral canthi. Electrode impedance was maintained below 5 kΩ throughout the experiment.

We used ASA software (www.ant-neuro.com) to analyze the data off-line. EEG data were re-referenced to the bi-mastoid average reference. EOG artifacts were corrected using the method proposed by Semlitsch et al. (1986). The EEG was segmented into the epoch from 200 ms pre-stimulus to 1000 ms post-stimulus. The EEG segment contaminated by amplifier clipping, bursts of electromyographic activity, or peak-to-peak deflection exceeding ±100 μV were excluded from averaging. The EEG segments were averaged separately for target and standard stimuli. The number of average trials left after removal of the artifacts was 60 (target) and 210 (standard) for normal controls and 64 (target) and 206 (standard) for patients, respectively.

The peak amplitudes and latencies of two ERP components, N2 and P3, were measured relative to the pre-stimulus baseline period (see Figure 1). The negative peak between 200 and 300 ms and the positive peak between 300 and 500 ms were used to define the N2 and

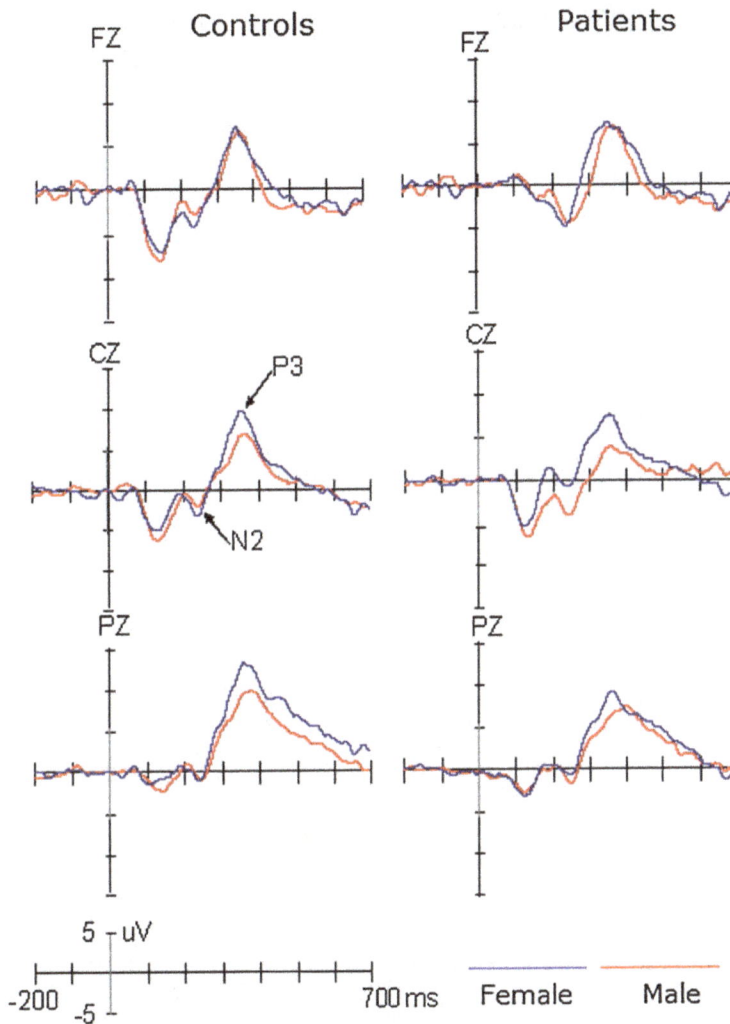

Figure 1 The grand averaged ERPs elicited by target stimuli in patients and controls, respectively.

P3 components, respectively. To reliably observe the target effect, the difference waveform was obtained by subtracting ERPs in response to standard stimuli from ERPs in response to target stimuli (see Figure 2). The mean amplitudes were measured between 200 and 300 ms for the N2d (i.e., the N2 target effect) and 300 and 500 ms for the P3d (i.e., the P3 target effect), respectively.

Data analysis

The measurements of N2 and P3 components were analyzed using repeated-measures analysis of variance (ANOVA), with Stimulus (target, standard) and Site (Fz, Cz, and Pz for P3; Fz and Cz for N2) as within-subject factors and with Gender (female, male) and Group (migraine, control) as between-subject factors.

For N2d and P3d components, the ANOVA was conducted with Site (Fz, Cz, and Pz for P3d; Fz and Cz for N2d) as within-subject factors and with Gender (female, male) and Group (migraine, control) as between-subject

factors. The degrees of freedom were corrected using the Greenhouse–Geisser epsilon.

Results

Behavioral data

For the accuracy, neither the group effect (control: 99%; patients: 99.25%) nor the gender effect (female: 99.25%; male: 99.11%) was significant (Fs < 1). The gender × group interaction was not significant ($F(1,53) < 1$).

The response speed was not affected by the group (323 ms and 333 ms for controls and patients, respectively; $F(1,53) < 1$), nor by the gender (331 ms and 345 ms for males and females, respectively; $F(1,53) < 1$). The gender × group interaction was not significant ($F(1,53) < 1$).

ERP data

N2 and N2d components

The amplitudes of N2 component showed significant main effect of Site ($F(1,53) = 10.184$, $p < 0.005$, $\eta2 = 0.16$),

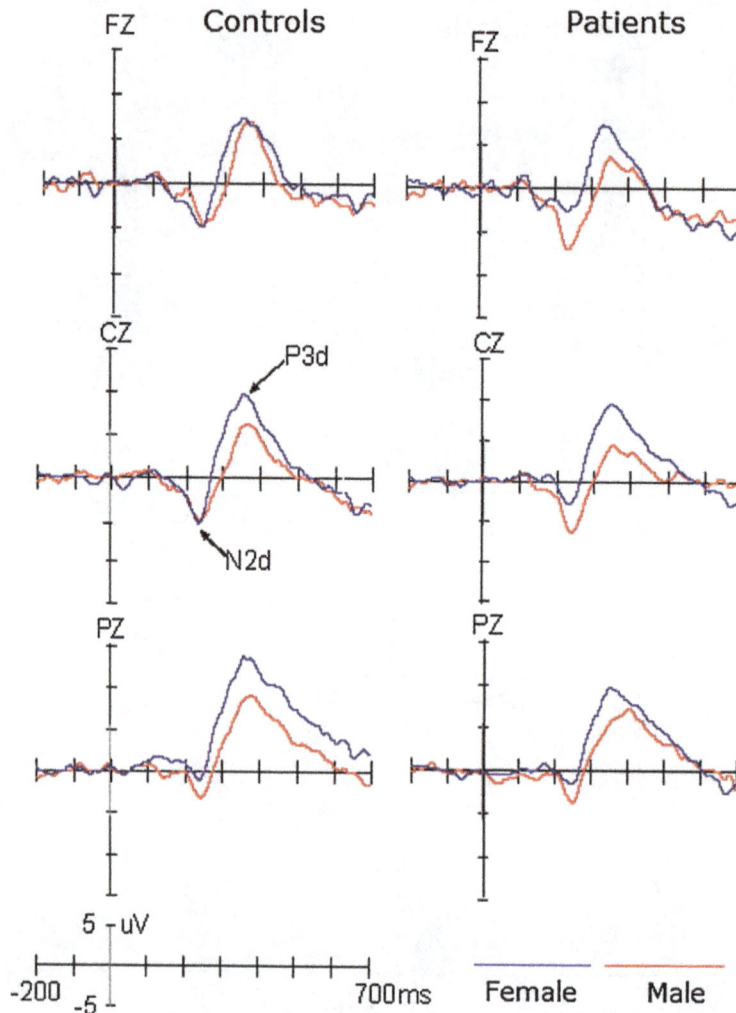

Figure 2 The difference waveforms by subtracting ERPs in response to standard stimuli from ERPs in response to target stimuli in patients and controls, respectively.

indicating larger N2 at Fz (-3.90 μV) than Cz (-2.16 μV) site. Although neither the group ($F(1,53) < 1$) nor the gender ($F(1,53) = 2.34$, $p > 0.05$) effect was significant, there was a significant interaction of Gender × Group ($F(1,53) = 5.785$, $p < 0.025$, $\eta2 = 0.398$). Post-hoc tests revealed that, while there was no significant difference between female patients and female controls ($p = 0.313$), the mean amplitude of N2 was larger for male patients (-6.06 μV) than male controls (-1.94 μV; $p < 0.025$, $\eta2 = 0.129$). In the control group the gender effect was not significant ($p = 0.532$), but for patients the N2 was larger for males than for females ($p < 0.01$). No other effects reached significant level ($ps > 0.1$).

The analysis of N2d amplitudes did not demonstrate the significant main effect of Site ($F(1,53) < 1$) or Group ($F(1,53) < 1$). The gender effect was marginally significant, $F(1,53) = 4.0$, $p = 0.051$, but qualified by the two-way interaction of Group × Gender, $F(1,53) = 4.467$,

$p < 0.05$, $\eta2 = 0.14$. Post-hoc tests revealed that the N2d was larger in male patients (-7.40 μV) than in male controls (-4.37 μV, $p < 0.05$) and that, although the gender effect was not significant in normal controls ($p = 0.907$), the N2d amplitude was larger for male patients than for female patients (-2.22 μV; $p < 0.01$). We did not observe any significant effects or interactions in the N2 or N2d latencies ($ps > 0.1$).

P3 and P3d components

Across conditions, both P3 and P3d showed significant main effects of Site ($F(2,106) = 16.52$, $p < 0.001$, $\eta2 = 0.388$ for P3 and $F(2,106) = 11.44$, $p < 0.001$, $\eta2 = 0.178$ for P3d), indicating a centro-parietal scalp distribution with a maximize of 8.77 μV for P3 and 8.81 μV for P3d at Pz. The amplitudes of P3 and P3d were smaller for patients (P3, 4.43 μV; P3d, 6.25 μV) than for controls (P3, 7.64 μV; P3d, 8.21 μV), $F(1,53) = 5.68$, $p < 0.025$,

$\eta 2 = 0.397$ for P3 and $F(1,53) = 4.22$, $p < 0.05$, $\eta 2 = 0.12$ for P3d, respectively. Although the amplitudes of P3 did not appear to be significantly affected by Gender ($F(1,53) = 2.92$, $p = 0.093$), across groups, the P3d were larger for female than for male participants ($F(1,53) = 5.73$, $p < 0.025$, $\eta 2 = 0.10$). No other effects reached significant level ($ps > 0.1$). The latencies of the P3 and P3d components did not show any significant effects ($ps > 0.1$).

Discussion

In this study, we used a traditional auditory oddball paradigm, in which participants were required to press a button for the infrequent target stimulus while ignoring the frequent non-target standard stimulus while ignoring the frequent non-target standard stimulus, and focused on P3 component, which is a generic name for a variety of relatively late positive components with a centro-parietal or centro-frontal midline distribution [17,18]. In addition, we will also investigate the N2, a frontal-central distributed negativity that reflects the stimulus evaluation response including action monitoring, the early target-selection and response preparation [19]. If there were gender effects on cognitive function in patients, it should be reflected by a modulation of the N2 and/or P3 components.

The present study found the P3 component was larger for female than for male participants, for both the patient and control groups. Compared with the control group, there was a decrease in the amplitude of P3 for patients, and this reduction was not modulated by gender. Although there was no gender effect on the amplitudes of N2 in the control group, they were larger for male than for female migraine patients and larger for healthy male participants.

This study replicated the results of previous studies by finding that females had larger P3 amplitudes than males, regardless of their migraine history. Importantly, the P3 amplitudes in migraine patients were significantly decreased in comparison with the control group, as was the case in previous studies [17]. It has been widely accepted that P3 is a neural signature of attention and/or the amount of working memory required for appropriately responding to environmental stimuli [20]. Using a similar paradigm to the present study, Wang et al. found smaller P3 for migraine patients than for control subjects. Interestingly, recent studies revealed that the reduction of the P3 amplitude was also evident when using the passive oddball paradigm, in which the infrequent novel stimuli were examined [13]. This indicates that migraine patients exhibit a deficit in the frontal function involved in automatic attention switching [14]. Overall, the present pattern of P3 components provided new evidence for the dysfunction of cognitive function in migraine patients.

Although we did not find an influence of gender on the P3 component, the N2 component was larger for male than for female patients (note that there were no gender effects in control participants) and was larger for male patients than for male controls. Generally, the target-related N2 component indicates action monitoring, early target-selection and response preparation [21-25]. Therefore, it is possible that male patients have a super-sensitive cerebral function that is relevant to early target-selection and response preparation. There have been neuroimaging studies providing some relevant evidences for the hypersensitivity of cortical function in patients with migraine. For example, Martín H, et al. studied light sensitivity and photophobia in migraineurs by assessing the response to light stimuli with fMRI-BOLD of the occipital cortex and found that migraineurs during interictal periods showed hyperxcitability of the visual cortex with a wider photoresponsive area [26]. Similarly, it was found that migraine patients showed significantly higher blood oxygen level-dependent siginal intensities in the brain areas including limbic structures and the rostral pons in response to olfactory stimulation during spontaneous and untreated attacks [27]. Recently, Woolf & Salter developed a conceptual framework for the contribution of plasticity in primary sensory and dorsal horn neurons to the pathogenesis of pain. They identified distinct forms of plasticity that elicit pain hypersensitivity by increasing gain [28,29]. However, it should be noted that the above studies did not investigate the gender effects of the hypersensitivity of the cortical function. In other word, to our knowledge there was no evidence for larger neutral plasticity of the brain in male than female migraineurs. Especially, the present findings showed that the N2 component, indeed, did not differ between female patients and control participants. Therefore, it is necessary in the future to determine whether the super neutral plasticity is specific to male participants, at least at the N2 level.

Interestingly, one recent neuroimaging study showed dysfunctional organization in the resting functional network of the brain that was more evident in female migraine patients [4]. In addition, the migraine may cause abnormal brain structure and brain function, which depends on the patients' gender. For example, compared with male migraineurs, female patients had thicker posterior insula and precuneus cortices [3]. To date, converging evidence shows that the incidence of migraine in females is about three times as high as in males, and that estrogen could be the main cause of this gender difference [30]. However, we did not observe gender differences in the P3 components and consequently, the differences of estrogen between male and female cannot account for the different cognitive function across patients' genders.

Conclusion

Before concluding, we would like to reiterate the procedural decisions that constrained the interpretation of the present findings. First, we did not measure ERPs in conjunction with other neuropsychological investigations. Second, the small cohort limited the examination of the effect of the age and the differences between migraine with and without aura. Nevertheless, we took steps to ensure that the sample was as homogeneous as possible by choosing only young participants, which undoubtedly reduced the impact of confounders on our analysis. Third, we did not check for the occurrence of an attack after the recording session. Finally, although the present study found group effects on the N2 and P3 components, the data were unable to reveal the spatial distribution of these abnormalities because of the limitation on recorded electrode sites (Fz, Cz, and Pz). Therefore, in order to reveal the gender differences of brain topographical distributions it is necessary to record multi-electrode sites with possible source analysis in the future.

These limitations notwithstanding, our findings emphasize the importance of considering gender when studying cognitive processing in migraine patients, and provide further empirical support that a gender effect exists.

Competing interests

All authors declare there are non-financial competing interests (political, personal, religious, ideological, academic, intellectual, commercial or any other) in relation to this manuscript.

Authors' contributions

M.D. RW, ZD, XC, MZ, FY, XZ and WJ carried out the studies. And RW drafted the manuscript. M.D. RW participated in the design of the study and performed the statistical analysis. Professor SY, the PI of this study, conceived of the study and participated in its design and helped to draft the manuscript. All authors read and approved the final manuscript.

Acknowledgments

The authors would like to thank all of the referring clinicians. This study was financially supported by the National Science Foundation Committee (NSFC) in China (no. 81171058). The funders had no role in study design, data collection and analysis, decision to publish, or preparation of the manuscript.

References

1. Steiner TJ, Stovner LJ, Birbeck GL (2013) Migraine: the seventh disabler. J Headache Pain 14:1
2. Yu S, Liu R, Zhao G, Yang X, Qiao X, Feng J, Fang Y, Cao X, He M, Steiner T (2012) The prevalence and burden of primary headaches in China: a population-based door-to-door survey. Headache 52:582–591
3. Maleki N, Linnman C, Brawn J, Burstein R, Becerra L, Borsook D (2012) Her versus his migraine: multiple sex difference in brain function and structure. Brain 135:2546–2559
4. Liu J, Qin W, Nan J, Li J, Yuan K, Zhao L, Zeng F, Sun J, Yu D, Dong M, Liu P, von Deneen KM, Gong Q, Liang F, Tian J (2011) Gender-related differences in the dysfunctional resting networks of migraine suffers. PLoS One 6:e27049
5. Mulder EJ, Linssen WH, Passchier J, Orlebeke JF, de Geus EJ (1999) Interictal and postictal cognitive changes in migraine. Cephalalgia 19:557–565
6. Riva D, Usilla A, Aggio F, Vago C, Treccani C, Bulgheroni S (2012) Attention in children and adolescents with headache. Headache 52:374–384
7. Koppen H, Palm-Meinders I, Kruit M, Lim V, Nugroho A, Westhof I, Terwindt G, van Buchem M, Ferrari M, Hommel B (2011) The impact of a migraine attack and its after-effects on perceptual organization, attention, and working memory. Cephalalgia 31:1419–1427
8. Le Pira F, Zappalà G, Giuffrida S, Lo Bartolo ML, Reggio E, Morana R, Lanaia F (2000) Memory disturbances in migraine with and without aura: a strategy problem? Cephalalgia 20:475–478
9. Calandre EP, Bembibre J, Arnedo ML, Becera D (2002) Cognitive disturbances and regional cerebral blood flow abnormalities in migraine patients: their relationship with the clinical manifestations of the illness. Cephalalgia 22:291–302
10. Coleston DM, Chronicle E, Ruddock KH, Kennard C (1994) Precortical dysfunction of spatial and temporal visual processing in migraine. J Neurol Neurosurg Psychiatry 57:1208–1211
11. Le Pira F, Lanaia F, Zappalà G, Morana R, Panetta MR, Reggio E, Reggio A (2004) Relationship between clinical variables and cognitive performances in migraineurs with and without aura. Funct Neurol 19:101–105
12. Riva D, Aggio F, Vago C, Nichelli F, Andreucci E, Paruta N, D'Arrigo S, Pantaleoni C, Bulgheroni S (2006) Cognitive and behavioural effects of migraine in childhood and adolescence. Cephalalgia 26:596–603
13. Wang W, Schoenen J, Timsit-Berthier M (1995) Cognitive functions in migraine without aura between attacks: a psychophysiological approach using the "oddball" paradigm. Neurophysiol Clin 25:3–11
14. Chen W, Shen X, Liu X, Luo B, Liu Y, Yu R, Sun G, Shen M, Wang W (2007) Passive paradigm single-tone elicited ERPs in tension-type headaches and migraine. Cephalalgia 27:139–144
15. Mazzotta G, Alberti A, Santucci A, Gallai V (1995) The event-related potential P300 during headache-free period and spontaneous attack in adult headache sufferers. Headache 35:210–215
16. Boćkowski L, Sobaniec W, Sołowiej E, Smigielska-Kuzia J (2004) Auditory cognitive event-related potentials in migraine with and without aura in children and adolescents. Neurol Neurochir Pol 38:9–14
17. Polich J (2007) Updating P300: an integrative theory of P3a and P3b. Clin Neurophysiol 118:2128–2148
18. Yuan J, He Y, Qinglin Z, Chen A, Li H (2008) Gender differences in behavioral inhibitory control: ERP evidence from a two-choice oddball task. Psychophysiology 45:986–993
19. Gaillard AWK, Lawson EA (1980) Mismatch negativity (N2) following the discrimination of consonant vowel stimuli. Psychophysiology 18:172–173
20. Pedroso RV, Fraga FJ, Corazza DI, Andreatto CA, Coelho FG, Costa JL, Santos-Galduróz RF (2012) P300 latency and amplitude in Alzheimer's disease: a systematic review. Braz J Otorhinolaryngol 78:126–132
21. Jamadar S, Hughes M, Fulham WR, Michie PT, Karayanidis F (2010) The spatial and temporal dynamics of anticipatory preparation and response inhibition in task-switching. Neuroimage 51:432–449
22. Hsieh S, Wu M (2011) Electrophysiological correlates of preparation and implementation for different types of task shifts. Brain Res 1423:41–52
23. Gajewski PD, Kleinsorge T, Falkenstein M (2010) Electrophysiological correlates of residual switch costs. Cortex 46:1138–1148
24. Botvinick MM, Cohen JD, Carter CS (2004) Conflict monitoring and anterior cingulate cortex: an update. Trends Cogn Sci 8:539–546
25. Carter CS, van Veen V (2007) Anterior cingulate cortex and conflict detection: an update of theory and data. Cogn Affect Behav Neurosci 7:367–379
26. Martín H, Sánchez del Río M, de Silanes CL, Álvarez-Linera J, Hernández JA, Pareja JA (2011) Photoreactivity of the occipital cortex measured by functional magnetic resonance imaging-blood oxygenation level dependent in migraine patients and healthy volunteers: pathophysiological implications. Headache 51:1520–1528
27. Stankewitz A, May A (2011) Increased limbic and brainstem activity during migraine attacks following olfactory stimulation. Neurology 77:476–482
28. Woolf CJ, Salter MW (2000) Neuronal plasticity: increasing the gain in pain. Science 288:1765–1769
29. Latremoliere A, Woolf CJ (2009) Central sensitization: a generator of pain hypersensitivity by central neural plasticity. J Pain 10:895–926
30. Brandes JL (2006) The influence of estrogen on migraine: a systematic review. JAMA 295:1824–1830

3

A common cause of sudden and thunderclap headaches: reversible cerebral vasoconstriction syndrome

Yu-Chen Cheng[1,4], Kuei-Hong Kuo[2,4] and Tzu-Hsien Lai[1,3,4*]

Abstract

Background: Thunderclap headache (TCH) is a sudden headache (SH) with accepted criteria of severe intensity and onset to peak within one minute. It is a well-known presentation for subarachnoid hemorrhage (SAH) but most patients with TCH or SH run a benign course without identifiable causes. Reversible cerebral vasoconstriction syndrome (RCVS), a recently recognized syndrome characterized by recurrent TCH attacks, has been proposed to account for most of these patients.

Methods: We recruited consecutive patients presenting with SH at our headache clinic. Computed tomography and/or magnetic resonance imaging with angiography were performed to exclude structural causes and to identify vasoconstriction. Catheter angiography and lumbar puncture were performed with patients consent. Reversibility of vasoconstriction was confirmed by follow-up study.

Results: From July 2010 to June 2013, 31 patients with SH were recruited. Twenty-four (72.7%) of these SH patients exhibited headache fulfilling the TCH criteria. The diagnosis of RCVS was confirmed in 14 (45.2%) of patients with SH and 11 (45.8%) of patients with TCH. Other diagnoses were as follows: primary headaches (SH: 41.9%, TCH: 45.8%) and other secondary causes (SH: 12.9%, TCH: 8.3%). Compared with non-RCVS patients, patients with RCVS were older (50.8 ± 9.3 years vs. 40.8 ± 10.0 years, $P = 0.006$) and less likely to experience short headache duration of < 1 hour (23.1% vs. 78.6%, $P = 0.007$). Patients with RCVS were more likely to cite bathing (42.9% vs. 0%, $P = 0.004$) and less likely to cite exertion (0% vs. 29.4%, $P = 0.048$) as headache triggers.

Conclusions: Reversible cerebral vasoconstriction syndrome is a common cause of SH and TCH. Considering the potential mortality and morbidity of RCVS, systemic examination of cerebral vessels should be performed in these patients.

Keywords: Bath-related thunderclap headache; Orgasmic headache; Primary cough headache; Primary exertional headache; Primary headache associated with sexual activity; Reversible cerebral vasoconstriction syndrome; Sentinel headache; Sudden headache; Subarachnoid hemorrhage; Thunderclap headache

Background

Thunderclap headache (TCH) is a well-known presentation of subarachnoid hemorrhage (SAH). The term was first used in a patient who had three episodes of "intense sentinel headache of sudden onset" before an unruptured aneurysm was found [1]. A later study following 71 patients for an average of 3.3 years reported no SAH, which led to the concept of "benign TCH" [2]. Other studies recruiting patients with similar sudden headache (SH) showed that 6-25% of these patients exhibited SAH [3-5]. More than one-half of the patients in these studies did not receive a definite diagnosis. The term "TCH" has been defined as a SH fulfilling criteria of both severe intensity and onset to peak within one minute [6]. Several possible causes of TCH have been reported, ranging from various vascular lesions of the brain to indolent headaches

---

* Correspondence: laitzuhsien@gmail.com
[1]Section of Neurology, Department of Internal Medicine, Far Eastern Memorial Hospital, No. 21, Sec. 2, Nanya S. Rd., Ban-Chiao Dist., New Taipei City 220, Taiwan
[3]Department of Neurology, Neurological Institute, Taipei Veterans General Hospital, Taipei, Taiwan

associated with sexual activity (HSA) or other triggers [7]. Nonetheless, most patients with SH are still categorized as having a "benign headache" [5].

Recently, reversible cerebral vasoconstriction syndrome (RCVS) has been added to the list of TCH differential diagnoses [8]. RCVS is a unifying term which encompasses a group of recurrent headache syndromes including: Call-Fleming syndrome, thunderclap headache with reversible vasospasm, benign angiopathy of the central nervous system, postpartum cerebral angiopathy, among others [8]. The clinical presentation of RCVS is characterized by recurrent TCH attacks and multifocal vasoconstriction which resolves within 2 to 3 months [8,9]. In contrast to "benign" causes of TCH, RCVS is linked with clinical (focal neurological deficits and seizure) and radiological (cortical SAH, intracranial hemorrhage, ischemic stroke, arterial dissection and posterior reversible encephalopathy syndrome) abnormalities, and sometimes increased morbidity and mortality [9-11]. After the term "RCVS" was coined in 2007, reports of this condition began accumulating rapidly, though most of these reports are sporadic cases. It has been postulated that RCVS is under-recognized and "accounts for most benign TCH" [12,13]. We aimed to test the hypothesis of RCVS as a common cause in patients presenting with TCH and similar SH.

Methods

Clinical settings

We recruited consecutive patients with SH at our headache clinic in Far Eastern Memorial Hospital from July 2010 to June 2013. The headache clinic has been operating since August 2009. Far Eastern Memorial Hospital is a 1012-bed medical center in Taipei, Taiwan. Under the local health care system, patients are free to call upon any hospital without a referral. Our patients are either self-referred or referred by our colleague neurologists. All patients presenting at this headache clinic are requested to fill out a detailed headache intake form, have their medical and headache histories recorded, receive a neurological examination and are suggested to keep a headache diary.

Diagnostic algorithm

Following previous studies, patients presenting with SH suggesting possible vascular origin, especially sentinel leakage or SAH, were included [3,4]. Patients were eligible for the study if they presented with a new type of headache within one month of onset and the duration of headache was at least > 1 minute. Patients with symptoms or signs indicating other primary (e.g. cranial autonomic symptoms, headache always occurring during sleep) or secondary causes of headache (e.g. trauma, meningitis, sinusitis) were excluded. Thunderclap headache

was defined following the ICHD-2 (International Classification of Headache Disorders, 2nd edition) criteria of onset to peak within one minute and severe intensity (≥7 on a 0–10 numerical rating scale) [6]. Patients were recorded as having TCH if they reported at least one, but not every, attack fulfilling the criteria. Neuroimaging studies, including brain computed tomography (CT) and/or magnetic resonance imaging (MRI) with 3-dimensional reformatting angiography (CTA and/or MRA), were arranged to exclude structural causes and to identify vasoconstriction. Catheter angiography and lumbar puncture were performed if patients agreed. All imaging data were interpreted by a neuroradiologist (Kuo KH), who was blinded to the diagnoses. The diagnosis of RCVS was made following ICHD-2 for headache attributed to benign (or reversible) angiopathy of the central nervous system (code 6.7.3) (Table 1) [6]. Follow-up neuroimaging studies (CTA or MRA) were performed approximately 3 months later to confirm the reversibility of vasoconstriction. Diagnoses of other primary headache disorders were made following ICHD-2, including primary cough headache (code 4.2), primary exertional headache (code 4.3), primary headache associated with sexual activity (HSA) (code 4.4), and primary TCH (code 4.7) [6].

Neuroimaging studies

All CT studies were scanned by a 64-detector CT system (Brilliance-64, Philips Healthcare) and a power injector was used to administer a bolus of 50 mL contrast at a 4 mL/s flow rate for CTA acquisition. All magnetic resonance (MR) studies were performed by two 1.5 T MR imaging systems (Tim CT and Avanto, Siemens) with 20 slices covering the entire brain (matrix 204-224 × 256-320; field of view 20-23 cm; slice thickness 5 mm, interslice gap 2 mm). Magnetic resonance angiography was obtained using a 3-dimensional time-of-flight MR technique with maximum intensity projection (MIP) (matrix 256 × 256; field of view 18 cm; 110 sections; total coverage 7 cm).

Treatment and follow up

All patients were suggested to avoid the possible headache triggers. Patients with primary headaches were given analgesics when needed. Patients with RCVS were treated with 30 mg nimodipine four times a day. No patient received intravenous nimodipine. In December 2013, we contacted each patient by telephone to determine whether or not any relapse had occurred. The study protocol was approved by the Institutional Review Board of the hospital.

Statistics

SPSS 18.0 for Windows (SPSS Inc., Chicago, IL, USA) was used for statistical analyses. Descriptive data were

Table 1 Diagnostic criteria of RCVS

ICHD-2 (code 6.7.3) [6]	Headache attributed to benign (or reversible) angiopathy of the CNS
	A. Diffuse, severe headache of abrupt or progressive onset, with or without focal neurological deficits and/or seizures and fulfilling criteria C and D
	B. 'Strings and beads' appearance on angiography and SAH ruled out by appropriate investigations
	C. One or both of the following:
	1. headache develops simultaneously with neurological deficits and/or seizures
	2. headache leads to angiography and discovery of 'strings and beads' appearance
	D. Headache (and neurological deficits, if present) resolves spontaneously within 2 months
ICHD-3, beta version (code 6.7.3) [14]	Headache attributed to RCVS
	A. Any new headache fulfilling criterion C
	B. RCVS has been diagnosed
	C. Evidence of causation demonstrated by at least one of the following:
	1. headache, with or without focal deficits and/or seizures, has led to angiography (with 'strings and beads' appearance) and diagnosis of RCVS
	2. headache has either or both of the following characteristics:
	a) recurrent during ≤1 month, and with thunderclap onset
	b) triggered by sexual activity, exertion, Valsalva maneuvers, emotion, bathing and/or showering
	3. no new significant headache occurs >1 month after onset
	D. Not better accounted for by another ICHD-3 diagnosis, and aneurysmal SAH has been excluded by appropriate investigations.
ICHD-3, beta version (code 6.7.3.1) [14]	Headache probably attributed to RCVS
	A. Any new headache fulfilling criterion C
	B. RCVS is suspected, but cerebral angiography is normal
	C. Probability of causation demonstrated by all of the following:
	1. at least two headaches within 1 month, with all three of the following characteristics:
	a) thunderclap onset, and peaking in <1 minute
	b) severe intensity
	c) lasting ≥5 minutes
	2. at least one thunderclap headache has been triggered by one of the following:
	a) sexual activity (just before or at orgasm)
	b) exertion
	c) Valsalva-like maneuver
	d) emotion
	e) bathing and/or showering
	f) bending
	3. no new thunderclap or other significant headache occurs >1 month after onset
	D. Not fulfilling ICHD-3 criteria for any other headache disorder
	E. Not better accounted for by another ICHD-3 diagnosis, and aneurysmal SAH has been excluded by appropriate investigations.

ICHD: International Classification of Headache Disorders; CNS: central nervous system; RCVS: reversible cerebral vasoconstriction syndrome; SAH: subarachnoid hemorrhage.

presented as mean ± standard deviation or percentages. Due to the relatively small sample size, non-parametric methods of Fisher's exact test for categorical data and the Mann Whitney U test for continuous measures were used. All calculated P-values were two-sided and significance was defined as a P-value < 0.05.

Results

From July 2010 to June 2013, 34 consecutive patients presented with SH to our headache clinic. Three patients were excluded for either withdrawal or refusing further diagnostic workup. Twenty-four (77.4%) of the 31 screened patients fulfilled the criteria of TCH (Figure 1). The final

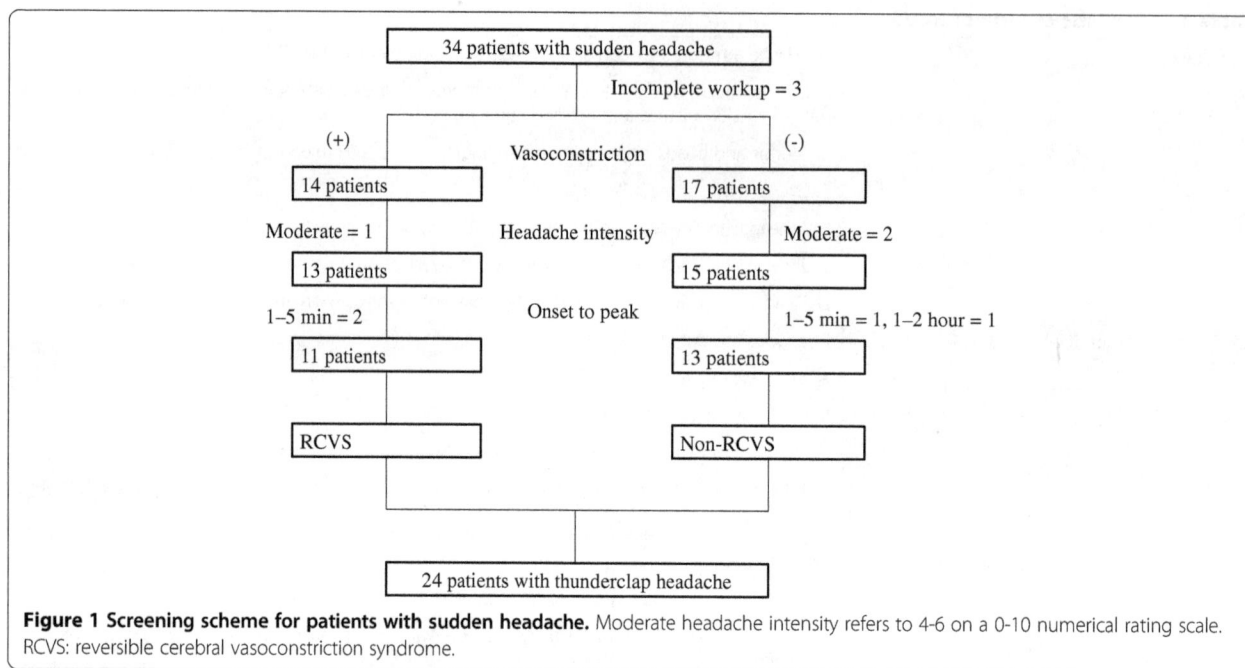

Figure 1 Screening scheme for patients with sudden headache. Moderate headache intensity refers to 4-6 on a 0-10 numerical rating scale. RCVS: reversible cerebral vasoconstriction syndrome.

diagnoses were listed in Table 2. Of note, 45.2% of SH patients and 45.8% of TCH patients exhibited RCVS. Secondary causes other than RCVS were recorded in 12.9% and 8.3% of patients in the SH and TCH groups, respectively. The ratios of RCVS in patients with "benign TCH", i.e., excluding patients with other secondary causes, were 51.9% (14 of 27 SH patients) and 50% (11 of 22 TCH patients). Of patients with primary headaches, patients with multiple triggers could not be categorized to any existing diagnoses of ICHD-2. These patients reported either sexual activity or bathing as triggers, and thus could not fulfill the ICHD-2 criteria of primary cough headache (triggered by cough, straining or Valsalva maneuver). We tested the new ICHD-3 criteria (beta version) in our patients (Table 1) (Figure 2).

Table 2 Final diagnoses of patients with SH and TCH

Diagnosis	Patient number (%)	
	SH, n = 31	TCH, n = 24
RCVS	14 (45.2%)	11 (45.8%)
Primary headaches	13 (41.9%)	11 (45.8%)
Multiple triggers	6 (19.4%)	5 (20.8%)
Primary HSA	4 (12.9%)	3 (12.5%)
Primary exertional headache	2 (6.5%)	2 (8.3%)
Primary TCH	1 (3.2%)	1 (4.2%)
Other secondary causes	4 (12.9%)	2 (8.3%)
Chiari malformation	1 (3.2%)	1 (4.2%)
Moyamoya syndrome	2 (6.5%)	1 (4.2%)
Subarachnoid hemorrhage	1 (3.2%)	0

SH: sudden headache; TCH: thunderclap headache; RCVS: reversible cerebral vasoconstriction syndrome; HSA: headache associated with sexual activity.

Of the six patients with multiple triggers, five (83.3%) could fulfill the criteria of probable RCVS. Nevertheless, these patients could be categorized as having probable RCVS by the ICHD-3, beta version (Table 1) [14]. The ratios of RCVS and probable RCVS in patients with "benign TCH" would thus be even higher (SH: 70.4%, TCH: 72.7%).

Demographics
The demographic and clinical profiles of both SH and TCH patients are listed in Table 3. A trend was observed of patients with RCVS being more likely female (SH: 85.7% vs. 52.9%, $P = 0.068$; TCH: 81.8% vs. 53.8%, $P = 0.211$). Patients with RCVS were older than non-RCVS patients (SH: 50.8 ± 9.3 years vs. 40.8 ± 10.0 years, $P = 0.006$; TCH: 49.4 ± 10.0 years vs. 42.6 ± 10.3 years, $P = 0.092$). In the RCVS group, female patients were significantly older than male patients, but the number of the latter group was very small (women: 53.8 ± 5.8 years, n = 12; men: 33.0 ± 4.2 years, n = 2; $P = 0.028$).

Precipitating factors
No patient in our study was in the postpartum state. The patients' medication history was carefully obtained but we did not observe any patient use of recreational drugs, selective serotonin reuptake inhibitors, triptans, immunosuppressants or even recent use of herbal medication. All patients using possible vasoactive substances had been using cough medication. For some patients, to determine which drugs they had used was simply not feasible. We thus adopted a loose guideline that use of any cough medication just before occurrence of headaches would be recorded. Since use of cough medication

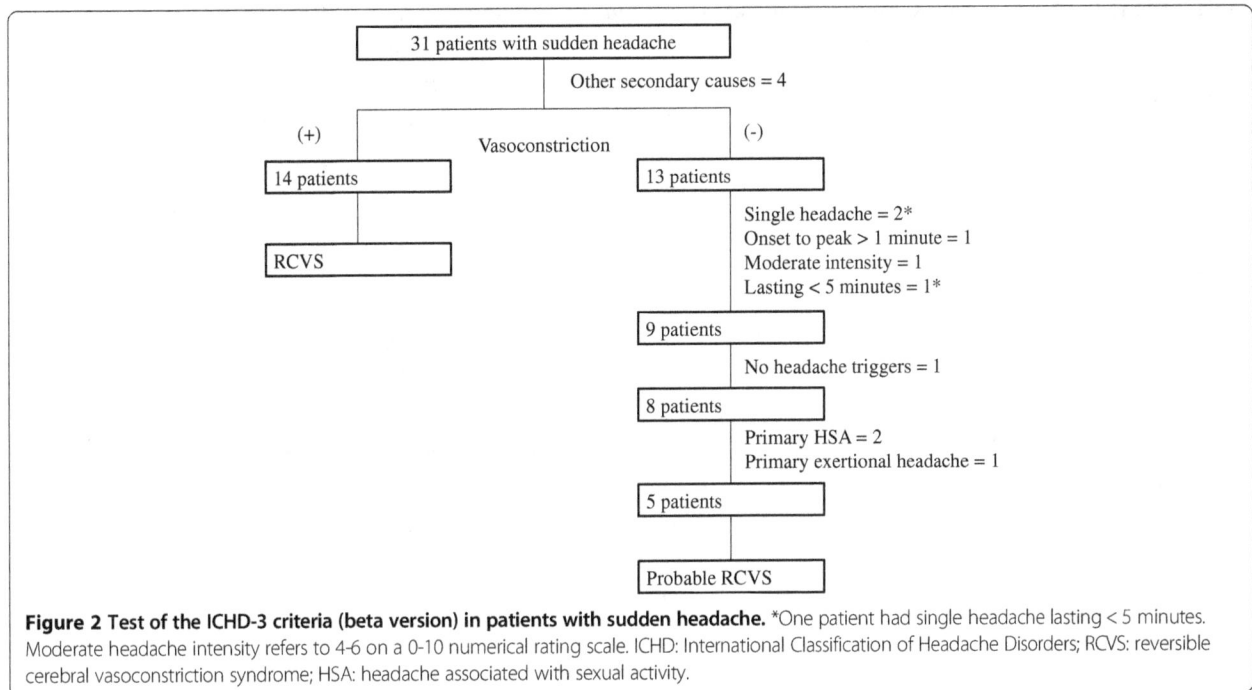

Figure 2 Test of the ICHD-3 criteria (beta version) in patients with sudden headache. *One patient had single headache lasting < 5 minutes. Moderate headache intensity refers to 4-6 on a 0-10 numerical rating scale. ICHD: International Classification of Headache Disorders; RCVS: reversible cerebral vasoconstriction syndrome; HSA: headache associated with sexual activity.

was very common, and not all cough medications precipitate RCVS, the percentage was likely over-estimated.

Headaches

As for the headache characteristics, patients with RCVS were less likely to exhibit short headache duration of < 1 hour (SH: 23.1% vs. 78.6%, $P = 0.007$; TCH: 10% vs. 75%, $P = 0.004$). The mean headache duration was not presented because most patients described their headache duration as a range e.g. several minutes (the shortest) or up to one day (the longest). We tried different cutoff points including half an hour and four hours but the best one to differentiate the two groups was one hour. Also, patients with RCVS were more likely to report bathing as their headache trigger (SH: 42.9% vs. 0%, $P = 0.004$; TCH: 36.4% vs. 0%, $P = 0.031$). On the other hand, patients with non-RCVS were more likely to report exertion as a trigger, but significance of this difference existed only in the SH sample (SH: 0% vs. 30.8%, $P = 0.098$; TCH: 0% vs. 29.4%, $P = 0.048$). Three patients complained of possible neurological symptoms during headache attacks (Table 3). This included bilateral leg numbness (RCVS), restlessness sensation of legs (RCVS with cortical SAH), and left palm numbness (moyamoya syndrome). All symptoms subsided before the patients called upon our clinic and no patients demonstrated abnormal neurological examination findings.

Diagnostic workup

Three patients with RCVS exhibited multifocal linear high-intensity signals along the cortical sulci and subarachnoid space (Figure 3). The neuroradiologist (Kuo KH) was more in favor of cortical SAH though the possibility of hyperintense vessels may not be excluded [15]. All of these patients received CT prior to their MRI exams and only one patient exhibited comparable hyperdense lesions. Catheter angiography was performed in each patient and no aneurysm was found. Follow-up MRI revealed resolution of the signals. One patient received lumbar puncture at emergency department two weeks before she presented to our clinic. The open and close pressures were 230/195 mmH$_2$O with the presence of red blood cells (143 cells/mm^3). The data were regarded as due to a traumatic tap and no further workup was performed. In our study, total three RCVS patients had received lumbar puncture while normal results were found in the other two patients.

Treatment and follow up

All patients recovered without neurological sequelae, including the patient with aneurysmal SAH received surgery. We also did not encounter any patients who develop new neurological symptoms or signs after their visits. The response to nimodipine in patients with RCVS was not presented because the adherence to headache diary was low. We contacted the patients by phone in December 2013; at this time, no patient had relapse of similar severe headaches or been diagnosed with SAH or sudden death. One patient with RCVS and one patient with primary exertional headache reported incomplete recovery and mild residual headache. Within the inclusion period, one patient reported relapse 22 months

Table 3 Demographic and clinical profiles of patients with sudden and thunderclap headaches

	Sudden headache				Thunderclap headache			
	Total (n = 31)	RCVS (n = 14)	Non-RCVS (n = 17)	P	Total (n = 24)	RCVS (n = 11)	Non-RCVS (n = 13)	P
Age (years)	45.3 ± 10.7	50.8 ± 9.3	40.8 ± 10.0	0.006	45.7 ± 10.5	49.4 ± 10.0	42.6 ± 10.3	0.092
Female	21 (67.7%)	12 (85.7%)	10 (58.8%)	0.132	16 (66.7%)	9 (81.8%)	8 (61.5%)	0.386
Previous headache	17 (54.8%)	10 (71.4%)	7 (41.2%)	0.149	14 (58.3%)	8 (72.7%)	6 (46.2%)	0.240
Precipitating factors				0.304				0.576
None	25 (80.6%)	9 (64.3%)	16 (94.1%)		19 (79.2%)	7 (63.6%)	12 (92.3%)	
Vasoactive substances	4 (12.9%)	3 (21.4%)	1 (5.9%)		3 (12.5%)	2 (18.2%)	1 (7.7%)	
Postpartum	0	0	0		0	0	0	
Headache characters								
Intensity	8.4 ± 1.7	8.6 ± 1.9	8.3 ± 1.6	0.375	8.7 ± 1.2	8.8 ± 1.5	8.5 ± 0.9	0.502
Location				1.0				1.0
Bilateral	17 (70.8%)	7 (70%)	10 (71.4%)		14 (70.0%)	6 (66.7%)	8 (72.7%)	
Duration				0.007				0.004
< 1 hour	14 (51.9%)	3 (23.1%)	11 (78.6%)		10 (45.5%)	1 (10.0%)	9 (75.0%)	
Single attack	4 (12.9%)	0	4 (23.5%)	0.107	2 (15.4%)	0	2 (8.3%)	0.482
Lingering pain	12 (38.7%)	6 (42.9%)	6 (35.3%)	0.724	10 (41.7%)	5 (45.5%)	5 (38.5%)	1.0
Triggers								
Sexual activity	9 (29.0%)	2 (14.3%)	7 (41.2%)	0.132	7 (29.2%)	2 (18.2%)	5 (38.5%)	0.386
Exertion[§]	5 (16.1%)	0	5 (29.4%)	0.048	4 (16.7%)	0	4 (30.8%)	0.098
Valsalva maneuver[§]	14 (45.2%)	8 (57.1%)	6 (35.3%)	0.289	10 (41.7%)	6 (54.5%)	4 (30.8%)	0.408
Emotion[§]	3 (9.7%)	1 (7.1%)	2 (11.8%)	1.0	3 (12.5%)	1 (9.1%)	2 (15.4%)	1.0
Bathing*	6 (19.4%)	6 (42.9%)	0	0.004	4 (16.7%)	4 (36.4%)	0	0.031
Cough[§]	2 (6.5%)	0	2 (11.8%)	1.0	1 (4.2%)	0	1 (7.7%)	1.0
Others	6 (19.4%)	5 (35.7%)	1 (5.9%)	0.067	4 (16.7%)	3 (27.3%)	1 (7.7%)	0.300
No triggers	3 (9.7%)	1 (7.1%)	2 (11.8%)	1.0	2 (8.3%)	0	2 (15.4%)	0.482
Possible neurological symptoms	3 (9.7%)	2 (14.3%)	1 (5.9%)	0.576	1 (4.2%)	1 (9.1%)	0	0.458
Abnormal CT or MRI[†]	5 (16.1%)	3 (21.4%)	2 (11.8%)	0.636	4 (16.7%)	3 (27.3%)	1 (7.7%)	0.300
Lumbar puncture	3 (9.7%)	3 (21.4%)	0	0.081	2 (8.3%)	2 (18.2%)	0	0.199
Angiography	8 (25.8%)	5 (35.7%)	3 (17.6%)	0.412	7 (29.2%)	5 (45.5%)	2 (15.4%)	0.182

Values presented are either mean ± standard deviation or number (%).
RCVS: reversible cerebral vasoconstriction syndrome; CT: computed tomography; MRI: magnetic resonance imaging.
[§]Valsalva maneuver includes defecation, urination, sneezing, bending, heavy lifting and related exercise. Laughing and crying are categorized as "emotion."
Exertion includes exercises not specifically involving Valsalva maneuvers. Cough includes only coughing but not straining or Valsalva maneuvers.
*Bathing includes also showering or exposure to water.
[†]Abnormal CT or MRI refers to changes other than vasospasm or moyamoya vessels.

after his first attack. This patient was diagnosed with primary HSA after the first attack; however, vasoconstriction was noted during the relapse and the diagnosis was subsequently changed to RCVS.

Discussion

In our study, 14 (45.2%) of the 31 patients with SH and 11 (45.8%) of the 24 patients with TCH had RCVS. Over past decades, several studies have recruited patients with SH, focusing on the identification of SAH and sentinel headache (Table 4). A significant proportion of patients exhibited SAH and other secondary causes, but more than one-half of the patients in these studies did not receive a definite diagnosis. It has been postulated that RCVS accounts for most of these "benign TCH" cases [13]. Our results show that about one-half of these patients exhibit RCVS. Due to a lack of similar studies, to the best of our knowledge, we compared our results with studies addressing related headache syndromes. In a study of 30 patients with HSA, 18 (60%) patients exhibited RCVS, 10 (33.3%) exhibited primary HSA and 2 (6.7%) exhibited other secondary causes (SAH and

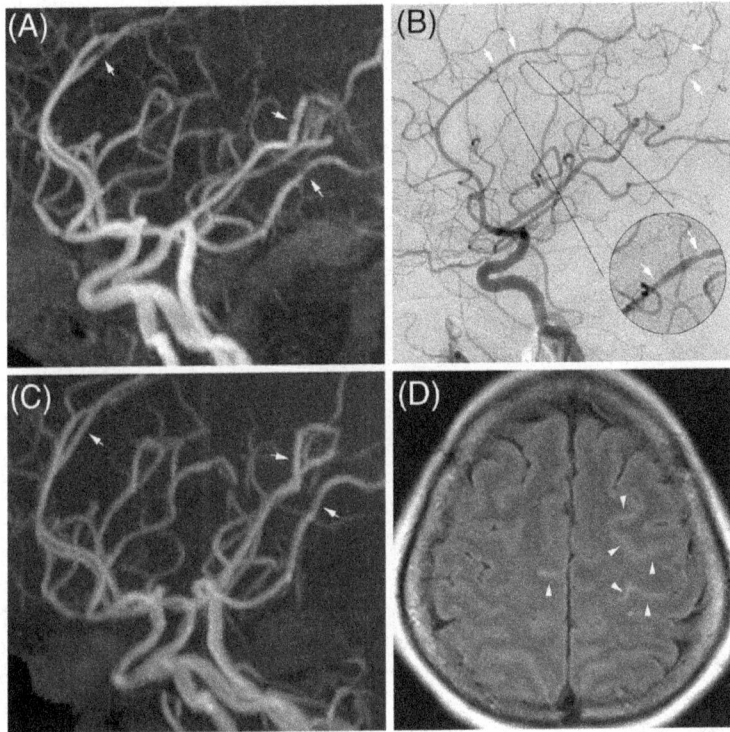

Figure 3 Imaging findings of reversible cerebral vasoconstriction syndrome. Multifocal vasoconstriction demonstrated by magnetic resonance angiography (MRA) **(A)** and catheter angiography **(B)**, involving the anterior, middle, and posterior cerebral arteries. Follow-up MRA **(C)** revealed significant interval resolution of the previous lesions. Axial fluid attenuated inversion recovery (FLAIR) imaging revealed linear hyperintensity lesions in the sulci of the bilateral frontal lobes **(D)**.

basilar artery dissection) [16]. In another study of 21 patients with bath-related TCH, 13 (62%) patients exhibited RCVS and no other secondary causes were identified [17]. The target populations in the above studies varied from that of our study: patients in the above studies were recruited mainly based on specific triggers (sexual activity and bathing, respectively), while our patients presented with SH or TCH, with or without triggers. In conclusion, our study provides direct evidence that RCVS is a common and likely under-recognized cause of SH and TCH.

Demographic data in our RCVS patients recaptured an obvious pattern reported in other studies with larger sample sizes: a majority of older female and a minority of younger male patients. In our study, around 80% of

Table 4 Summary of studies on patients with sudden headache

	Current study	Perry [5]	Landtblom [4]	Linn [3]	Harling [26]
SAH	3.3%	6.2%	11.3%	25%	71.4%
No diagnosis	19.4%	57.7%	73.0%	62.8%	2.0%
	(3.3%)*				
Onset	sudden	< 1 hour	sudden	< 1 minute	sudden
Intensity	NS	NS	NS	Severe	NS
Duration	> 1 minute	NS	NS	> 1 hour	NS
Onset to visit	< 30 days	< 14 days	NS	NS	NS
Settings	Clinic	Emergency department	Emergency department	Clinic and emergency	In-hospital
Follow up	6-42 months	6 months	12 months	12 months	18-30 months
Further SAH	0	0	0	0	0

SAH: subarachnoid hemorrhage; NS: not specified.
*When we conducted the study, patients with multiple triggers could not be classified by the criteria of International Classification of Headache Disorders, 2nd edition (ICHD-2) (Table 1). However, five of these six patients may be categorized as probable reversible cerebral vasoconstriction syndrome by the criteria of ICHD-3, beta version (Table 1) (Figure 2).

patients with RCVS were female, compared with 64.2% to 89.6% in previous studies [9,11,18]. Female RCVS patients were typically aged in their late forties or fifties, while male patients were aged in their thirties (women: 53.8 ± 5.8 years, men: 33.0 ± 4.2 years). The mean age of our female RCVS patients seemed slightly older than those in other studies (women: 44.2-49.7 years, men: 34.7-34.9 years) [9-11]. We propose that this difference is due to the absence of a third group of RCVS patients in our study: younger women in the postpartum state. This proposition is likely supported by the larger standard deviation in studies with higher ratios of postpartum female [9,11].

The clinical profiles of our RCVS patients differed from previous studies in several aspects. First, our patients demonstrated more favorable outcomes. Only a few patients presented with subtle neurological symptoms, and no patients exhibited focal neurological signs or seizure throughout the course of the study. We did not observe any complications of cerebral infarction, intracerebral hemorrhage, or posterior reversible encephalopathy syndrome. Second, most of our RCVS patients were spontaneous (78.6%), i.e., without precipitants. There was no patient in the postpartum state. All patients with possible vasoactive substances used cough medicine and the percentage was probably over-estimated (please refer to Precipitating factors paragraph of Results). We encountered only one Vietnamese patient who reported use of ecstasy one month after childbirth but she was seen before the initiation of the study and thus not included [19]. This was in contrast with the use of recreational drugs (especially cannabis) in French study or serotonergic drugs (selective serotonin reuptake inhibitors and triptans) in American study [9,11]. In general, the above clinical profiles were similar to another Taiwanese study but differed from French and American cohorts [9-11]. The discrepancy may be attributed to the clinic-based settings of both Taiwanese studies, in comparison with emergency or inpatient settings of other studies, i.e. patients with complications were more likely to call upon emergency service and to be admitted. It is also possible that the benign course of our RCVS patients were related to the absence of postpartum state and cannabis use, as both have been associated with stroke and poorer outcome [20,21]. However, another study from the same French group reported women and migraine history, instead of postpartum or vasoactive substances, were associated with intracranial hemorrhage in RCVS patients [22]. Two recent retrospective studies of RCVS do not identify any precipitants as predictors of outcome. Of note, the target in one study was clinical worsening (rather than final outcome), while the other study was small in sample size (n = 10) [23,24].

In our study, patients with RCVS were less likely to have short headache duration < 1 hour (Table 3). The duration of RCVS ranges from 5 minutes to 36 hours with a mean of 5 hours in one study, and a median of 3 hours in another study [9,10]. The duration of primary headaches vary in a wide span, by the definition of ICHD-2 [6]. For primary TCH, the duration range is 1 hour to 10 days and for primary exertional headache, the duration range is 5 minutes to 48 hours. Nevertheless, a study of 596 adolescent patients with primary exertional headache reported 467 (78.4%) patients had headache duration < 1 hour [25]. The duration of primary cough headache (1 second to 30 minutes) is significantly shorter than the duration of RCVS; however, only two (11.8%) of the non-RCVS patients in our study reported cough as the trigger (Table 3). Another study of HSA showed no difference in headache characteristics, including duration, between patients with primary HSA and RCVS [16]. In general, fewer patients with RCVS had short headache duration (< 1 hour) compared to non-RCVS patients; however, the headache duration may vary significantly in the latter group.

Among the various triggers, bathing (including showering and water exposure) was more frequently associated with RCVS in both SH and TCH cohorts. It has been reported that RCVS was noted in 13 (62%) of 21 patients with bath-related TCH [17]. In our study, all patients reported bathing as a trigger were in the RCVS group (100%, n = 6). Bathing is unique among RCVS triggers, in that it is not associated with the Valsalva maneuver or emotion. In contrast to bathing, exertion was associated with non-RCVS diagnoses, but the significance of this association was borderline, and only in the SH sample (SH: $P = 0.048$; TCH: $P = 0.098$). Further studies are necessary to validate the associations between different triggers and RCVS.

Although TCH was first used to describe the headache associated with an unruptured aneurysm [1], only one (3.1%) patient with SAH was noted in our study. The studies focused on SAH and sentinel headache on patients with SH showed that 6.2-25% of them exhibited SAH, except for the earliest study, which identified 71.4% of patients exhibiting SAH (Table 4) [3-5,26]. Compared with a very modest decline of SAH incidence over recent decades, the dramatic decrease of SAH ratios in these studies was confusing [27]. We proposed that the low ratio of SAH in our patients may be due to the following reasons. First, the definition of SH, unlike that of TCH, was not well-determined and varied with each study (Table 4). Second, previous studies either recruited patients from an emergency department only or from both emergency and outpatient clinics, while our study was strictly clinic-based. Given the low rates of patients receiving lumbar puncture and catheter angiography in our study, the possibility of missed SAH may not be excluded. Nevertheless, based on the high sensitivity of the modern CT to detect SAH and CTA/MRA to detect aneurysm and the fact that no patients developed SAH during at least 6 months of follow-up, the contribution of missed SAH to the low SAH percentage in our study may be minor [17,28,29].

This study has limitations. First, the sample size is relatively small and further study with a larger population is needed. Second, as stated above, the definition of SH and the clinical setting were not consistent across studies and the ratios of RCVS in these patients may change accordingly. In this study, we included patients with a new SH of possible vascular origins while excluded those with typical clinical presentations suggesting other primary or secondary headaches. This may carry a potential risk of missing SAH or RCVS patients presenting with typical features of other headaches. We also excluded patients with recurrent SH or TCH. Interpretation and generalization of the data should be handled with caution. Third, the percentage of patients receiving catheter angiography was low. Although CTA and MRA have been widely accepted for detection of vasoconstriction in patients with RCVS, catheter angiography is still the gold standard [7,18]. Besides, vasoconstriction has been reported to elude primary detection, and serial repetition may be necessary [9,18]. Therefore, the percentage of RCVS may be underestimated. This observation did not change—and may perhaps strengthen—our conclusion that RCVS is a common cause of SH and TCH. The low angiography rate may also contribute to the result that arterial dissection in patients with RCVS was not observed [30]. Fourth, the percentage of RCVS patients receiving lumbar puncture was also low (SH: 21.4%, TCH: 18.2%). As stated above, we could not exclude the possibility of missed SAH, but the chance may be low. Fifth, several rare causes of TCH were not excluded properly. Without MR venography, cerebral venous sinus thrombosis may be ignored, but the neuroradiologist denied any related findings by CT or MRI in all patients. Without routine lumbar puncture, meningitis may be undetected; however, none of the patients exhibited fever or neck stiffness. We did not screen pheochromocytoma, though no patients exhibited uncontrolled hypertension. Altogether, these diseases were rare in patients with isolated TCH, and we were convinced that the ratio of RCVS may not change significantly [13].

Conclusions

In this study, we provided direct evidence of RCVS as a common cause of SH and TCH. Demographic data in our RCVS patients recaptured a typical pattern reported in other studies: a majority of older female and a minority of younger male patients. The clinical profiles were similar to another clinic-base study from Taiwan but differed from other studies with emergency or inpatient settings. Compared to non-RCVS patients, patients with RCVS were older and had longer headache duration. They were more likely to cite bathing but less likely to cite exertion as triggers. Reversible cerebral vasoconstriction syndrome is a clinical emergency linked with potential clinical worsening, morbidity and even mortality [23,24]. Systemic examination of cerebral vessels should be adopted in these patients, so that they may benefit from potential treatments such as avoidance of triggers and use of nimodipine.

Abbreviations
CT: Computed tomography; CTA: Computed tomography angiography; HSA: Headache associated with sexual activity; ICHD: International Classification of Headache Disorders; MR: Magnetic resonance; MRA: Magnetic resonance angiography; MRI: Magnetic resonance imaging; RCVS: Reversible cerebral vasoconstriction syndrome; SAH: Subarachnoid hemorrhage; SH: Sudden headache; TCH: Thunderclap headache.

Competing interests
The authors declare that they have no competing interests.

Authors' contributions
CYC collected the data, analyzed the data and participated in manuscript preparation. KKH was responsible for the imaging protocols, interpretation and preparation of Figure 3. LTH took charge of the whole study, especially the ideation, recruitment of patients and manuscript preparation. All authors read and approved the final manuscript.

Acknowledgements
The study was supported in part by grants from the National Science Council (NSC) of Taiwan (NSC 99-2314-B-418-007, 100-2314-B-418-001, 101-2314-B-418-007), and Far Eastern Memorial Hospital (FEMH 2011-C-016, 2012-C-050).

Author details
[1]Section of Neurology, Department of Internal Medicine, Far Eastern Memorial Hospital, No. 21, Sec. 2, Nanya S. Rd., Ban-Chiao Dist., New Taipei City 220, Taiwan. [2]Department of Radiology, Far Eastern Memorial Hospital, New Taipei, Taiwan. [3]Department of Neurology, Neurological Institute, Taipei Veterans General Hospital, Taipei, Taiwan. [4]Department of Neurology, National Yang-Ming University School of Medicine, Taipei, Taiwan.

References
1. Day JW, Raskin NH (1986) Thunderclap headache: symptom of unruptured cerebral aneurysm. Lancet 2:1247–1248
2. Wijdicks EF, Kerkhoff H, van Gijn J (1988) Long-term follow-up of 71 patients with thunderclap headache mimicking subarachnoid hemorrhage. Lancet 9:68–70
3. Linn FH, Wijdicks EF, van der Graaf Y, Weerdesteyn-van Vliet FA, Bartelds AI, van Gijn J (1994) Prospective study of sentinel headache in aneurysmal subarachnoid hemorrhage. Lancet 344:590–593
4. Landtblom AM, Fridriksson S, Boivie J, Hillman J, Johansson G, Johansson I (2002) Sudden onset headache: a prospective study of features, incidence and causes. Cephalalgia 22:354–360
5. Perry JJ, Stiell IG, Sivilotti ML, Bullard MJ, Hohl CM, Sutherland J, Emond M, Worster A, Lee JS, Mackey D, Pauls M, Lesiuk H, Symington C, Wells GA (2013) Clinical decision rules to rule out subarachnoid hemorrhage for acute headache. JAMA 310:1248–1255

6. Headache Classification Committee of the International Headache Society (2004) The international classification of headache disorders, 2nd edition. Cephalalgia 24(suppl 1):9–160

7. Ducros A (2012) Reversible cerebral vasoconstriction syndrome. Lancet Neurol 11:906–917

8. Calabrese LH, Dodick DW, Schwedt TJ, Singhal AB (2007) Narrative review: reversible cerebral vasoconstriciton syndromes. Ann Intern Med 146:34–44

9. Ducros A, Boukobza M, Porcher R, Sarov M, Valade D, Bousser MG (2007) The clinical and radiological spectrum of reversible cerebral vasoconstriction syndrome: a prospective series of 67 patients. Brain 130:3091–3101

10. Chen SP, Fuh JL, Chang FC, Lirng JF, Shia BC, Wang SJ (2008) Transcranial color doppler study for reversible cerebral vasoconstriction syndromes. Ann Neurol 63:751–757

11. Singhal AB, Hajj-Ali RA, Topcuoglu MA, Fok J, Bena J, Yang D, Calabrese LH (2011) Reversible cerebral vasoconstriction syndromes: analysis of 139 cases. Arch Neurol 68:1005–1012

12. Chen SP, Fuh JL, Wang SJ (2010) Reversible cerebral vasoconstriction syndrome: an under-recognized clinical emergency. Ther Adv Neurol Disord 3:161–171

13. Ducros A, Bousser MG (2013) Thunderclap headache. BMJ 346:e8557

14. Headache Classification Committee of the International Headache Society (2013) The International Classification of Headache Disorders, 3rd edition (beta version). Cephalalgia 33:629–808

15. Chen SP, Fuh JL, Lirng JF, Wang SJ (2012) Hyperintense vessels on flair imaging in reversible cerebral vasoconstriction syndrome. Cephalalgia 32:271–278

16. Yeh YC, Fuh JL, Chen SP, Wang SJ (2010) Clinical features, imaging findings, and outcomes of headache associated with sexual activity. Cephalalgia 30:1329–1335

17. Wang SJ, Fuh JL, Wu ZA, Chen SP, Lirng JF (2008) Bath-related thunderclap headache: a study of 21 consecutive patients. Cephalalgia 28:524–530

18. Chen SP, Fuh JL, Wang SJ, Chang FC, Lirng JF, Fang YC, Shia BC, Wu JC (2010) Magnetic resonance angiography in reversible cerebral vasoconstriction syndromes. Ann Neurol 67:648–656

19. Hu CM, Lin YJ, Fan YK, Chen SP, Lai TH (2010) Isolated thunderclap headache during sex: orgasmic headache or reversible cerebral vasoconstriction syndrome? J Clin Neurosci 17:1349–1351

20. Fugate JE, Ameriso SF, Ortiz G, Schottlaender LV, Wijdicks EF, Flemming KD, Rabinstein AA (2012) Variable presentations of postpartum angiopathy. Stroke 43:670–676

21. Wolff V, Lauer V, Rouyer O, Sellal F, Meyer N, Raul JS, Sabourdy C, Boujan F, Jahn C, Beaujeux R, Marescaux C (2011) Cannabis use, ischemic stroke, and multifocal intracranial vasoconstriction: a prospective study in 48 consecutive young patients. Stroke 42:1778–1780

22. Ducros A, Fiedler U, Porcher R, Boukobza M, Stapf C, Bousser MG (2010) Hemorrhagic manifestation of reversible cerebral vasoconstriction syndrome: frequency, features and risk factors. Stroke 41:2505–2511

23. Katz BS, Fugate JE, Ameriso SF, Pujol-Lereis VA, Mandrekar J, Flemming KD, Kallmes DF, Rabinstein AA (2014) Clinical worsening in reversible cerebral vasoconstriction syndrome. JAMA Neurol 71:68–73

24. Robert T, Kawkabani Marchini A, Oumarou G, Uske A (2013) Reversible cerebral vasoconstriction syndrome identification of prognostic factors. Clin Neurol Neurosurg 115:2351–2357

25. Chen SP, Fuh JL, Lu SR, Wang SJ (2009) Exertional headache–a survey of 1963 adolescents. Cephalalgia 29:401–407

26. Harling DW, Peatfield RC, van Hille PT, Abbott RJ (1989) Thunderclap headache: is it migraine? Cephalalgia 9:87–90

27. de Rooij NK, Linn FH, van der Plas JA, Algra A, Rinkel GJ (2007) Incidence of subarachnoid hemorrhage: a systematic review with emphasis on region, age, gender and time trends. J Neurol Neurosurg Psychiatry 78:1365–1372

28. Gee C, Dawson M, Bledsoe J, Ledyard H, Phanthavady T, Youngquist S, McGuire T, Madsen T (2012) Sensitivity of newer-generation computed tomography scanners for subarachnoid hemorrhage: a Bayesian analysis. J Emerg Med 43:13–18

29. Brunell A, Ridefelt P, Zelano J (2013) Differential diagnostic yield of lumbar puncture in investigation of suspected subarachnoid hemorrhage: a retrospective study. J Neurol 260:1631–1636

30. Mawet J, Boukobza M, Franc J, Sarov M, Arnold M, Bousser MG, Ducros A (2013) Reversible cerebral vasoconstriction syndrome and cervical arterial dissection in 20 patients. Neurology 81:821–824

4

Measurement precision and biological variation of cranial arteries using automated analysis of 3 T magnetic resonance angiography

Faisal Mohammad Amin[1], Elisabet Lundholm[1], Anders Hougaard[1], Nanna Arngrim[1], Linda Wiinberg[1], Patrick JH de Koning[2], Henrik BW Larsson[3] and Messoud Ashina[1*]

Abstract

Background: Non-invasive magnetic resonance angiography (MRA) has facilitated repeated measurements of human cranial arteries in several headache and migraine studies. To ensure comparability across studies the same automated analysis software has been used, but the intra- and interobserver, day-to-day and side-to-side variations have not yet been published. We hypothesised that the observer related, side-to-side, and day-to-day variations would be less than 10%.

Methods: Ten female participants were studied using high-resolution MRA on two study days separated by at least one week. Using the automated LKEB-MRA vessel wall analysis software arterial circumferences were measured by blinded observers. Each artery was analysed twice by each of the two different observers. The primary endpoints were to determine the intraclass correlation coefficient (ICC) and intra- an inter-observer, the day-to-day, and side-to-side variations of the circumference of the middle meningeal (MMA) and middle cerebral (MCA) arteries.

Results: We found an excellent intra- and interobserver agreement for the MMA (ICC: 0.909-0.987) and for the MCA (ICC: 0.876-0.949). The coefficient of variance within observers was $\leq1.8\%$ for MMA and $\leq3.1\%$ for MCA; between observers $\leq3.4\%$ (MMA) and $\leq4.1\%$ (MCA); between days $\leq6.0\%$ (MMA) and $\leq8.0\%$ (MCA); between sides $\leq9.4\%$ (MMA) and $\leq6.5\%$ (MCA).

Conclusion: The present study demonstrates a low (<5%) inter- and intraobserver variation using the automated LKEB-MRA vessel wall analysis software. Furthermore, the study also suggests that the day-to-day and side-to-side variations of the MMA and MCA circumferences are less than 10%.

Keywords: Magnetic resonance angiography; Middle meningeal artery; Middle cerebral artery; Migraine

Background

The three-dimensional time-of-flight magnetic resonance angiography (3D-TOF-MRA) method has enabled *in vivo* investigation of the human cranial arteries with a relatively high spatial resolution. The 3D-TOF-MRA method is simple to use and requires no intravenous contrast to visualize the arteries [1]. Thus, it is possible to detect changes of the luminal size of larger and smaller arteries relatively precise. This method has been employed in several headache and migraine studies to measure arterial changes before and after infusion of different vasoactive drugs and during versus outside attacks of migraine headache [2-8]. Most recently, using this method we compared the arterial circumferences on the headache side with the non-headache side and a migraine attack day with a non-headache day in patients with migraine. Surprisingly, we found intracranial but *not* extracranial arterial dilatation on the headache-side relative to the non-headache-side [6]. In a previous MRA study of drug-induced migraine attacks the middle cerebral artery (intracranial) and middle meningeal artery (extracranial) were both dilated on the pain-side versus the non-pain side [4], while another MRA study

* Correspondence: ashina@dadlnet.dk
[1]Danish Headache Center and Department of Neurology, Glostrup Hospital, Faculty of Health and Medical Sciences, University of Copenhagen, Nordre Ringvej 57, DK-2600 Glostrup, Denmark

of drug-induced migraine attacks reported no side-to-side changes at all [2]. Although, the differences were ascribed different drug effects, it raised the question about the biological variations in day-to-day and side-to-side arterial circumference in migraine patients. In addition, these variations may also be affected by the observer related variability. Automated analysis of the acquired MRA images may reduce observer related variability and may also ensure better repeatability across different studies. The LKEB-MRA vessel wall analysis software [9], which has been used in several headache and migraine studies [2-8], provides an automated method to detect the vessel lumen contour accurately. The required user interaction is limited to placing only a proximal and a distal point in the vessel of interest [9]. In the present study, we therefore initially investigated the intra- and inter-observer variations and then the day-to-day, and side-to-side variations of the MMA and MCA using LKEB-MRA vessel wall analysis software [9]. We hypothesized that the observer related variability would be less than 5% using automated analysis software and the biological variations, including observer variation, would be less than 10%.

Methods

Participants

This study included 10 female migraine patients without aura who were recruited between July 2011 and February 2012 via a Danish website for recruitment of participants for biomedical research projects (www.forsoegsperson.dk). Exclusion criteria were: a history of neurological disorder (except migraine without aura or infrequent tension-type headache less than 5 days per month), a history of cardiovascular disease, any daily medication intake (except oral contraceptives), any other somatic or psychiatric disease, pregnant or breast feeding, and any contraindication for magnetic resonance imaging. The regional Ethical Committee of Copenhagen (Denmark) approved the study. All participants gave their written informed consent and the study was conducted in accordance with the Helsinki Declaration. This study was a part of a larger study investigating physiological effects of vasoactive drugs [8].

Study design

Magnetic resonance angiography (MRA) was performed in all participants on two different study days with at least one week between the study days. None of the participants had a headache or an intake of any type of medication during or 48 h prior to the MRA scans. All participants were abstinent from tobacco, alcohol and caffeine-containing food or drinks for 8 h, and totally fasting in 4 h prior to the MRA scans. Moreover, heart rate, blood pressure, respiratory frequency, end-tidal pressure of carbon dioxide (CO_2), haematocrit, and haemoglobin levels were measured on both days.

MRA acquisition

We used a 3.0 Tesla Philips Achieva machine (Philips Medical Systems, Best, Netherlands) with an eight-element phased-array receiver head coil to acquire single-slab three-dimensional time-of-flight MRA of the middle cerebral artery (MCA [FOV, $200 \times 200 \times 74$ mm^3; matrix size, 800×406; acquired voxel resolution, $0.25 \times 0.49 \times 1.00$ mm^3; reconstructed resolution, $0.20 \times 0.20 \times 0.50$ mm^3; TR, 25 ms; TE, 3.5 ms; flip angle 20°; sense factor 2; four chunks; acquisition time, 9 min 3 seconds]) and the middle meningeal artery (MMA [FOV, $200 \times 200 \times 16$ mm^3; matrix size, 800×571; acquired voxel resolution, $0.25 \times 0.35 \times 0.70$ mm^3; reconstructed resolution, $0.20 \times 0.20 \times 0.35$ mm^3; TR, 25 ms; TE, 3.5 ms; flip angle 20°; sense factor 3; four chunks; acquisition time, 5 min 29 seconds]). We used the MCA location and the branching point of the MMA as references to plan the MRA slabs on the same position on both days. It would have been most optimal to use the same scan for both arteries, but as the MMA is smaller than MCA, small circumference changes would not have been detected. We therefore used a smaller voxel size for the MMA. However, if the MMA scan was used to record both MMA and MCA it would have consumed much more time, increasing the risk of movement artefacts. Even though, we used a higher resolution for the MMA scan it was not enough to capture the intracranial part of the MMA, because the artery size decreases and vary much in location inside the cranial cavity.

Data analysis

The MRA data were transferred from the scanner computer to a remote workstation in DICOM format and then analysed by the LKEB-MRA vessel wall analysis software (version 6.2007). The MMA was identified by marking the branch from the main trunk of the maxillary artery (Figure 1). The MCA was identified by marking the branch from the main trunk of the internal carotid artery (Figure 2). The software calculated a path line and measured the diameter and circumference of the selected vessel segment every 0.2 mm perpendicular to the centre line, from which the average circumference of a 5 mm long vessel segment was finally obtained. To determine intra- and inter-observer variations, all images were analysed twice by two different investigators, who were blinded to the experimental day. Each observer analysed a total of 40 MMAs (EL and LW) and 40 MCAs twice (NA and LW) (10 right-sided and 10 left-sided arteries for day 1 and 2). The only manual input by the observer was selection of a start and an end point on each image (Figures 1 and 2). The results for the

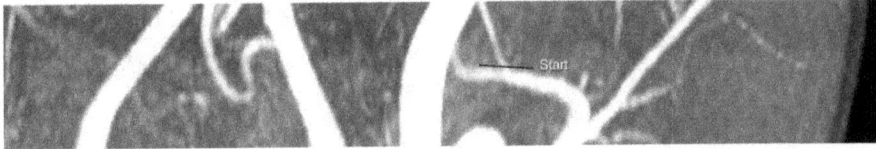

Figure 1 The start of the middle meningeal artery segment was selected by marking the branch from the main trunk of the maxillary artery. The black line indicates the start point.

investigator who had the best intra-observer variation were used to analyse the biological variations.

Statistics

All absolute values are presented as mean (SD). Age, height, weight, and days between the experiments are presented as mean (range).

The primary endpoints of the study were to determine the 1) intra-observer, 2) inter-observer, 3) day-to-day, and 4) side-to-side variations of the circumference of the MCA and the MMA.

We initially assessed the intra- and inter-observer measurement reliability by determining the Intraclass Correlation Coefficient (two-way mixed; absolute agreement). Coefficient of variance was then determined for all four endpoints using the Cfvar function in IBM SPSS Statistics software (version 20). We tested for differences in mean arterial circumferences within observers and between observers, days and sides using the paired samples t test. Differences in the physiological and biochemical data were also tested using the paired samples t test.

We used IBM SPSS Statistics (version 20) for all statistical analyses. No adjustment for multiple analyses was made. Thus, the level of significance at 0.05 was accepted for each comparison.

Results

All ten participants (10 female [6 right-handed, 4 left-handed], mean age 24 [range 19–31], height 165 cm [range 157–174], weight 58 kg [range 52–68] were scanned on two different experimental days (mean time between the scans 17 days [range 7–29]). There was no difference in the heart rate, the respiratory frequency, end-tidal pressure of CO_2, hematocrit, and hemoglobin levels between the two days. However, the blood pressure was slightly higher on the first day (Table 1).

Intra- and inter-observer agreements and variations

The intraclass correlation coefficients for average measures were excellent for the MMA and the MCA measurements. MMA: EL 0.936 (95% CI 0.879 to 0.966) and LW 0.985 (95% CI 0.971 to 0.992). MCA: NA 0.949 (95% CI 0.904 to 0.973) and for LW 0.938 (95% CI 0.884 to 0.967).

The coefficient of variance was smaller in the MMA (observer EL, 1.8% and observer LW, 1.8%) than in the MCA (observer NA, 3.0% and observer LW, 3.1%) (Figure 3).

The agreement between observers was also very high for the MMA measurements (first 0.909 (95% CI 0.827 to 0.952) and second 0.987 (95% CI 0.976 to 0.993)).

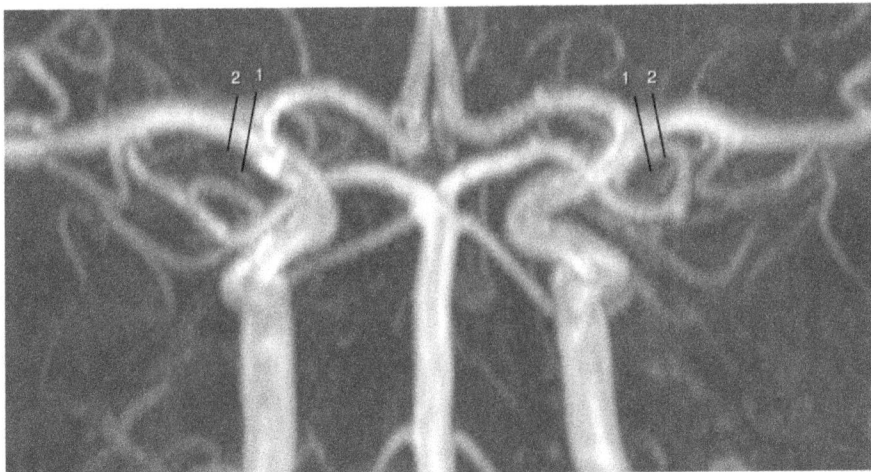

Figure 2 The start point of the middle cerebral artery (MCA) segment was identified at the point where artery branches from the main trunk of the internal carotid artery. It is difficult to choose where exactly the MCA starts. The black lines marked with 1 and 2 show two different start points. If it is chosen that MCA starts from line number 1, the MCA in every analysis in this patients should start from number 1.

Table 1 Mean values (±SD) of physiological variables between the two days

Variable	Day 1	Day 2	P-value
Heart rate (beats/min)	63 (5)	64 (5)	0.250
Systolic blood pressures (mmHg)	121 (10)	116 (11)	0.028
Diastolic blood pressure (mmHg)	68 (8)	65 (8)	0.093
Mean arterial blood pressure (mmHg)	85 (7)	82 (8)	0.038
Respiratory frequency (breaths/min)	15 (3)	15 (3)	0.343
End-tidal pressure of CO2 (kPa)	4.8 (0.2)	4.7 (0.3)	0.348
Hematocrit	0.38 (0.03)	0.39 (0.03)	0.333
Hemoglobin (mmol/L)	8.1 (0.5)	8.2 (0.5)	0.264

P-value: The paired samples t-test.

The MCA measurements also showed high interobserver agreement (first 0.876 (95% CI 0.768 to 0.934) and second 0.929 (95% CI 0.827 to 0.967). We found a smaller coefficient of variation when we compared an observer's second analysis with the other observer's second analysis (MMA, 1.7% and MCA, 3.3%) compared to the variance in their first analyses (MMA, 3.4% and MCA, 4.1%) (Figure 3).

Day-to-day variations
The right MMA circumference varied 6.0% and left 5.9% between the two days. There was an 8.0% variation in the right MCA circumference and 7.1% in the left sided MCA circumference (Table 2).

Side-to-side variations
We found almost the same variations between the right- and left-sided MMAs and MCAs on both experimental

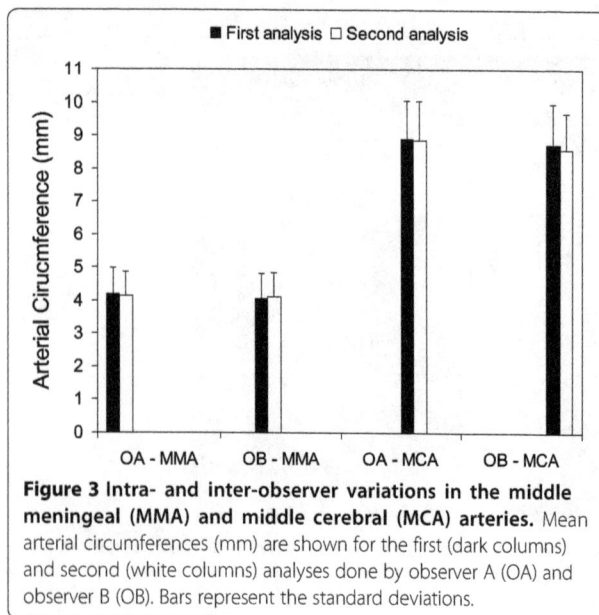

Figure 3 Intra- and inter-observer variations in the middle meningeal (MMA) and middle cerebral (MCA) arteries. Mean arterial circumferences (mm) are shown for the first (dark columns) and second (white columns) analyses done by observer A (OA) and observer B (OB). Bars represent the standard deviations.

Table 2 Day-to-day differences of the mean arterial circumference (±SD) and the coefficient of variance

Artery	Side	Day 1	Day 2	P-value	Variance
MMA	Right	4.17 mm (0.77)	4.03 mm (1.00)	0.327	6.0%
	Left	4.18 mm (0.54)	4.15 mm (0.65)	0.810	5.9%
MCA	Right	9.35 mm (1.36)	8.68 mm (0.80)	0.106	8.0%
	Left	8.83 mm (1.44)	8.61 mm (0.94)	0.583	7.1%

MMA = middle meningeal artery; MCA = middle cerebral artery; P-value: The paired samples t-test.

days. On day 1 MMA varied 9.3% and 9.4% on day 2. The coefficient of variance for the MCA was 6.4% on day 1 versus 6.5% on day 2 (Table 3).

Discussion
This is the first MRA based study of experimental and biological variations in the circumference of human middle cerebral and meningeal arteries. Using the automated LKEB-MRA vessel wall software [9], we found an excellent intra- and interobserver agreements and relatively small variations within (<3.1%) and between (<4.1%) observers, as well as between the days (<8.0%) and sides (<9.4%).

Observer variations
The variation in the MCA was higher than in the MMA for both observers. Identification of the start points are complicated by the anatomy of the vessel. An identical start point of the MMA is more plausible to determine consistently as there is a marked decrease in vessel size where the MMA branches out from the maxillary artery (Figure 1). However, in some cases the MMA branches directly from the external carotid artery, where a starting point is more difficult to select. On the contrary, the size difference between the distal part of the internal carotid artery and the MCA very small, which makes it challenging to identify the exact same starting point within and between observers (Figure 2). Unlike the main trunk of the extracranial MMA, the MCA circumference decreases along its main trunk, making it more susceptible to differences in the starting point. For instance, if the

Table 3 Side-to-side differences of the mean arterial circumference (±SD) values and the coefficient of variance in 10 subjects

Artery	Day	Right	Left	P-value	Variance
MMA	1	4.17 mm (0.77)	4.18 mm (0.54)	0.958	9.3%
	2	4.03 mm (1.00)	4.15 mm (0.65)	0.613	9.4%
MCA	1	9.35 mm (1.36)	8.83 mm (1.44)	0.155	6.4%
	2	8.68 mm (0.80)	8.61 mm (0.94)	0.076	6.5%

MMA = middle meningeal artery; MCA = middle cerebral artery; P-value: The paired samples t-test.

start is selected 2–3 mm more distally on one image, it results in a smaller circumference of that MCA.

The variation of the second analyses was almost the same between the observers as it was within the observers. In contrast, comparison of the first analyses showed varied slightly more, indicating that some exercise is necessary to analyse the arteries accurately. Observers in this study (EL, LW, NA) had no previous experience with the software or analysis of MRA images. They received the same 15 min instruction by an experienced observer (FMA) before they started the measurements. The gold standard to assess MCA diameter changes before the advent of MRI was the contrast agent based arteriography. Intravenous contrast based methods are not optimal for repeated measurements. Therefore, many studies of vascular mechanisms of drug-induced and spontaneous headache and migraine used the transcranial Doppler (TCD) method. The TCD methods is based on recordings of the velocity changes of the MCA, which can be calculated to diameter changes given that the cerebral blood flow is constant [10]. However, the variations of the TCD methods are expected to be large due to several factors, such as different angles of insonation, heart rate variability, and those caused by different observers (13%) [11]. To the best of our knowledge, no such study of the MMA exits.

Biological variations of the cranial arteries

The day-to-day and side-to-side variations in the MCA circumference found in the present study were smaller than the previously reported variation in the blood velocity (BV) of MCA using TCD [11]. An increase in the BV indicates vasoconstriction, whereas decreased velocity represents increased vessel diameter, provided that the cerebral blood flow is constant. Different factors have been demonstrated to influence the BV and thereby the day-to-day variation in the vessel size. These factors include age [12-16], haematocrit [17], and the end-tidal pressure of CO_2 [18]. In addition, intake of alcohol or caffeine-containing food or drinks, use of medication, and headache [6,19] may also play a role in the day-to-day variation. The age is unlikely to play any role in the present study, as all participants rescanned within 30 days (mean 17 days). The haematocrit and end-tidal pressure of CO_2 were determined on both days and showed no statistical differences between the days in our study, suggesting a minimal input to the day-to-day differences seen in the present study. The participants were abstinent from tobacco, alcohol, and caffeine for at least 8 hours, and they had no medication use or headache for 48 h prior to the experiment starts. While there was a small difference in the day-to-day variation, the side-to-side differences were almost same on both days. The side-to-side differences may be explained by anatomical differences of the arteries. These data provide a possibility to calculate sufficient sample size in future studies (Figure 4). However, these data also suggest that only circumference changes higher than 10% in headache and migraine studies can be considered clinical relevant using this method.

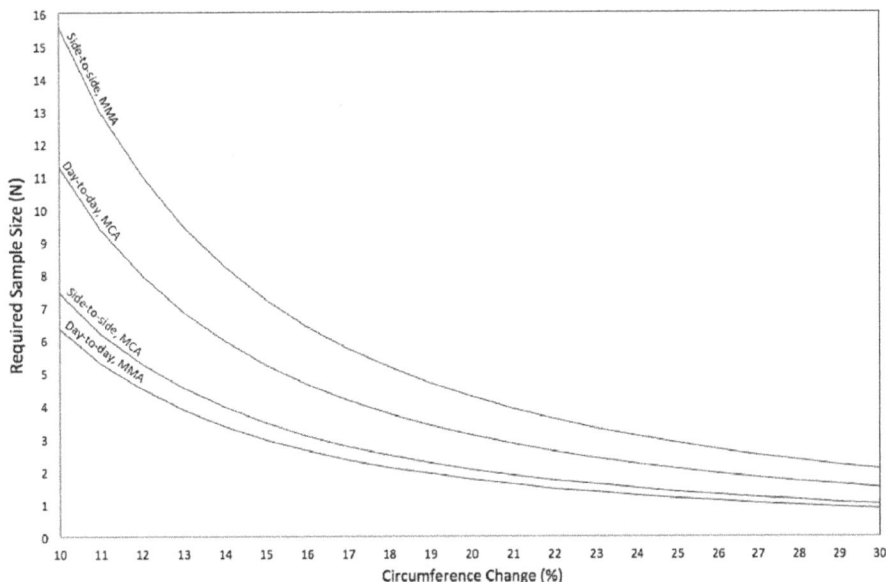

Figure 4 Sample size determination using the coefficient of variance for unpaired data in 3D-TOF-MRA studies where day-to-day and side-to-side differences of the middle meningeal (MMA) and middle cerebral (MCA) arterial calibre are desired (5% significance, 90% power). For paired data, the sample size is half of the required sample size should be used: N = 21*(coefficient of variance)^2 / (lnμ_0 − lnμ_1)^2.

Methodological considerations

Although, the present day-to-day variations are relatively small, there are some methodological considerations, which have to be mentioned. First, we are not able to exactly sort out how much of the found biological variation is real and how much is influenced by the observer, but it is certainly less than 10%. However, the 3D-TOF-MRA method itself can affect the measurements (i.e. two MRA's obtained in the same scan session, may also play a role). Even small body movement during the scan can result in blurred MRA images. Blurred images makes the arteries appear larger, but at the moment, there is no way to detect the image quality for motion of the 3D-TOF-MRA other than visual assessment by the observer or calculation of signal-to-noise ratios, when comparing two different MRA images. Another important consideration when comparing different segments with each other is that signal obtained from arteries located in-plane decrease the more distally the selected segments are. It is therefore crucial that exact the same segment is selected across different images, when comparison between two days or conditions is desired. A possible difference between the MCA and MMA variations could also be related to the fact that the MMA is running along the plane of acquisition with possible increased risk of flow artefacts.

Conclusion

The present study demonstrates a low (<5%) inter- and intraobserver variation using the automated LKEB-MRA vessel wall analysis software. Furthermore, the study also suggests that the day-to-day and side-to-side variations of the MMA and MCA circumferences are less than 10%.

Abbreviations

3D-TOF: Three-dimensional time-of-flight; BV: Blood velocity; CO_2: Carbon monoxide; DICOM: Digital Imaging and Communcations in Medicine; FOV: Field-of-view; MCA: Middle cerebral artery; MMA: Middle meningeal artery; MRA: Magnetic resonance angiography; SD: Standard deviation; TCD: Transcranial Doppler; TE: Echo time; TR: Repetition time.

Competing interests

The authors declare that they have no competing interests in relation to this study.

Authors' contributions

FMA and AH carried out the scans, designed the study, performed statistical tests, and drafted the manuscript. EL, NA, and LW analysed the images, were involved in study design, and participated in manuscript drafting. PJHdK and HBWL were involved in interpretation of data and revising the manuscript critically for important intellectual content. MA designed the study, was involved in interpretation and drafting, and revised the manuscript critically. All authors have given final approval of the version to be published.

Acknowledgements

We gratefully thank Professor Lene T. Skovgaard for statistical advice, Dr. Stephen W. Pedersen for scientific advises, all participants in the study, radiographers Bente S. Møller and Helle J. Simonsen for help with the scans.

Funding

The study was supported by grants from the University of Copenhagen, the Lundbeck Foundation through the Center for Neurovascular Signalling (LUCENS), the Research Foundation of the Capital Region of Denmark, Danish Council for Independent Research-Medical Sciences, the Novo Nordisk Foundation, and the IMK Almene Foundation.

Author details

[1]Danish Headache Center and Department of Neurology, Glostrup Hospital, Faculty of Health and Medical Sciences, University of Copenhagen, Nordre Ringvej 57, DK-2600 Glostrup, Denmark. [2]Division of Image Processing, Department of Radiology, Leiden University Medical Center, Leiden, Netherlands. [3]Functional Imaging Unit, Diagnostic Department, Glostrup Hospital, Faculty of Health and Medical Sciences, University of Copenhagen, Copenhagen, Denmark.

References

1. Davis WL, Blatter DD, Harnsberger HR, Parker DL (1994) Intracranial MR angiography: comparison of single-volume three-dimensional time-of-flight and multiple overlapping thin slab acquisition techniques. AJR Am J Roentgenol 163:915–920
2. Schoonman GG, van der Grond J, Kortmann C, van der Geest RJ, Terwindt GM, Ferrari MD (2008) Migraine headache is not associated with cerebral or meningeal vasodilatation–a 3 T magnetic resonance angiography study. Brain 131:2192–2200
3. Asghar MS, Hansen AE, Kapijimpanga T, van der Geest RJ, de Koning P, Larsson HBW, Olesen J, Ashina M (2010) Dilatation by CGRP of middle meningeal artery and reversal by sumatriptan in normal volunteers. Neurology 75:1520–1526
4. Asghar MS, Hansen AE, Amin FM, van der Geest RJ, van der Koning P, Larsson HBW, Olesen J, Ashina M (2011) Evidence for a vascular factor in migraine. Ann Neurol 69:635–645
5. Amin FM, Asghar MS, Guo S, Hougaard A, Hansen AE, Schytz HW, van der Geest RJ, de Koning PJH, Larsson HBW, Olesen J, Ashina M (2012) Headache and prolonged dilatation of the middle meningeal artery by PACAP38 in healthy volunteers. Cephalalgia 32:140–149
6. Amin FM, Asghar MS, Hougaard A, Hansen AE, Larsen VA, de Koning PJH, Larsson HB, Olesen J, Ashina M (2013) Magnetic resonance angiography of intracranial and extracranial arteries in patients with spontaneous migraine without aura: a cross-sectional study. Lancet Neurol 12:454–461
7. Amin FM, Asghar MS, Ravneberg JW, de Koning PJH, Larsson HBW, Olesen J, Ashina M (2013) The effect of sumatriptan on cephalic arteries: A 3 T MR-angiography study in healthy volunteers. Cephalalgia 33:1009–1016
8. Amin FM, Hougaard A, Schytz HW, Asghar MS, Lundholm E, Parvaiz AI, de Koning PJ, Andersen MR, Larsson HB, Fahrenkrug J, Olesen J, Ashina M (2014) Investigation of the pathophysiological mechanisms of migraine attacks induced by pituitary adenylate cyclase-activating polypeptide-38. Brain 137:779-794.
9. de Koning PJH, Schaap JA, Janssen JP, Westenberg JJM, van der Geest RJ, Reiber JHC (2003) Automated segmentation and analysis of vascular structures in magnetic resonance angiographic images. Magn Reson Med 50:1189–1198
10. Aaslid R, Markwalder TM, Nornes H (1982) Noninvasive transcranial Doppler ultrasound recording of flow velocity in basal cerebral arteries. J Neurosurg 57:769–774
11. Thomsen LL, Iversen HK (1993) Experimental and biological variation of three-dimensional transcranial Doppler measurements. J Appl Physiol 75:2805–2810
12. Ackerstaff RGA, Keunen RWM, van Pelt W, van Swijndregt ADM, Stijnen T (1990) Influence of biological factors on changes in mean cerebral in mean cerebral blood flow velocity in normal ageing: a transcranial Doppler study. Neurol Res 12:187–191
13. Arnolds BJ, von Reutern GM (1986) Transcranial doppler-sonography. Examination technique and normal reference values. Ultrasound Med Biol 12:115–123
14. Grolimund P, Seiler RW (1988) Age dependence of the flow velocity in the basal cerebral arteries—a transcranial Doppler ultrasound study. Ultrasound Med Biol 14:191–198

15. Lindegaard KF, Bakke SJ, Grolimund P, Aaslid R, Huber P, Nornes H (1985) Assessment of intracranial hemodynamics in carotid artery disease by trancranial doppler ultrasound. J Neurosurg 63:890–898
16. Vriens EM, Kraaier V, Musbach M, Wrienke GH, Huffelen AC (1989) Transcranial pulsed Doppler measurements of blood velocity in the middle cerebral artery: reference values at rest and during hyperventilation in healthy volunteers in relation to age and sex. Ultrasound Med Biol 15:1–8
17. Brass LM, Pavlakis SG, de Vivo D, Piomelli S, Mohr JP (1988) Transcranial doppler measurements of the middle cerebral artery effect of hematocrit. Stroke 19:1466–1469
18. Markwalder TM, Grolimund P, Seiler RF, Roth F, Aaslid R (1984) Dependency of blood flow velocity in the middle cerebral artery on end-tidal carbon dioxide partial pressure—a transcranial ultrasound Doppler study. J Cereb Blood Flow Metab 4:368–372
19. Thomsen LL, Iversen HK, Olesen J (1995) Cerebral blood flow velocities are reduced during attacks of unilateral migraine without aura. Cephalalgia 15:109–116

5

Prolonged acute migraine with aura and reversible brain MRI abnormalities after liquid sclerotherapy

Yassine Zouitina[1], Mathilde Terrier[1], Marie Hyra[2], Djohar Seryer[3], Jean-Marc Chillon[4,5] and Jean-Marc Bugnicourt[1,6*]

Abstract

Transient visual disturbances constitute the most commonly reported neurological side effect during and immediately after sclerotherapy. A few studies, based on clinical and diffusion-weighted MRI assessments, have suggested that these transient neurological symptoms correspond to migraine with aura. Recently, it has been reported that brain magnetic resonance imaging can reveal transient T2*-weighted abnormalities during the acute phase of migraine with aura. We reported a 36-year-old man who presented with transient neurological symptoms and concomitant T2*-weighted abnormalities on brain magnetic resonance imaging immediately after liquid sclerotherapy. We hypothesize that the reversible nature of the patient's T2*-weighted abnormalities may indicate a relationship with the post-sclerotherapy migraine with aura attack.

Keywords: Migraine; Migraine aura; Sclerotherapy; Magnetic resonance imaging; Gradient-echo T2*-weighted imaging

Background

Transient visual disturbances constitute the most commonly reported neurological side effect during and immediately after sclerotherapy, with an incidence of 1.4%s [1]. Furthermore, foam sclerotherapy appears to be associated with a higher incidence of transient visual disturbances than liquid sclerotherapy [2]. Research has suggested that these transient neurological symptoms (which are more frequent in patients with patent foramen ovale (PFO) and/or a history of migraine) correspond to migraine with aura (MA) [3-5].

More recently, it has been reported that brain magnetic resonance imaging (MRI) can reveal transient T2*-weighted abnormalities during the acute phase of MA [6-8].

Here, we report on a patient who presented with transient neurological symptoms and concomitant T2*-weighted abnormalities on MRI immediately after liquid sclerotherapy. We hypothesize that the reversible nature of the patient's T2*-weighted abnormalities may indicate a relationship with the post-sclerotherapy MA attack.

* Correspondence: bugnicourt.jean-marc@chu-amiens.fr
[1]Department of Neurology, Amiens University Hospital, 1 Place Victor Pauchet, F-80054 Amiens cedex, France
[6]Laboratory of Functional Neuroscience and Pathology (EA 4559), Department of Neurology, Amiens University Hospital, Amiens, France

Case presentation

A 36-year-old man presented with symptomatic but moderate varicosity of the left small saphenous vein. The patient had no vascular risk factors, no history of venous diseases, no family history of migraine and no reported migraine comorbidities. He reported a few episodes of headache, the description of which was compatible with migraine without aura. In February 2014, he underwent liquid sclerotherapy (carried out in accordance with the European consensus statement) [9]. After contraindications to treatment were ruled out and the patient had given his written, informed consent, the first sclerotherapy session (with a total of 2 ml of 0.25% lauromacrogol solution) was not followed by any complications. Two weeks later, the patient received a second injection of 4 ml of 0.25% lauromacrogol solution. Immediately following the injection, the patient reported flickering lights in his right eye and several minutes of photopsiae, followed by right hemianopsia. These symptoms disappeared after two hours. Two weeks later, the patient underwent a third sclerotherapy (with 4 ml of 0.25% lauromacrogol solution). Immediately following injection of the liquid, the patient again reported flickering lights in his right eye, followed by right hemianopsia and (two hours later) the progressive onset of aphasia and psychomotor slowing. Comprehension was not affected. An evaluation by a neurologist revealed headache, right hemianopia, mild word-finding difficulties and a slowly progressing disturbance of consciousness. The National Institutes of Health Stroke Scale (NIHSS) score was 4 out of 42 [10]. Brain MRI (performed three hours after symptom onset) was normal. However, gradient-echo T2*-weighted images revealed several hypointense areas in both hemispheres of the brain (though predominantly in the left hemisphere) (Figure 1A). The patient's movement prevented us from interpreting the results of magnetic resonance angiography of the Circle of Willis. Since the acute symptoms persisted, acute encephalopathy was suspected. Although the results of a cerebrospinal fluid analysis were normal, treatment with acyclovir was initiated. The chest radiography was unremarkable. The electrocardiogram, carotid ultrasonography, transcranial Doppler ultrasound and transthoracic echocardiography results were normal. The laboratory test results (including thyroid function, arterial blood gas measurement, and syphilis screening tests) were also normal. The coagulation work-up did not show any factor V Leiden or prothrombin gene G20210A mutations, and protein C, protein S, antithrombin III, factor VIII and homocysteine levels were normal. Antibody screening was negative. Transoesophageal echocardiography revealed a PFO with an associated atrial septal aneurysm. A color flow duplex scan revealed a moderate right-to-left shunt but only during provocation tests. The cardiac valves were normal, and there was no evidence of aortic atheroma or pulmonary arterial hypertension. The colour duplex ultrasonography results for the lower limbs were normal. After 48 h, the symptoms (including the headache) resolved spontaneously and the patient was diagnosed with probable migraine with aura (on the basis of this first episode of migraine with prolonged aura). Brain MRI was repeated five days after symptom onset and the T2* images were normal (Figure 1B). The patient was discharged six days after admission, with a favourable outcome (NIHSS score: 0). Following hospitalisation, the patient suffered from to other episodes of migraine with aura lasting for less than 1 hour.

Conclusions

In migraine with aura, visual disturbances may comprise additional features (such as flickering lights and spots), or the loss of features (such as hemianopia and loss of vision) and may be associated with sensory disturbance and speech impairment (depending on the extent of cortical spreading depression (CSD) [1,11]. These complications appear to be more frequent after foam sclerotherapy than after liquid sclerotherapy [2]. Although the degree to which the injected volume of sclerotic agent contributes to the development of neurological side effects is subject to debate, it appears reasonable to decrease the volume when (i) neurological symptoms occurs after sclerotherapy and (ii) another sclerotherapy session is required [11]. Recent clinical and brain MRI studies have shown that these transient neurological symptoms (which are more frequent in patients with PFO) correspond to MA rather than to transient ischemic events [5,12].

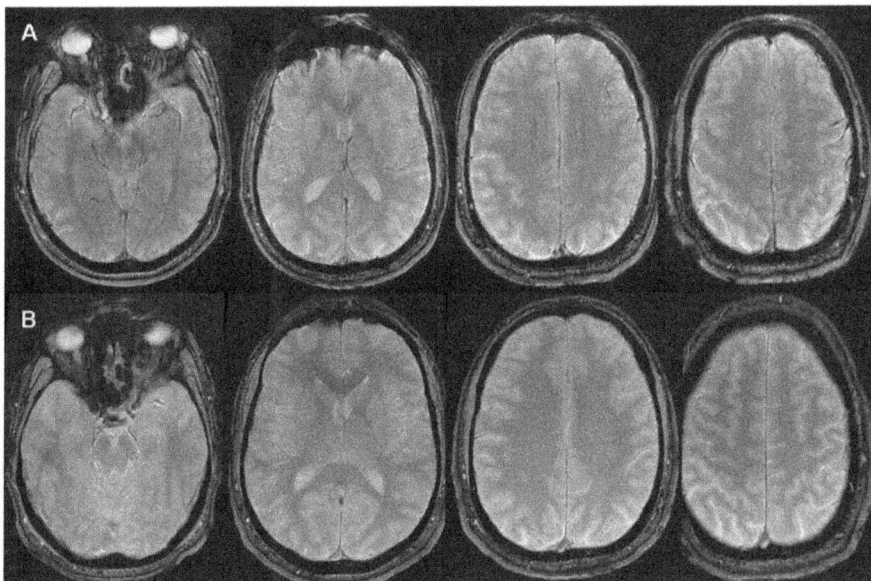

Figure 1 A gradient-echo T2*-weighted magnetic resonance image showing hypointense signals in both hemispheres of the brain but especially in the left hemisphere (A) and a normal gradient-echo T2*-weighted magnetic resonance image acquired five days after the migraine attack (B).

Migraine with aura occurs in about one third of migraine sufferers [13]. It is clinically defined by at least two recurrent episodes of fully reversible symptoms (the most frequent of which are visual disturbances, sensory disturbances and speech and/or language impairment). The aura symptom spreads gradually over a period of 5 minutes and (for each individual aura) lasts between 5 and 60 minutes (although this upper limit was set arbitrarily). Indeed, it has been reported that aura lasts for more than one hour in up to 37% of patients [14]. This epidemiological reality has been recently taken into consideration in the third edition of the International Classification of Headache Disorders, in which aura lasting more than an hour but less than a week (in the absence of radiologically confirmed brain ischemia) was defined as "probable migraine with aura (prolonged aura)" [15]. These atypical clinical presentations always warrant a thorough work-up, since cerebrovascular disease must be always considered [16]. As such, brain MRI is usually required to carefully screen for the underlying cause during the acute phase. Recently, transient T2*-weighted imaging abnormalities on brain MRI have been reported during the acute phase of MA [6-8]. The occurrence of these transient T2*-weighted imaging abnormalities after sclerotherapy lends support to the hypothesis whereby endothelin release and microembolization trigger CSD [17]. The two most likely explanations for these T2* findings relate to (i) increased oxygen consumption and a subsequent increase in the intravenous deoxyhaemoglobin concentration [18] and (ii) venous dilatation following the release of vasoactive factors (such as endothelin). In murine models, systemic levels of endothelin-1 (ET-1, one of the most potent vasoconstrictors and a CSD inducer) are significantly elevated one and five minutes after the initiation of foam sclerothapy [19]. Furthermore, Lemos et al.'s study of a population of Portuguese patients revealed a possible role for the endothelin receptor type A in migraine without aura [20]. Nevertheless, the prevalence and significance of these phenomena merit further investigation.

In conclusion, the present observation suggests that the transient nature of the T2*-weighted imaging abnormalities is associated with a CSD caused by migraine aura after sclerotherapy.

Competing interests
The authors declare that they have no competing interests.

Authors' contributions
YZ conceived the study, participated in its design and coordination and helped to draft the manuscript. MT has made substantial contributions to conception and design, acquisition of data, analysis and interpretation of data. MH has made substantial contributions to conception and design, acquisition of data, analysis and interpretation of data. DS participated in the design of the study, and helped to draft the manuscript. JMC has made substantial contributions to conception and design, acquisition of data, analysis and interpretation of data. JMB conceived the study, participated in its design and coordination, helped to draft the manuscript, and has been involved in revising it for important intellectual content. All the authors have participated sufficiently in the work to take public responsibility for appropriate portions of the content. All authors read and approved the final manuscript.

Acknowledgments
We thank David Fraser PhD for providing medical writing services on behalf of Amiens University Hospital.

Author details
[1]Department of Neurology, Amiens University Hospital, 1 Place Victor Pauchet, F-80054 Amiens cedex, France. [2]Department of Physical Medicine and Rehabilitation, Amiens University Hospital, Amiens, France. [3]Department of Radiology, Amiens University Hospital, Amiens, France. [4]INSERM U1088, Amiens, France. [5]Department of Clinical Pharmacology, Amiens University Hospital, Amiens, France. [6]Laboratory of Functional Neuroscience and Pathology (EA 4559), Department of Neurology, Amiens University Hospital, Amiens, France.

References
1. Jia X, Mowatt G, Burr JM, Cassar K, Cook J, Fraser C (2007) Systematic review of foam sclerotherapy for varicose veins. BJS 94:925–936
2. Guex JJ, Allaert FA, Gillet JL, Chleir F (2005) Immediate and mid-term complications of sclerotherapy: report of a prospective multi-centric registry of 12,173 sclerotherapy sessions. Dermatol Surg 31:123–128
3. Ratinahirana H, Benigni JP, Bousser MG (2003) Injection of polidocanol foam in varicose veins as a trigger for attacks of migraine with aura. Cephalalgia 23:850–885
4. Coleridge SP (2006) Chronic venous disease treated by ultrasound guided foam sclerotherapy. Eur J Vasc Endovasc Surg 32:577–583
5. Gillet JL, Donnet A, Lausecker M, Guedes JM, Guex JJ, Lehmann P (2010) Pathophysiology of visual disturbances occurring after foam sclerotherapy. Phlebology 25:261–266
6. Karaarslan E, Ulus S, Kürtüncü M (2011) Susceptibility-weighted imaging in migraine with aura. Am J Neuroradiol 32:e5–e7
7. Shimoda Y, Kudo K, Kuroda S, Zaitsu Y, Fujinma N, Terae S, Sasaki M, Houkin K (2011) Susceptibility weighted imaging and magnetic resonance angiography during migraine attack: a case report. Magn Reson Med Sci 10:49–52
8. Bugnicourt JM, Canaple S, Lamy C, Deramond H, Godefroy O (2013) T2*-weighted findings in prolonged acute migraine aura. Chin Med J 126:20
9. Breu FX, Guggenbichler S (2004) European consensus meeting on foam sclerotherapy. Dermatol Surg 30:709–717
10. Kasner SE, Chalela JA, Luciano JM, Cucchiara BL, Raps EC, McGarvey ML, Conroy MB, Localio AR (1999) Reliability and validity of estimating the NIH stroke scale score from medical records. Stroke 30:1534–1537
11. Sarvananthan T, Shepherd AC, Willenberg T, Davies AH (2012) Neurological complications of sclerotherapy for varicose veins. J Vasc Surg 55:243–251
12. Gillet JL, Guedes JM, Guex JJ, Hamel-Desnos C, Schadeck M, Lauseker M, Allaert FA (2009) Side effects and complications of foam sclerotherapy of the great and small saphenous veins: a controlled multicentre prospective study including 1025 patients. Phlebology 34:131–138
13. International Headache Society Classification Subcommittee (2004) International classification of headache disorders, 2nd edition. Cephalalgia 24(suppl 1):1–160
14. Viana M, Sprenger T, Andelova M, Goadsby PJ (2013) The typical duration of migraine aura: a systematic review. Cephalalgia 33:483–490
15. Headache Classification Committee of the International Headache Society (2013) The international classification of headache disorders, 3rd edition (beta version). Cephalalgia 33:629–808

16. Schoene J, Sandor PS (2004) Headache with focal neurological signs or symptoms: a complicated differential diagnosis. Lancet Neurol 3:237–245
17. Dreier JP, Kleeberg J, Petzold G, Priller J, Windmüller O, Orzechowski HD, Lindauer U, Heinemann U, Einhäupl KM, Dirnagl U (2002) Endothelin-1 potently induces Leaˉo's cortical spreading depression in vivo in the rat: a model for an endothelial trigger of migrainous aura? Brain 125:102–112
18. Zagami AS, Goadsby PJ, Edvinsson L (1990) Stimulation of the superior sagittal sinus in the cat causes release of vasoactive peptides. Neuropeptides 16:69–75
19. Frullini A, Felice F, Burchielli S, Di Stefano R (2011) High production of endothelin after foam sclerotherapy: a new pathogenetic hypothesis for neurological and visual disturbances after sclerotherapy. Phlebology 26:203–208
20. Lemos C, Neto JL, Pereira-Monteiro J, Mendonça D, Barros J, Sequeiros J, Alonso I, Sousa A (2011) A role for endothelin receptor type A in migraine without aura susceptibility? A study in Portuguese patients. Eur J Neurol 18:649–655

6

Cognitive processing of cluster headache patients: evidence from event-related potentials

Rongfei Wang[1], Zhao Dong[1], Xiaoyan Chen[1], Ruozhuo Liu[1], Mingjie Zhang[1,2], Jinglong Wu[3*] and Shengyuan Yu[1*]

Abstract

Background: The peripheral and central origins of pain in cluster headache (CH) have been a matter of much debate. The development and application of functional imaging techniques have provided more evidence supporting the hypothesis that CH is not a disorder exclusively peripheral in origin, and in fact central regions might be more important. Event-related potentials confer advantages in the functional evaluation of the cortex, but few studies thus far have employed this method in cluster headache.

Methods: Seventeen cluster patients (15 males; mean age = 35.4 years) and 15 age-matched healthy participants (13 males; mean age = 34.6 years) were recruited. A visual oddball paradigm was employed to analyze target processing using event-related potentials. We investigated the P3/P3d components in the experiment.

Results: P3/P3d amplitudes were decreased in CH patients (P3, 3.82 μV; P3d, 5.8 μV) compared with controls (P3, 7.28 μV; P3d, 8.95 μV), $F(1,30) = 4.919$, $p < 0.05$, $\eta 2 = 0.141$ for P3 and $F(1,30) = 8.514$, $p < 0.05$, $\eta 2 = 0.221$ for P3d, respectively). Moreover, the amplitudes of P3/P3d were no significantl difference in the side of pain as compared to contralateral one ($p > 0.05$).

Conclusions: These results provide evidence of dysfunction in the cognitive processing of CH patients, which may also contribute to the pathophysiology of CH.

Keywords: Cluster headache; ERPs; P3/P3d; Cognitive processing

Background

Cluster headache (CH) causes severe unilateral temporal or periorbital pain, usually lasting between 15 and 180 minutes, and is accompanied by autonomic symptoms in the nose, eyes, and face. Headaches often recur at the same time each day during the cluster period, which can last for weeks or even months. CH is more prevalent in men, and its typical onset is 20–40 years of age. A Chinese clinic-based study, approximately 1 year in duration, estimated that trigeminal autonomic cephalalgia accounts for 5.3% of primary headaches, of which 84.7% are CH [1]. However, the pathophysiology of CH is not yet understood fully.

Central structures play an important role in the etiology of CH. The development of functional imaging techniques has been invaluable for the development of theories pertaining to the central mechanisms of CH. Several functional imaging studies have demonstrated the involvement of the hypothalamus [2-4]; in addition, activation in certain areas of the pain neuromatrix, which includes the thalamus, anterior cingulate cortex (ACC), insula, basal ganglia, cingulum, frontal cortex, and the cerebellar hemispheres, has also been reported during the acute pain state [4-7]. Cognitive processing studies employing event-related potentials (ERPs) support the hypothesis that CH cannot be exclusively peripheral in origin [8-11]. Many researchers report that brain structures involved in cognitive processing also underlie the pathophysiology of CH [8].

ERPs reveal coherent stimulus-related postsynaptic activity in the cortices, with a temporal resolution measurable in milliseconds. Accordingly, ERPs are ideally suited for investigation of the cortical activation time course during cognitive processing and also confer advantages during functional cortical evaluation. Several ERP studies have

* Correspondence: wu@mech.okayama-u.ac.jp; yushengyuan301@yahoo.com
[3]Biomedical Engineering Laboratory, Graduate School of Natural Science and Technology, Okayama University, 3-1-1 Tsushima-Naka, Okayama 700-8530, Japan
[1]Department of Neurology, Chinese PLA General Hospital, Fuxing Road 28, Haidian District, Beijing 100853, China

been conducted in CH patients in an effort to understand certain higher brain abnormalities. For example, Evers et al. [9,10] reported an increase in P3 latency in CH patients during the cluster period in a visual ERP test. Because P3 latency is an indicator of cognitive performance [11], the authors concluded that cognitive processing is impaired during the cluster period, lending credence to the notion that CH has a central origin. However, other neuropsychological tasks did not reveal significant abnormalities in CH patients (pertaining to their cognitive processing) [12]. Furthermore, personality studies have implied that CH patients do not experience learning disabilities [13,14]. The above studies also failed to demonstrate changes in the amplitude of P3, mainly because of the type of patients recruited and the difficulty involved in effecting stimulations.

In the present study, we used a traditional visual oddball paradigm, in which participants were required to press a button for the infrequent target stimulus, while ignoring the frequent non-target standard stimulus. We focused on P3 (a generic name for a variety of relatively late positive components [15,16]).

Methods

Participants

We recruited 17 cluster patients (15 males; mean age, 35.4 years; range, 20–45 years) from the Chinese PLA General Hospital according to the diagnostic criteria of the International Classification of Headache Disorders (3rd ed., beta version; ICHD-3 beta). The CH duration among patients ranged from 5 to 15 years, and the cluster period ranged from 1 to 6 months. The frequency of CH attacks during previous cluster periods was 1–3 attacks per day. Patients were not receiving prophylactic therapy, were drug-free for at least 24 hours, and were in bout but not in headache when recruited. We also recruited 15 healthy age-matched participants (13 males; mean age, 34.6 years; range, 22–43 years) with no history of headache or drug/alcohol abuse. Patients and controls had normal or corrected-to-normal vision and normal hearing capabilities. No participants had notable motor or sensory dysfunction or deep tendon reflexes. We excluded participants who were illiterate or suffering from depression, stroke, or brain injuries. The study was approved by the Ethical Committee of the Chinese PLA General Hospital in accordance with the ethical principles of the Declaration of Helsinki. All participants provided written and informed consent prior to commencement of the experiment.

The following clinical data of the CH patients were included: 1) past history of CH; 2) frequency of headaches over the previous year; 3) ratings for the most severe headache experienced during the previous year using a visual analog scale (VAS); and 4) position of the

headache. The exclusion criteria were as follows: 1) taking prophylactic medications for CH; 2) history of analgesic drug overuse; 3) history of general neurological or psychiatric disease; 4) history of drug abuse or dependency, including alcohol and cigarettes; 5) history of mixed-type headache; and 6) past history of neurological disorder or abnormal findings on a neurological examination.

The evaluation of the Montreal Cognitive Assessment (MoCa) and Mini-Mental Status Examination (MMSE) scores were carried out in all the participants.

Stimuli and procedures

The experiment was performed in a sound-attenuated room with a dim light. Stimuli comprised target stimuli (Figure 1, 20% probability of presentation) and standard stimuli (Figure 2, 80% probability of presentation). The duration of both stimuli was 105 ms. The inter-stimulus interval (ISI) varied randomly between 1,000 and 1,500 ms (mean = 1,200 ms). Two separate blocks, each comprising 160 stimuli, were presented. All the stimuli were showed out by the E-prime software.

Participants were instructed to focus on a fixation cross in the center of the screen and to press the button as quickly and accurately as possible when they viewed the target stimuli (Figure 1). The accuracy was the rate of pressing the button when viewed the target stimuli. The appropriate reaction time was the length between viewing the target stimuli and pressing the button accurately. The accuracy and appropriate reaction time were recorded by the E-prime software.

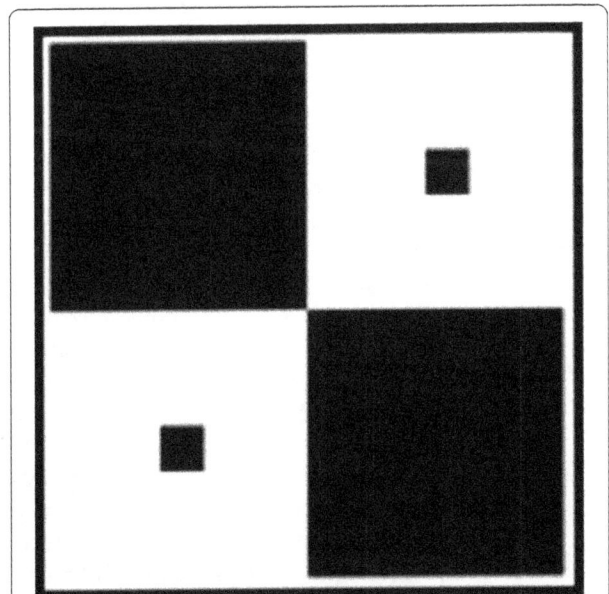

Figure 1 The picture showed the appearance of the target stimulus.

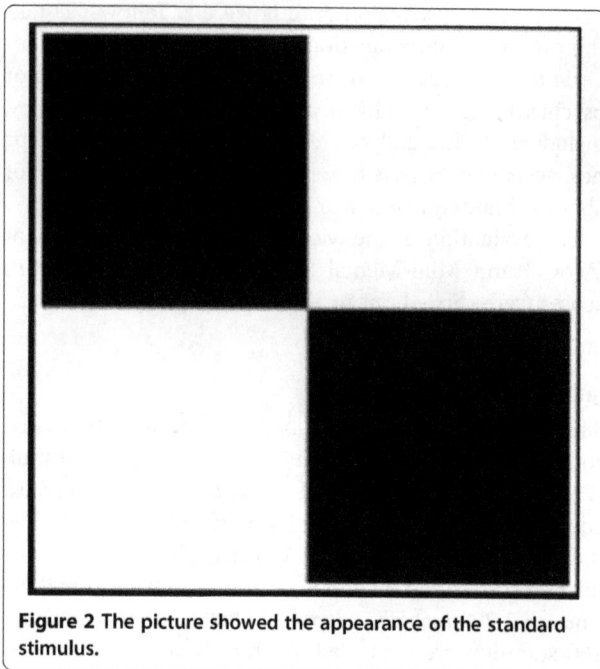

Figure 2 The picture showed the appearance of the standard stimulus.

EEG recording and analysis

An electroencephalogram (EEG) was recorded continuously (band pass 0.05-100 Hz, sampling rate 500 Hz) at the F3, F4, Fz, C3, C4, Cz, P3, P4, and Pz electrode sites, according to the international 10–20 system and using an ASA-Lab EEG/ERP 64-channel amplifier (www.ant-neuro.com) referenced to the left mastoid (right mastoid was used as the recording site). vertical electroculogram (VEOG) and horizontal electroculogram (HEOG) were recorded using two pairs of electrodes, one pair placed above and below the right eye, and the other placed 10 mm from the lateral canthi. Electrode impedance was maintained below 5 kΩ throughout the experiment.

We used ASA software (www.ant-neuro.com) to analyze the data offline. EEG data were re-referenced to the bi-mastoid average reference. EOG artifacts were corrected using the method proposed by Semlitsch et al. (1986). EEG was segmented into the epoch running from 200 ms pre-stimulus to 1,000 ms post-stimulus. EEG segments contaminated by amplifier clipping, bursts of electromyographic activity, or peak-to-peak deflection exceeding ± 100 μV were excluded from the average calculation. EEG segments were averaged separately for the target and standard stimuli. The EEG segments were averaged separately for target and standard stimuli. The number of average trials left after removal of the artifacts was 60 (target) and 240 (standard) for normal controls and 60 (target) and 240 (standard) for patients, respectively.

The peak amplitudes and latencies for one ERP component, P3, were measured relative to the pre-stimulus baseline period (Figure 3). The positive peak between 300–500 ms was used to define the P3 components. To

reliably observe the target effect, P3d was obtained by subtracting the ERPs in response to standard stimuli from those in response to target stimuli (Figure 4). The mean amplitudes of the P3d were measured between 300 and 500 ms.

P3 components were analyzed using repeated-measures analysis of variance (ANOVA), with Stimulus (target, standard) and Site (F$_3$, F$_4$, Fz, C$_3$, C$_4$, Cz, P$_3$, P$_4$, and Pz) as the within-subject factors and Group (CH, control) as the between-subjects factor.

For P3d components, ANOVA was conducted with Site (F$_3$, F$_4$, Fz, C$_3$, C$_4$, Cz, P$_3$, P$_4$, and Pz) as the within-subject factor and Group (CH, control) as the between-subjects factor. Degrees of freedom were corrected using the Greenhouse–Geisser epsilon.

Results

MoCa and MMSE scores

The mean MMSE scores did not differ between CH patients (28.32 ± 1.48) and control subjects (29.03 ± 0.57; $p > 0.05$); this also applied to the mean MoCa scores (patients, 27.71 ± 1.35; control subjects, 28.06 ± 1.63; $p > 0.05$).

Behavioral data

There was no significant group difference in accuracy (control, 99.33%; patients, 96.65%; $F(1, 30) < 1$). There was also no significant difference in the appropriate reaction time between CH patients (460.32 ms) and controls (446.91 ms; $F(1, 30) < 1$).

ERP data: P3 and P3d components

Across conditions, a significant main effect of Site for P3 was observed ($F(2,60) = 12.70$, $p < 0.001$, $\eta2 = 0.297$), indicating a centro-parietal scalp distribution with a maximum of 9.16 μV at Pz. Post-hoc tests revealed that, while there was significant difference between patients and controls (p = 0.034), the mean amplitude of P3 was larger for controls (7.28 μV) than patients (3.82 μV; $p < 0.05$, $\eta2 = 0.141$). No other effects reached significant level (ps > 0.1).

There was a significant main effect of Site for P3d was observed ($F(2,60) = 40.53$, $p < 0.001$, $\eta2 = 0.575$), indicating a centro-parietal scalp distribution with a maximum of 11.00 μV for P3d at Pz. Post-hoc tests revealed that, while there was significant difference between patients and controls (p = 0.007), the mean amplitude of P3d was larger for controls (8.95 μV) than patients (5.78 μV; $p < 0.05$, $\eta2 = 0.221$). No other effects reached significant level (ps > 0.1).

The latencies of the P3 and P3d components did not show any significant effects (ps > 0.1).

Eight CH patients had pain on the left side of the head and seven patients on the right side. The amplitudes of

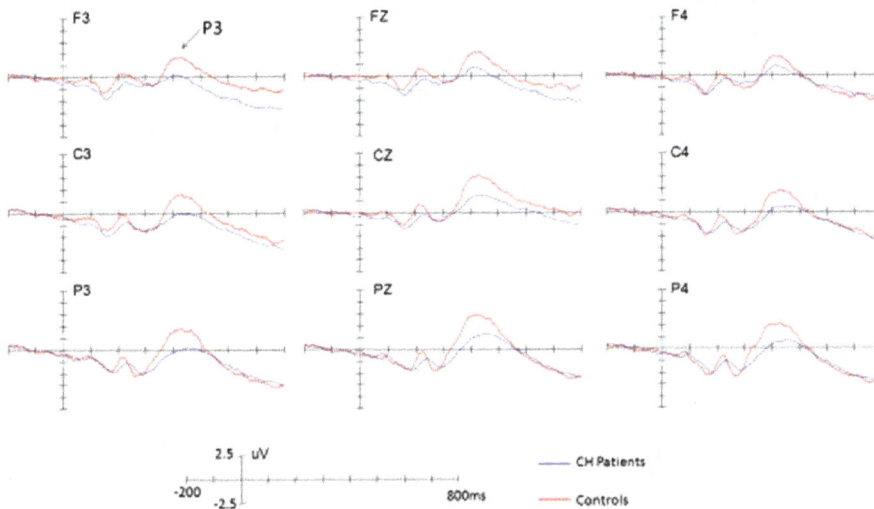

Figure 3 The grand averaged ERPs elicited by target stimuli in patients and controls, respectively.

P3 were similar between the pain and no pain sides ($F(1,30) = 1.807$, $p > 0.05$). This also applied to the P3d ($F(1,30) = 0.057$, $p > 0.05$).

Discussion

The present study investigated possible impairments in the cognitive processing of CH, using target processing and a visual oddball paradigm. Compared with the control group, there was a decrease in the amplitude of P3/P3d in the patients. Before, there were no experiments investigate the reduced P3 amplitude in the cluster headache patients during the cluster bout period but outside an attack. Many studies focused on the latencies of P3 during an attack. For example, Evers et al. reported that latencies for the endogenous ERP components were significantly increased during the cluster bout period compared with outside the cluster bout period. In healthy subjects [9,10], P3 latencies in particular were longer [17]. Positive findings regarding the amplitude of ERP components have been observed infrequently; the instances in which they were observed owed principally to a lower CH incidence and a reduced impairment in cognitive ability.

The P3 component will now be discussed. P3 is a generic name for a variety of relatively late, positive components with a centro-parietal or centro-frontal midline distribution [16,18]. Initially discovered in response to task-relevant, infrequent oddball stimuli [19] and found to be sensitive to the subjective probability assigned to the occurrence of the eliciting event [20], many cognitive

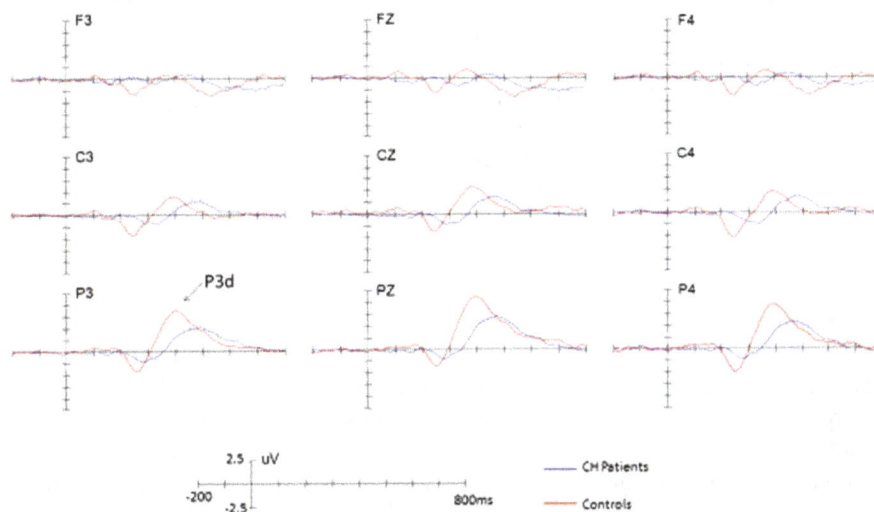

Figure 4 The difference waveforms by subtracting ERPs in response to standard stimuli from ERPs in response to target stimuli in patients and controls, respectively.

mechanism models underlying this neural event have been proposed [21-24]. Notwithstanding these controversies, it is widely accepted that P3 latency reflects the length of stimulus evaluation processes, when a two-choice reaction time (RT) is required [25] and its amplitude is largely determined by stimulus relevance [26], the amount of attention allocated to the stimulus [27] and the task's complexity [28].

There is a low abundance of early research pertaining to correlations of hypothalamus, cingulate cortex and frontal lobe activations with the thought, comprehension, memory and other cognitive function domains. However, Honda, et al. [29], who recorded auditory ERP using the standard oddball paradigm, reported a low-amplitude P300 in a patient with a hypothalamic lesion. May et al. [5] also reported that the right anterior cingulate cortex and hypothalamus were involved in the exchange process between pain and cognition. Knight et al. [30] compared electrophysiological indices of auditory selective attention between control subjects and patients with unilateral dorsolateral frontal lobe lesions; they observed that lesions in the frontal lobes reduced attention-related negativity and impaired behavioral performance. Accordingly, decreased P3/P3d amplitudes in CH patients are likely due to functional and structural changes in hypothalamus, frontal lobe and cingulate cortex.

Many functional neuroimaging studies have confirmed abnormalities in structures such as the hypothalamus, cingulate gyrus, prefrontal lobe, and insular lobe. For example, May et al. [7] also investigated CH patients using PET and reported that activation occurred in the ipsilateral posterior inferior hypothalamic gray, the contralateral ventroposterior thalamus, the anterior cingulate cortex, the ipsilateral basal ganglia, the right anterior frontal lobe, and both insulae during an acute CH attack triggered by nitroglycerin (NTG). Qiu et al. [6,31], who employed resting-state functional magnetic resonance imaging (RS-fMRI), reported altered regional homogeneity in the anterior cingulate cortex, posterior cingulate cortex, prefrontal cortex, and insular cortex; recently, they also confirmed the presence of abnormal brain functional connectivity of the hypothalamus. Morelli et al. [2] used fMRI to show that during typical pain attacks in CH patients, significant activation occurs in the hypothalamic region ipsilateral to the side in which pain is being experienced.

The occurrence of abnormal functions in CH were due to the plasticity and hypersensitization of the cortics, this theory was well confirmed by many fundamental researches such as above mentioned [32]. Furthermore, the plasticity and hypersensitization of the cortics were also the reasons for the lack of habituation in electrophysiological examination of CH [33]. For instance, during the

bout but not outside, cluster headache patients were chrarcterized by a pronounced lack of habituation of the brainstem blink reflex and a general sensitization of pain processing on the headache side. All of these could be due to the descending metabolism of the dopamine [34]. And the dopamine agonist, such as rotigotine had proven to be effective in treating chronic cluster headache [35]. Then in the related intracranial structure,hypothalamus as a part of a supraspinal network involved in the descending control of pain was payed close attention for all the time. The hypothalamus in cluster headache might be characterized not only by a neuronal dysfunction but even by changes in the membrane lipids [36]. Studies with the proton MR spectroscopy (1H-MRS) demonstrated that the NAA and the Cho/Cr metabolite ratio were reduced in the hypothalamus in CH patients when compared to healthy subjects [37,38]. Armando Perrotta, et al. [39] studied the functional activity of the diffuse noxious inhibitory control by evaluating the effect of the cold pressor test on the temporal summation threshold of the nociceptive withdrawal reflex, found that CH revealed a significant facilitation in temporal processing of pain stimuli during the active phase. So they hypothesized that there was a dysfunction of the supraspinal control of pain in CH, and possibly supported by an abnormal hypothalamic function. Furthermore, the P3/P3d amplitudes were dysfunctioning equally in both affected and not affected sides. These phenomena revealed that the influences on the cognitive processing of affected sides were same as the not affected. These phenomena supported that the cognitive processing of cluster headache patients was damaged whatever the headache on the right or left. The hypothalamus played the key role in above mentioned processes, not only involved in human cognitive processing, but also participate in the occurs of cluster headache.

In accordance with the above discussion, we conclude that the hypothalamus is the central site involved in CH development, and that it communicates with other brain structures, such as the frontal lobe, parietal lobe, and cingulate gyrus (Figure 5). The metabolic disorders play the key role in these procedures. In ERP studies, these can manifest as disorders of the P3/P3d and many other components, and in neuroimaging studies, these can manifest as disorders in all the above mentioned regions. However, we have to admit that the evidences support the conclusion above-mentioned are poor, and our conclusion is in the preliminary stage. So in the future we need to conduct the further researches such as observing the patients with hypothalamic lesions by ERP.

In closing, we would like to restate the procedural decisions that can somewhat constrain interpretation of the present findings. First, we did not employ other neuropsychological indices in conjunction with ERPs. Second, CH patients out of bout were not included in

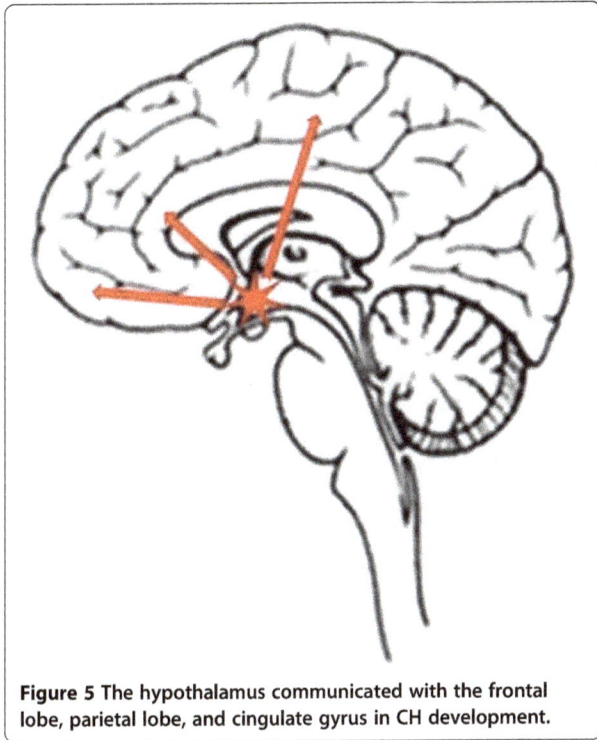

Figure 5 The hypothalamus communicated with the frontal lobe, parietal lobe, and cingulate gyrus in CH development.

our study. Third, if we had observed patients with hypothalamic lesions, then our results would have been more comprehensive; as such, there are many avenues via which future studies could expand upon our findings.

Conclusion

Our results pertaining to P3/P3d provide evidence for dysfunction in the cognitive processing of CH patients. Furthermore, our findings emphasize the involvement of the hypothalamus in the pathophysiology of CH.

Competing interests
The authors declare that they have no competing interests.

Authors' contributions
MD RW, ZD, XC, MZ and LR carried out the studies. And RW drafted the manuscript. MD RW participated in the design of the study and performed the statistical analysis. Professor JW participated in the design of the study. Professor SY, the PI of this study, conceived of the study and participated in its design and helped to draft the manuscript. All authors read and approved the final manuscript.

Acknowledgments
The authors would like to thank all of the referring clinicians.

Funding
This study was financially supported by the National Science Foundation Committee (NSFC) in China (no. 81171058). The funders had no role in study design, data collection and analysis, decision to publish, or preparation of the manuscript.

Author details
[1]Department of Neurology, Chinese PLA General Hospital, Fuxing Road 28, Haidian District, Beijing 100853, China. [2]Medical school, Nankai University, Tianjin, China. [3]Biomedical Engineering Laboratory, Graduate School of Natural Science and Technology, Okayama University, 3-1-1 Tsushima-Naka, Okayama 700-8530, Japan.

References
1. Dong Z, Di H, Dai W, Liang J, Pan M, Zhang M, Zhou Z, Li Z, Liu R, Yu S (2012) Application of ICHD-II criteria in a headache clinic of China. PLoS One 7:e50898
2. Morelli N, Rota E, Gori S, Guidetti D, Michieletti E, De Simone R, Di Salle F (2013) Brainstem activation in cluster headache: an adaptive behavioural response? Cephalalgia 33:416–420
3. Morelli N, Pesaresi I, Cafforio G, Maluccio MR, Gori S, Di Salle F, Murri L (2009) Functional magnetic resonance imaging in episodic cluster headache. J Headache Pain 10:11–14
4. Sprenger T, Boecker H, Tolle TR, Bussone G, May A, Leone M (2004) Specific hypothalamic activation during a spontaneous cluster headache attack. Neurology 62:516–517
5. May A, Bahra A, Büchel C, Frackowiak RS, Goadsby PJ (1998) Hypothalamic activation in cluster headache attacks. Lancet 352:275–278
6. Qiu EC, Yu SY, Liu RZ, Wang Y, Ma L, Tian LX (2012) Altered regional homogeneity in spontaneous cluster headache attacks: a resting-state functional magnetic resonance imaging study. Chin Med J 125:705–709
7. May A, Bahra A, Büchel C, Frackowiak RS, Goadsby PJ (2000) PET and MRA findings in cluster headache and MRA in experimental pain. Neurology 55:1328–1335
8. Evers S (2005) Cognitive processing in cluster headache. Curr Pain Headache Rep 9:109–112
9. Evers S, Bauer B, Suhr B, Voss H, Frese A, Husstedt IW (1999) Cognitive processing is involved in cluster headache but not in chronic paroxysmal hemicrania. Neurology 53:357–363
10. Evers S, Bauer B, Suhr B, Husstedt IW, Grotemeyer KH (1997) Cognitive processing in primary headache: a study on event-related potentials. Neurology 48:108–113
11. Braverman ER, Blum K (2003) P300 (latency) event-related potential: an accurate predictor of memory impairment. Clin Electroenceph 34:124–139
12. Sinforiani E, Farina S, Mancuso A, Manzoni GC, Bono G, Mazzucchi A (1987) Analysis of higher nervous functions in migraine and cluster headache. Funct Neurol 2:69–77
13. Levi R, Edman GV, Ekbom K, Waldenlind E (1992) Episodic cluster headache I: personality and some neuropsychological characteristics in male patients. Headache 32:119–125
14. Blomkvist V, Hannerz J, Orth Gomér K, Theorell T (1997) Coping style and social support in women suffering from cluster headache or migraine. Psychother Psychosom 66:150–154
15. Yuan J, He Y, Qinglin Z, Chen A, Li H (2008) Gender differences in behavioral inhibitory control: ERP evidence from a two-choice oddball task. Psychophysiology 45:986–993
16. Polich J (2007) Updating P300: an integrative theory of P3a and P3b. Clin Neurophysiol 118:2128–2148
17. Sandrini G, Proietti Cecchini A, Pucci E, Milanov I, Nappi G (1999) Neurophysiological approach to the study of cluster headache. Italian J Neurol Sci 20:531–533
18. Donchin E (1981) Presidential address, 1980. Surprise! …Surprise? Psychophysiology 18:493–513
19. Sutton S, Braren M, Zubin J, John ER (1965) Evoked-potential correlates of stimulus uncertainty. Science 150:1187–1188
20. Duncan J, Donchin (1977) On quantifying surprise: the variation of event-related potentials with subjective probability. Psychophysiology 14:456–467
21. Donchin E (1987) The P300 as a metric for mental workload. Electroencephalogr Clin Neurophysiol Suppl 39:338–343
22. Donchin E, Coles MGH (1988) Is the P300 component a manifestation of context updating? Behav Brain Sci 11:357–374
23. Verleger R (1988) The true P3 is hard to see: some comments on Kok's (1986) paper on degraded stimuli. Biol Psychol 27:45–50
24. Verleger R, Görgen S, Jaśkowski P (2005) An ERP indicator of processing relevant gestalts in masked priming. Psychophysiology 42:677–690
25. McCarthy G, Donchin E (1981) A metric for thought: a comparison of P300 latency and reaction time. Science 211:77–80
26. Chiu P, Ambady N, Deldin P (2004) Contingent negative variation to emotional in- and out-group stimuli differentiates high- and low-prejudiced individuals. J Cogn Neurosci 16:1830–1839

27. Kok A (2001) On the utility of P3 amplitude as a measure of processing capacity. Psychophysiology 38:557–577

28. Johnson R Jr (1986) A triarchic model of P300 amplitude. Psychophysiology 23:367–384

29. Honda M, Suwazono S, Nagamine T, Yonekura Y, Shibasaki H (1996) P300 abnormalities in patients with selective impairment of recent memory. J Neurol Sci 139:95–105

30. Knight RT, Hillyard SA, Woods DL, Neville HJ (1981) The effects of frontal cortex lesions on event-related potentials during auditory selective attention. Electroencephalogr Clin Neurophysiol 52:571–582

31. Qiu E, Wang Y, Ma L, Tian L, Liu R, Dong Z, Xu X, Zou Z, Yu S (2013) Abnormal brain functional connectivity of the hypothalamus in cluster headaches. PLoS One 8:e57896

32. Dirks A, Groenink L, Schipholt MI, van der Gugten J, Hijzen TH, Geyer MA, Olivier B (2002) Reduced startle reactivity and plasticity in transgenic mice overexpressing corticotropin-releasing hormone. Biol Psychiatry 51:583–590

33. Coppola G, Di Lorenzo C, Schoenen J, Pierelli F (2013) Habituation and sensitization in primary headaches. J Headache Pain 14:65

34. Palmieri A (2006) Chronic cluster headache responsive to pramipexole. Cephalalgia 26:761–762

35. Di Lorenzo C, Coppola G, Pierelli F (2013) A case of cluster headache treated with rotigotine: clinical and neurophysiological correlates. Cephalalgia 33:1272–1276

36. Iacovelli E, Coppola G, Tinelli E, Pierelli F, Bianco F (2012) Neuroimaging in cluster headache and other trigeminal autonomic cephalalgias. J Headache Pain 13:11–20

37. Lodi R, Pierangeli G, Tonon C, Cevoli S, Testa C, Bivona G, Magnifico F, Cortelli P, Montagna P, Barbiroli B (2006) Study of hypothalamic metabolism in cluster headache by proton MR spectroscopy. Neurology 66:1264–1266

38. Wang SJ, Lirng JF, Fuh JL, Chen JJ (2006) Reduction in hypothalamic ^{1}H-MRS metabolite ratios in patients with cluster headache. J Neurol Neurosurg Psychiatry 77:622–625

39. Perrotta A, Serrao M, Ambrosini A, Bolla M, Coppola G, Sandrini G, Pierelli F (2013) Facilitated temporal processing of pain and defective supraspinal control of pain in cluster headache. Pain 154:1325–1332

7

Reduced circulating endothelial progenitor cells in reversible cerebral vasoconstriction syndrome

Shih-Pin Chen[1,2,3], Yen-Feng Wang[1,2,3], Po-Hsun Huang[1,5], Chin-Wen Chi[6,7], Jong-Ling Fuh[1,2,3,4*†] and Shuu-Jiun Wang[1,2,3,4*†]

Abstract

Background: The pathophysiology of reversible cerebral vasoconstriction syndrome (RCVS) remains elusive. Endothelial dysfunction might play a role, but direct evidence is lacking. This study aimed to explore whether patients with RCVS have a reduced level of circulating circulating endothelial progenitor cells (EPCs) to repair the dysfunctional endothelial vasomotor control.

Methods: We prospectively recruited 24 patients with RCVS within one month of disease onset and 24 healthy age- and sex-matched controls. Flow cytometry was used to quantify the numbers of circulating EPCs, defined as KDR^+CD133^+, $CD34^+CD133^+$, and $CD34^+KDR^+$ double-positive mononuclear cells. The Lindegaard index, an index of vasoconstriction, was calculated by measuring the mean flow velocity of middle cerebral arteries and distal extracranial internal carotid arteries via color-coded sonography on the same day as blood drawing. A Lindegaard index of 2 was chosen as the cutoff value for significant vasoconstriction of middle cerebral arteries based on our previous study.

Results: Patients with RCVS had a reduced number of $CD34^+KDR^+$ cells ($0.009 \pm 0.006\%$ vs. $0.014 \pm 0.010\%$, $p = 0.031$) but not KDR^+CD133^+ cells or $CD34^+CD133^+$ EPCs, in comparison with controls. The number of $CD34^+KDR^+$ cells was inversely correlated with the Lindegaard index ($rs = -0.418$, $p = 0.047$). Of note, compared to controls, patients with a Lindegaard index > 2 (n = 13) had a reduced number of $CD34^+KDR^+$ cells ($0.007 \pm 0.005\%$ vs. $0.014 \pm 0.010\%$, $p = 0.010$), but those with a Lindegaard index ≤ 2 did not.

Conclusions: Patients with RCVS had reduced circulating $CD34^+KDR^+$ EPCs, which were correlated with the severity of vasoconstriction. Endothelial dysfunction might contribute to the pathogenesis of RCVS.

Keywords: Reversible cerebral vasoconstriction syndrome; Thunderclap headaches; Endothelial progenitor cells; Endothelial dysfunction; Cerebral arteries

Background

Reversible cerebral vasoconstriction syndrome (RCVS) is clinical-radiological syndrome characterized by recurrent thunderclap headaches and reversible segmental vaso-constrictions of cerebral arteries [1,2]. Large case series have demonstrated that RCVS is not uncommon [3-5], but rather an under-recognized clinical emergency [6]. Patients with RCVS exhibit substantial risks of devastating complications such as posterior reversible encephalopathy syndrome (PRES), ischemic stroke, and intracranial hemorrhages (including cortical subarachnoid, intracerebral, and even subdural hemorrhage) [3-5,7-9].

RCVS can be either idiopathic or secondary. For some secondary RCVS cases, the use of cocaine or marijuana is the inciting factor responsible for the pathogenesis. However, the pathogenesis of idiopathic RCVS is enigmatic. Sympathetic overactivity [10], oxidative stress [11] and genetic predisposition [12] might play certain roles. We suspect that endothelial dysfunction in RCVS is also highly plausible because both sympathetic overactivity and oxidative stress are detrimental to the endothelium [13-15]. Recent studies showed that bone marrow-derived endothelial progenitor cells (EPCs) are the main source that contributes to the regeneration and maintenance of the endothelium [16,17]. The number of circulating EPCs

* Correspondence: jlfuh@vghtpe.gov.tw; sjwang@vghtpe.gov.tw
†Equal contributors
¹Faculty of Medicine, School of Medicine, National Yang-Ming University, Taipei, Taiwan

has been reported to be a surrogate biologic marker of vascular function and to correlate inversely with the endothelial repair capacity and cardiovascular risks [17-19]. We hypothesized that patients with RCVS might have decreased circulating EPCs during the course of vasoconstriction.

Methods

Ethics

The study protocol was approved by the Institutional Review Board of Taipei Veterans General Hospital. All participants provided written informed consent before entering the study. All clinical investigations were conducted according to the principles expressed in the Declaration of Helsinki. The corresponding authors had full access to all of the data in the study and had final responsibility for the decision to submit the results for publication.

Participants and clinical settings

Patients with RCVS were recruited from the Neurology Department of Taipei Veterans General Hospital, a 2,909-bed national medical center located in Taipei City from 2011 to 2013. Age- and sex-matched volunteer participants who had neither headache history nor severe medical illness were recruited as normal controls. The inclusion criteria for the participants (both patients and controls) were the following: (1) age between 20 and 65 years, and (2) subjects could fully understand the purpose of the research and voluntarily join the study. Because many intrinsic or exogenous factors could influence the number of circulating EPCs, we applied very strict exclusion criteria and selectively enrolled matched controls to eliminate the influence of these confounders. Subjects were excluded if they met the following criteria: (1) had a smoking history, (2) had a major systemic illness such as uncontrolled hypertension (systolic blood pressure > 160 mmHg, diastolic blood pressure > 100 mmHg) at baseline, diabetes mellitus, cardiovascular or cerebrovascular disease, chronic hepatic or renal disease, or malignancies, (3) used illicit drugs; or (4) women who were pregnant or within 3 months postpartum. Subjects with a history of migraine and grade 1 hypertension (systolic blood pressure 140–159 mmHg, diastolic blood pressure 90–99 mmHg) were permitted to enroll because some patients with RCVS may have migraine and hypertension.

The diagnosis of RCVS was based on the following criteria: (1) at least two acute-onset severe headaches (thunderclap headaches), with or without focal neurological deficits; (2) vasoconstrictions demonstrated on magnetic resonance angiography (MRA); (3) reversibility of vasoconstrictions, as demonstrated by at least one follow-up MRA within 3 months; and (4) aneurysmal subarachnoid hemorrhage or other intracranial disorders were ruled out by appropriate investigations, but cortical subarachnoid hemorrhage in RCVS was allowed. The diagnostic criteria were adapted from the criteria of "benign (or reversible) angiopathy of the central nervous system" proposed by the International Classification of Headache Disorders, second edition (ICHD-2) (Code 6.7.3) [20] with the exception of the duration criterion D as well as the essential diagnostic elements of RCVS proposed by Calabrese et al. [1]. In this study, only patients with idiopathic RCVS within one month of headache onset were eligible to minimize potential confounders.

Clinical evaluations

Basic demographic information and anthropometric measurements including height, body weight, and body mass index (BMI) [21] were collected. All enrolled subjects received comprehensive clinical and neurological examinations, and provided detailed medical, headache, and drug histories upon entering the study. Lipid profiles were obtained from general serological surveys. Diagnostic investigations including the first MRA, transcranial color-coded sonography and/or spinal taps were performed within the first two days after the patient was seen. Control subjects did not receive neuroimaging studies. The protocols have been reported previously [3,7,8]. In brief, brain MRI, MRA and MR venography (MRV) studies were performed with a 3-Tesla MR scanner. Intracranial lesions were carefully evaluated with adequate MR sequences, for example, subarachnoid hemorrhage with susceptibility weighted imaging (SWI) and intracranial aneurysms with three-dimensional time-of flight (TOF) MRA. Sequential MRAs were performed in all subjects with RCVS until the normalization of vasoconstrictions. The mean flow velocity of the major cerebral arteries was detected by transcranial color-coded sonography and recorded; the protocols were detailed elsewhere [7]. The following data were analyzed: mean flow velocity of middle cerebral artery (MCA) (V_{MCA}) and the Lindegaard index (LI), which is calculated by dividing the V_{MCA} by the mean flow velocity of the ipsilateral distal extracranial internal carotid artery. The LI was selected to evaluate the vasoconstrictions to avoid possible misreading of hyperemia as vasospasm. For computational purposes, the average V_{MCA} and LI derived from the bilateral MCAs in each patient were calculated. We analyzed only V_{MCA} and LI because MCA is the most widely studied and validated vessel for vasoconstrictions using transcranial color-coded sonography (TCCS) and there have been no validated sonographic criteria of vasoconstrictions for the other cerebral vessels with adequate sensitivity [7]. In addition, our previous studies showed a good correlation of V_{MCA} and LI with the severity of vasoconstrictions detected by MRA.

Because the severity of vasoconstriction of the MCA could vary between patients at the time of blood sampling, we further stratified the patients according to their LI values. Based on our previous study [7], an LI value of 2, the upper limit of our normal controls, was chosen to stratify the patients into two groups: those having either significant or insignificant vasoconstrictions of the MCA. An LI value of 3 was also used to evaluate whether patients at risk of ischemic complications [7] could have lower EPCs. Of note, the cut-off values of LI used here were based on our previous study in RCVS patients using TCCS [7] and should not be translated to the same severity of vasopasm in SAH based on studies using transcranial Doppler (TCD) [22]. In patients with SAH, the LI is disproportionately amplified because of low extracranial ICA flow velocity due to cerebral hypoperfusion caused by increased intracranial pressure (IICP) [22,23], while patients with RCVS usually have normal ICP [1-3]. Patients with RCVS who fulfilled the mild vasospasm criteria for SAH already had high risks of developing PRES (75%) or ischemic stroke (50%) [7].

Flow cytometric analysis of circulating EPCs
The flow cytometric analysis of circulating EPCs was performed based on our previously established methods [24]. Peripheral blood was collected from the antecubital vein on the same day of transcranial color-coded sonography, before administration of any therapeutics. The samples were processed immediately after blood drawing. A volume of 100 μL blood was incubated for 15 minutes in the dark with monoclonal antibodies against human kinase insert domain receptor (KDR; R&D, Minneapolis, MN, USA) followed by phycoerythrin (PE)-conjugated secondary antibody, with the fluorescein isothiocyanate (FITC)-labeled monoclonal antibodies against human CD45 (Becton Dickinson, Franklin Lakes, NJ, USA), with the PE-conjugated monoclonal antibody against human CD133 (Miltenyi Biotec, Germany), and with FITC-conjugated or PE-conjugated monoclonal antibodies against human CD34 (Serotec, Raleigh, NC, USA). Isotype-identical antibodies were used as controls (Becton Dickinson, Franklin Lakes, NJ, USA). After incubation, cells were lysed, washed with phosphate-buffered saline (PBS), and fixed in 2% paraformaldehyde before analysis. Each analysis included 100,000 events. Flow cytometry was used to quantify the numbers of circulating EPCs defined as KDR^+CD133^+, $CD34^+CD133^+$, and $CD34^+KDR^+$ double-positive mononuclear cells (Additional file 1: Figure S1). To assess the reproducibility of the EPC measurements, circulating EPCs were measured from two separate blood samples in 20 subjects (10 controls and 10 patients each). Mature circulating endothelial cells, which are generally recognized as cells expressing endothelial markers (CD 144, CD 146, vWF, VEGFR-2) in the absence of hematopoietic (CD 14, CD 45) and progenitor (CD 34, CD 133) markers (despite the lack of a clear concensus on their phenotypic definitions) [25,26], were excluded with this method.

Statistics
Descriptive statistics are presented as the mean ± standard deviation or as the number (percentage). For normally distributed variables, continuous ones were compared by the Student's t-test, and categorical ones were compared by the Chi-square or Fisher exact tests. For variables that don't have a normal distribution, Kruskal-Wallis test and Mann–Whitney U test were used as appropriate. For correlations between EPC counts with other variables, Spearman correlation coefficient r_s was applied because EPC counts were not normally distributed (by Shapiro-Wilk test). All calculated p-values were two-tailed. Statistical significance was defined as $p < 0.05$. Because there was collinearity between the number of KDR^+CD133^+, $CD34^+CD133^+$, and $CD34^+KDR^+$ cells (the correlation coefficients were 0.666 for $CD34^+CD133^+$ and $CD34^+KDR^+$ cells (p < 0.001), 0.735 for KDR^+CD133^+ and $CD34^+CD133^+$ cells (p < 0.001), and 0.570 for KDR^+CD133^+ and $CD34^+KDR^+$ cells (p < 0.001)), corrections for multiple comparisons were not applied in this study. All analyses were performed with the IBM SPSS Statistics software package, version 18.0.

Results
Participants and their characteristics
During the two-year study period, we prospectively recruited 31 patients with RCVS. After excluding one patient with a previous history of intracerebral hemorrhage, one patient with previous cerebral infarction, two patients who used psueodephedrine, one patient who had a history of marijuana use, one patient who was postpartum, and one heavy smoker, 24 patients were eligible for study. Another 24 age- and sex-matched controls were recruited during the study period. There was no difference in the demographics, BMIs, medical illnesses, and serum cholesterol levels between the two groups (Table 1). Most of the patients (91.7%) had identifiable triggers for their thunderclap headaches, with defecation (58.3%) and bathing (29.2%) being the most common. The cerebrospinal fluid was studied in 12 (50%) patients, and their results were all normal.

Neuroimaging findings
None of the patients had posterior reversible encephalopathy syndromes, ischemic stroke, intracerebral hemorrhage or intracranial arterial dissection on the initial or follow-up MR studies, but one patient had cortical subarachnoid hemorrhage confined to right anterior high frontal cortex without identifiable aneurysm. None of the patients had aneurysmal subarachnoid hemorrhage in consecutive MR studies.

EPC measurements
The blood samples were taken at a mean of 5.4 ± 3.7 days (range 2–13) after headache onset. Of the 20 subjects

Table 1 Basic demongraphics, body mass index, and medical illness of participants

	Controls(n = 24)	RCVS(n = 24)	P value
Age, y (mean ± SD)	45.0 ± 11.9	48.8 ± 9.5	0.229
Gender (M/F)	4/20	4/20	1.000
Menopause, n (%)	6 (12%)	7 (14%)	0.906
Body mass index (kg/m^2)	25.3 ± 1.7	24.0 ± 3.0	0.525
Hypertension, n (%)	0 (0%)	1 (4.2%)	0.312
Diabetes, n (%)	0 (%)	0 (0%)	1.000
Coronary artery disease, n (%)	0 (%)	0 (0%)	1.000
Migraine, n (%)	2 (8.3%)	4 (16.7%)	0.663
Cholesterol (mg/dL)	193.6 ± 35.3	183.7 ± 28.7	0.370

who had two separate blood samples, there was a strong correlation between the two measurements suggesting high reproducibility (CD34$^+$CD133$^+$: rs = 0.973, $p < 0.001$; CD34$^+$KDR$^+$: rs = 0.972, $p < 0.001$; and KDR$^+$CD133$^+$: rs = 0.976, $p < 0.001$). There were no correlations between the EPC counts and age, gender, BMI, menopausal status, migraine, hypertension, or serum cholesterol level.

In comparison to the controls, patients with RCVS had reduced numbers of CD34$^+$KDR$^+$ cells (0.009 ± 0.006% vs. 0.014 ± 0.010%, $p = 0.031$), but they had no reduction in KDR$^+$CD133$^+$ cells (0.031 ± 0.015% vs. 0.039 ± 0.020%, $p = 0.176$) or CD34$^+$CD133$^+$ EPCs (0.045 ± 0.028% vs. 0.060 ± 0.041%, $p = 0.140$). The EPC counts in patients with comorbid migraine (n = 4) did not differ from that in patients without comorbid migraine (n = 20) (CD34$^+$KDR$^+$ cells (0.007 ± 0.006% vs. 0.009 ± 0.006%, $p = 0.751$), KDR$^+$CD133$^+$ cells (0.027 ± 0.010% vs. 0.032 ± 0.015%, $p = 0.642$), CD34$^+$CD133$^+$ EPCs (0.042 ± 0.007% vs. 0.045 ± 0.030%, $p = 0.781$)).

In comparison with the controls, patients with an LI > 2 (n = 13) had fewer CD34$^+$KDR$^+$ cells (0.007 ± 0.005% vs. 0.014 ± 0.010%, $p = 0.010$), but there was no difference in the number of KDR$^+$CD133$^+$ cells (0.032 ± 0.014% vs. 0.039 ± 0.020%, $p = 0.186$) or CD34$^+$CD133$^+$ EPCs (0.042 ± 0.023% vs. 0.060 ± 0.041%, $p = 0.087$).The EPC counts of patients with LI ≤ 2 did not differ from those of the controls (CD34$^+$KDR$^+$ cells: 0.012 ± 0.006% vs. 0.014 ± 0.010%, $p = 0.392$; KDR$^+$CD133$^+$ cells: 0.036 ± 0.016% vs. 0.039 ± 0.020%, $p = 0.404$; CD34$^+$CD133$^+$ cells: 0.052 ± 0.032% vs. 0.060 ± 0.041%, $p = 0.534$.) (Figure 1)

In patients with LI > 3 (n = 3), the trend was similar: Their CD34$^+$KDR$^+$ cell counts were lower than the controls (0.006 ± 0.002% vs. 0.014 ± 0.010%, $p = 0.015$), but there was no difference in the numbers of KDR$^+$CD133$^+$ cells (0.023 ± 0.008% vs. 0.039 ± 0.020%, $p = 0.070$) or CD34$^+$CD133$^+$ EPCs (0.032 ± 0.012% vs. 0.060 ± 0.041%, $p = 0.054$).

Correlations between EPCs and clinical variables

The number of CD34$^+$KDR$^+$ cells was negatively correlated with the LI (rs = −0.418, $p = 0.047$) (Figure 2), whereas there was no significant correlation of LI with the number of KDR$^+$CD133$^+$ (rs = −0.265, $p = 0.221$) or CD34$^+$CD133$^+$ cells (rs = −0.207, $p = 0.344$). None of the other clinical variables such as triggers (including defecation, bathing, exertion, cough, rage, or sex) or the number and duration of thunderclap headaches before blood drawing had significant correlations with the EPCs counts (data not shown).

Discussions

Our study demonstrated that patients with RCVS had reduced circulating CD34$^+$KDR$^+$ EPCs in comparison with controls, especially in those with more severe vasoconstrictions (LI > 2) and those at risk of ischemic complications (LI > 3). The number of CD34$^+$KDR$^+$ EPCs was negatively correlated with the severity of vasoconstrictions evaluated with the LI. In contrast, the KDR$^+$CD133$^+$ and CD34$^+$CD133$^+$ EPCs did not show any associations with RCVS.

Circulating EPCs are capable of patching sites of denuding injury, and they serve as a cellular reservoir for the replacement of dysfunctional endothelium [27,28]. However, it is unclear which antigenic profiles best identify progenitor cells with the potential for endothelial repair [29]. Cells expressing CD34 (an adhesion molecule expressed on hematopoietic stem cells) and KDR (a type 2 vascular endothelial growth factor receptor that indicates early endothelial differentiation) might be the main constituent of the circulating EPCs responsible for re-endothelialization [30]. The identification of fewer circulating CD34$^+$KDR$^+$ EPCs was consistent with our hypothesis that patients with RCVS had a reduced capacity for endothelial repair. The inverse correlation between the CD34$^+$KDR$^+$ EPC count and the severity of vasoconstriction further supports the hypothesis that the reduced endothelial repair capability might be associated with the overwhelmed vasomotor control in RCVS. The reason why the KDR$^+$CD133$^+$ and CD34$^+$CD133$^+$ EPCs were not correlated with severity of vasoconstrictions was unknown, but these findings might suggest that not all the EPC phenotypes were associated with vasomotor control.

It is unclear whether there is a causal relationship between reduced EPC counts and vasoconstrictions in RCVS. Whether patients with RCVS have already had reduced circulating EPCs before disease onset could never be proved since it's almost impossible to have pre-morbid EPC measurement. We put forth the following hypotheses. First, it is possible that when an unknown insult ignites the vicious cycle of sympathetic overactivity [10] and oxidative stress [11], which damages the endothelium of the cerebral vasculature, EPCs will be mobilized from the bone marrow into the circulation to repair the endothelial damage.

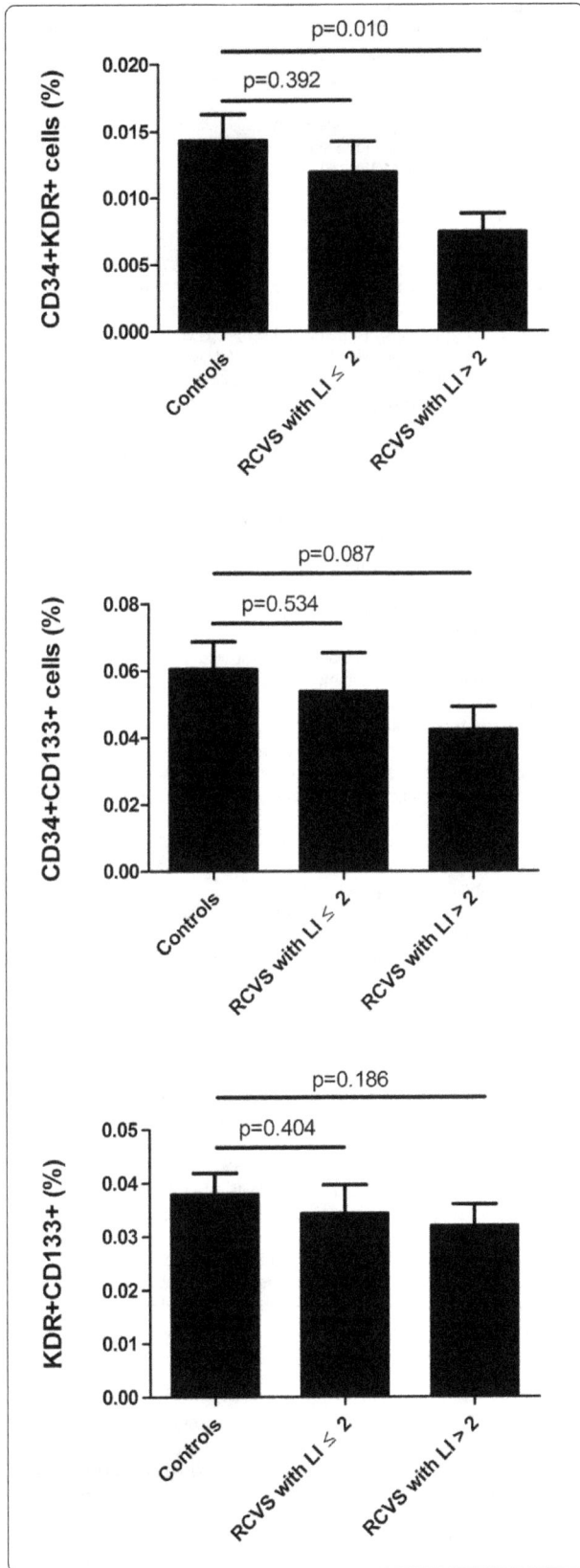

Figure 1 Comparison of the numbers of endothelial progenitor cells between patients with reversible cerebral vasoconstriction syndrome and controls. (column: mean, error bars: standard errors). RCVS: reversible cerebral vasoconstriction syndrome; LI: Lindegaard index.

When patients have low baseline EPCs or a compromised capacity of EPC mobilization, they are likely to develop more severe vasoconstriction. In contrast, patients with sufficient EPCs might have less severe vasoconstrictions. Second, sympathetic overactivity and oxidative stress may accelerate the consumption or senescence of circulating EPCs [31,32], which could further hamper the numbers and function of EPCs. However, this was purely speculative because we did not perform functional assays on EPCs in this study. Previous studies have shown that headache disorders such as migraine or cluster headache could be modulated by immunological cells that migrate from peripheral blood circulation into central nervous system, via an altered expression of adhesion molecules and chemotactic cytokines. Although mechanistically different, this neuroimmunological interplay might serve as a model for us to envision the mechanism of EPCs in RCVS [33,34].

Our study has limitations. First, to eliminate the influence of potential confounders that might interfere EPC counts, we applied very strict exclusion criteria and selectively enrolled matched controls. Hence, it is not possible to conclude whether the study results are generalizable to patients who have multiple vascular risk factors or obvious secondary causes of RCVS, such as illicit drug users. In addition, the number of participants was limited in this study partially due to the exclusion and matching criteria. However, considering the prevalence of RCVS, the possible interassay variability during the prolonged study duration (which could be due to machines, operators, and reagents, etc.), and the significant study results, we believe that the

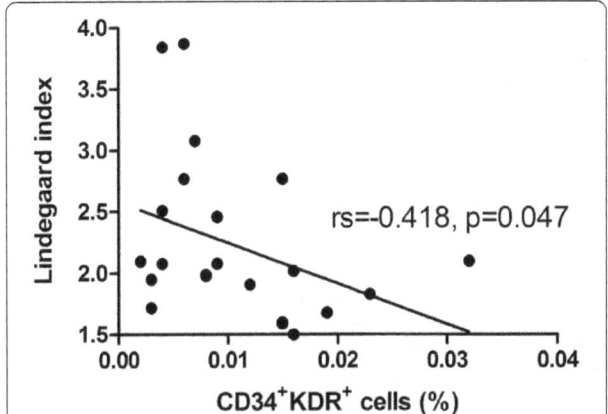

Figure 2 Correlation between the numbers of CD34+KDR+ endothelial progenitor cells and Lindegaard index.

current case numbers are appropriate for our research purposes. Finally, as mentioned above, we did not perform functional assays on EPCs. Further mechanistic approaches are required.

Conclusions

Patients with RCVS had reduced circulating CD34$^+$KDR$^+$ EPCs, which were inversely correlated with the severity of vasoconstrictions. A reduced capacity of circulating EPCs to repair dysfunctional endothelial vasomotor control might contribute to the pathogenesis of vasoconstrictions in patients with RCVS. The potential of therapies targeting the restoration of endothelial function deserves exploration.

Abbreviations

BMI: Body mass index; EPC: Endothelial progenitor cell; ICHD-2: International Classification of Headache Disorders, second edition; IICP: Increased intracranial pressure; LI: Lindegaard index; MCA: Middle cerebral artery; MRA: Magnetic resonance angiography; MRV: Magnetic resonance venography; PRES: Posterior reversible encephalopathy syndrome; RCVS: Reversible cerebral vasoconstriction syndrome; SAH: Subarachnoid hemorrhage; TCCS: Transcranial color-coded sonography; TCD: Transcranial Doppler; V$_{MCA}$: Mean flow velocity of middle cerebral artery.

Competing interests

The authors declare that they have no competing interests.

Authors' contributions

Dr. SPC - Study concept and design, patient recruitment, acquisition of data, analysis and interpretation, manuscript writing. Dr. JLF - Study concept and design, patient recruitment, study supervision, critical revision of the manuscript for important intellectual content. Dr. SJW - Study concept and design, patient recruitment, study supervision, critical revision of the manuscript for important intellectual content. Dr. YFW - patient recruitment, acquisition of data, analysis and interpretation. Dr. PHH - technical support, critical revision of the manuscript for important intellectual content. Dr. CWC - technical support, critical revision of the manuscript for important intellectual content. All authors read and approved the final manuscript.

Study funding

This study was supported by grants from the National Science Council of Taiwan (99-2314-B-075-036-MY3, 100-2314-B-010-019-MY2, 100-2314-B-010-018-MY3), Taipei-Veterans General Hospital (V100B-007, VGHUST101-G7-1-1, V101C-106, V101E7-003), NSC support for Center for Dynamical Biomarkers and Translational Medicine, National Central University, Taiwan (NSC 100-2911-I-008-001), Brain Research Center, National Yang-Ming University and a grant from Ministry of Education, Aim for the Top University Plan. No additional external funding received for this study. The funders had no role in study design, data collection and analysis, decision to publish, or preparation of the manuscript.

Author details

[1]Faculty of Medicine, School of Medicine, National Yang-Ming University, Taipei, Taiwan. [2]Department of Neurology, Neurological Institute, Taipei Veterans General Hospital, Taipei, Taiwan. [3]Brain Research Center, National Yang-Ming University, Taipei, Taiwan. [4]Institute of Brain Science, National Yang-Ming University, Taipei, Taiwan. [5]Department of Internal Medicine, Division of Cardiology, Taipei Veterans General Hospital, Taipei, Taiwan. [6]Department and Institute of Pharmacology, School of Medicine, National Yang-Ming University, Taipei, Taiwan. [7]Department of Medical Research & Education, Taipei Veterans General Hospital, Taipei, Taiwan.

References

1. Calabrese LH, Dodick DW, Schwedt TJ, Singhal AB (2007) Narrative review: reversible cerebral vasoconstriction syndromes. Ann Intern Med 146(1):34–44
2. Ducros A (2012) Reversible cerebral vasoconstriction syndrome. Lancet Neurol 11(10):906–917
3. Chen SP, Fuh JL, Lirng JF, Chang FC, Wang SJ (2006) Recurrent primary thunderclap headache and benign CNS angiopathy: spectra of the same disorder? Neurology 67(12):2164–2169
4. Ducros A, Boukobza M, Porcher R, Sarov M, Valade D, Bousser MG (2007) The clinical and radiological spectrum of reversible cerebral vasoconstriction syndrome. A prospective series of 67 patients. Brain 130(Pt 12):3091–3101
5. Singhal AB, Hajj-Ali RA, Topcuoglu MA, Fok J, Bena J, Yang D, Calabrese LH (2011) Reversible cerebral vasoconstriction syndromes: analysis of 139 cases. Arch Neurol 68(8):1005–1012
6. Chen SP, Fuh JL, Wang SJ (2010) Reversible cerebral vasoconstriction syndrome: an under-recognized clinical emergency. Ther Adv Neurol Disord 3(3):161–171
7. Chen SP, Fuh JL, Chang FC, Lirng JF, Shia BC, Wang SJ (2008) Transcranial color doppler study for reversible cerebral vasoconstriction syndromes. Ann Neurol 63(6):751–757
8. Chen SP, Fuh JL, Wang SJ, Chang FC, Lirng JF, Fang YC, Shia BC, Wu JC (2010) Magnetic resonance angiography in reversible cerebral vasoconstriction syndromes. Ann Neurol 67(5):648–656
9. Ducros A, Fiedler U, Porcher R, Boukobza M, Stapf C, Bousser MG (2010) Hemorrhagic manifestations of reversible cerebral vasoconstriction syndrome: frequency, features, and risk factors. Stroke 41(11):2505–2511
10. Chen SP, Yang AC, Fuh JL, Wang SJ (2013) Autonomic dysfunction in reversible cerebral vasoconstriction syndromes. J Headache Pain 14(1):94, doi:10.1186/1129-2377-14-94
11. Chen SP, Chung YT, Liu TY, Wang YF, Fuh JL, Wang SJ (2013) Oxidative stress and increased formation of vasoconstricting F2-isoprostanes in patients with reversible cerebral vasoconstriction syndrome. Free Radic Biol Med 61C:243–248
12. Chen SP, Fuh JL, Wang SJ, Tsai SJ, Hong CJ, Yang AC (2011) Brain-derived neurotrophic factor gene Val66Met polymorphism modulates reversible cerebral vasoconstriction syndromes. PLoS One 6(3):e18024, doi:10.1371/journal.pone.0018024
13. Zalba G, Fortuno A, San Jose G, Moreno MU, Beloqui O, Diez J (2007) Oxidative stress, endothelial dysfunction and cerebrovascular disease. Cerebrovasc Dis 24(Suppl 1):24–29
14. Faraci FM (2006) Reactive oxygen species: influence on cerebral vascular tone. J Appl Physiol (1985) 100(2):739–743
15. Bruno RM, Ghiadoni L, Seravalle G, Dell'oro R, Taddei S, Grassi G (2012) Sympathetic regulation of vascular function in health and disease. Front Physiol 3:284, doi:10.3389/fphys
16. Asahara T, Masuda H, Takahashi T, Kalka C, Pastore C, Silver M, Kearne M, Magner M, Isner JM (1999) Bone marrow origin of endothelial progenitor cells responsible for postnatal vasculogenesis in physiological and pathological neovascularization. Circ Res 85(3):221–228
17. Hill JM, Zalos G, Halcox JP, Schenke WH, Waclawiw MA, Quyyumi AA, Finkel T (2003) Circulating endothelial progenitor cells, vascular function, and cardiovascular risk. N Engl J Med 348(7):593–600
18. Werner N, Kosiol S, Schiegl T, Ahlers P, Walenta K, Link A, Bohm M, Nickenig G (2005) Circulating endothelial progenitor cells and cardiovascular outcomes. N Engl J Med 353(10):999–1007
19. Ghani U, Shuaib A, Salam A, Nasir A, Shuaib U, Jeerakathil T, Sher F, O'Rourke F, Nasser AM, Schwindt B, Todd K (2005) Endothelial progenitor cells during cerebrovascular disease. Stroke 36(1):151–153
20. Headache Classification Subcommittee of the International Headache Society (2004) The International Classification of Headache Disorders: 2nd edition. Cephalalgia 24(Suppl 1):9–160
21. MacEneaney OJ, Kushner EJ, Van Guilder GP, Greiner JJ, Stauffer BL, DeSouza CA (2009) Endothelial progenitor cell number and colony-forming capacity in overweight and obese adults. Int J Obes (Lond) 33(2):219–225
22. Lindegaard KF, Nornes H, Bakke SJ, Sorteberg W, Nakstad P (1989) Cerebral vasospasm diagnosis by means of angiography and blood velocity measurements. Acta Neurochir (Wien) 100(1–2):12–24
23. Lindegaard K (1999) The role of transcranial Doppler in the management of patients with subarachnoid hemorrhage- a review. Acta Neurochir Suppl 72:59–71
24. Huang PH, Chen YH, Tsai HY, Chen JS, Wu TC, Lin FY, Sata M, Chen JW, Lin SJ (2010) Intake of red wine increases the number and functional capacity of

circulating endothelial progenitor cells by enhancing nitric oxide bioavailability. Arterioscler Thromb Vasc Biol 30(4):869–877

25. Jacques N, Vimond N, Conforti R, Griscelli F, Lecluse Y, Laplanche A, Malka D, Vielh P, Farace F (2008) Quantification of circulating mature endothelial cells using a whole blood four-color flow cytometric assay. J Immunol Methods 337(2):132–143

26. Khan SS, Solomon MA, McCoy JP Jr (2005) Detection of circulating endothelial cells and endothelial progenitor cells by flow cytometry. Cytometry B Clin Cytom 64(1):1–8

27. Hristov M, Erl W, Weber PC (2003) Endothelial progenitor cells: mobilization, differentiation, and homing. Arterioscler Thromb Vasc Biol 23(7):1185–1189

28. Schmidt-Lucke C, Rossig L, Fichtlscherer S, Vasa M, Britten M, Kamper U, Dimmeler S, Zeiher AM (2005) Reduced number of circulating endothelial progenitor cells predicts future cardiovascular events: proof of concept for the clinical importance of endogenous vascular repair. Circulation 111(22):2981–2987

29. Ingram DA, Caplice NM, Yoder MC (2005) Unresolved questions, changing definitions, and novel paradigms for defining endothelial progenitor cells. Blood 106(5):1525–1531

30. Urbich C, Dimmeler S (2004) Endothelial progenitor cells: characterization and role in vascular biology. Circ Res 95(4):343–353

31. Imanishi T, Hano T, Nishio I (2005) Angiotensin II accelerates endothelial progenitor cell senescence through induction of oxidative stress. J Hypertens 23(1):97–104

32. Imanishi T, Moriwaki C, Hano T, Nishio I (2005) Endothelial progenitor cell senescence is accelerated in both experimental hypertensive rats and patients with essential hypertension. J Hypertens 23(10):1831–1837

33. Martelletti P, Giacovazzo M (1996) Putative neuroimmunological mechanisms in cluster headache. An integrated hypothesis. Headache 36(5):312–315

34. Martelletti P, Stirparo G, Morrone S, Rinaldi C, Giacovazzo M (1997) Inhibition of intercellular adhesion molecule-1 (ICAM-1), soluble ICAM-1 and interleukin-4 by nitric oxide expression in migraine patients. J Mol Med (Berl) 75(6):448–453

8

High sensitivity C-reactive protein and cerebral white matter hyperintensities on magnetic resonance imaging in migraine patients

Aynur Yilmaz Avci[1*], Hatice Lakadamyali[2], Serap Arikan[3], Ulku Sibel Benli[1] and Munire Kilinc[1]

Abstract

Background: Migraine is a common headache disorder that may be associated with vascular disease and cerebral white matter hyperintensities (WMHs) on magnetic resonance imaging (MRI) scan. High sensitivity C-reactive protein (hs-CRP) is a marker of inflammation that may predict subclinical atherosclerosis. However, the relation between migraine, vascular risks, and WMHs is unknown. We evaluated hs-CRP levels and the relation between hs-CRP level and WMHs in adult migraine patients.

Methods: This case–control study included 432 subjects (216 migraine patients [without aura, 143 patients; with aura, 73 patients]; 216 healthy control subjects without migraine; age range 18–50 y). Migraine diagnosis was determined according to the International Classification of Headache Disorders II diagnostic criteria. The migraine patients and control subjects had no known vascular risk factors, inflammatory disease, or comorbid disease. The presence and number of WMHs on MRI scans were determined, and serum hs-CRP levels were measured by latex-enhanced immunoturbidimetry.

Results: Mean hs-CRP level was significantly greater in migraine patients (1.94 ± 2.03 mg/L) than control subjects (0.82 ± 0.58 mg/L; $P \leq .0001$). The mean number of WMHs per subject and the presence of WMHs was significantly greater in migraine patients (69 patients [31.9%]; 1.68 ± 3.12 mg/dL) than control subjects (21 subjects [9.7%]; 0.3 ± 1.3; $P \leq .001$). However, there was no correlation between hs-CRP level and WMHs in migraine patients ($r = 0.024$; not significant). The presence of WMHs was increased 4.35-fold in migraine patients (odds ratio 4.35, $P \leq .001$).

Conclusions: High hs-CRP level may be a marker of the proinflammatory state in migraine patients. However, the absence of correlation between hs-CRP level and WMHs suggests that hs-CRP is not causally involved in the pathogenesis of WMHs in migraine patients. The WMHs were located mostly in the frontal lobe and subcortical area.

Keywords: Headache; Inflammation; Vascular disease; Pathophysiology

Background

Migraine is a common neurologic disorder, typically characterized by recurrent attacks of debilitating headache and symptoms of autonomic nervous system dysfunction. In one third patients, migraine attacks are accompanied by transient focal neurologic aura symptoms. The frequency of migraine is 3-fold greater in women than men [1]. Migraine prevalence is 8.6% in males, 17.5% in females, and 13.2% overall in the United States [2]. In Turkey, migraine prevalence is 8.5% in males and 24.6% in females, and the 1-year prevalence of migraine (16.4%) is similar or higher than the prevalence worldwide [3]. The risk of having migraine is greater in women aged < 45 years, and hormonal effects may be a causal factor for this female predominance [4]. Migraine is associated with an increased risk of developing cardiovascular disease and a 2-fold increased risk of developing ischemic stroke [4-7]. The relation between migraine and the risk of vascular disease may be explained, in part, by the higher prevalence of multiple risk factors in migraine patients [4-6]. Additionally, the association between migraine with aura and ischemic stroke is more apparent for individuals

* Correspondence: yilmazaynur@yahoo.com
[1]Department of Neurology, Baskent University, Saray Mah, Yunusemre cad, No. 1, Alanya-Antalya 07400 Ankara, Turkey

without vascular risk factors [8-10]. Migraine also has also been associated with hemorrhagic stroke [11].

Migraine is a neurovascular disorder associated with cortical spreading depression, neurogenic inflammation, and cranial vascular contractile dysfunction. Activation of brain tissue causes release of peptides from the perivascular trigeminal regions that cause inflammation and dilation of extraparenchymal vessels. Repeated migraine attacks are associated with inflammatory arteriopathy of the cranial vessels [12,13]. In migraine, specific abnormalities of inflammatory marker levels in the systemic circulation have been observed, including increased levels of C-reactive protein (CRP), interleukins, and adhesion molecules [13-15].

Migraine is a risk factor for white matter hyperintensities (WMHs), which are infarct-like lesions associated with volume changes in the brain (grey matter and white matter regions) [16]. Incidental findings on brain magnetic resonance imaging (MRI) scans are common, and incidental findings detection is more likely using high resolution MRI sequences than standard resolution sequences [17-20]. The pathophysiology of WMHs is unknown. Increased age and atherosclerosis may be the main risk factors for the development of WMHs [17,20,21]. In migraine, the duration of disease and attack frequency are important in the development of WMHs, and comorbid disease also may contribute to the development of WMHs [18,20,21]. In migraine, cumulative effects of repeated intracerebral hemodynamic changes may contribute to the development of WMHs, including oligemia, focal hypoperfusion with ischemia, and hypoxia below the ischemic threshold [22].

High sensitivity C-reactive protein (hs-CRP) is a marker of inflammation, and hs-CRP levels may increase in vascular diseases such as myocardial infarction and ischemic stroke or in healthy individuals who have no cardiovascular disease [23]. The hs-CRP level has prognostic use in the Framingham coronary risk score, severity of metabolic syndrome, severity of hypertension, and patients who have or do not have subclinical atherosclerosis [23,24]. The association of CRP level with migraine has been shown in small case–control studies of migraine with vascular risk factors and a large prospective cohort study of women aged > 45 years [15,25-27]. Higher CRP levels were associated with the presence and progression of periventricular and subcortical WMHs, independent of cardiovascular risk factors and carotid atherosclerosis, in old nondemented patients [28-30].

The complex mechanisms involved in migraine and mechanisms linking migraine and vascular risks are incompletely understood [4,5]. The distribution of brain WMHs in patients who have migraine is unclear, and limited information is available about the complex relation between migraine, ischemia, and WMHs [18-20].

We hypothesized that hs-CRP levels may be associated with migraine disease, and that high hs-CRP levels also may be associated with the presence and distribution of cerebral WMHs on brain MRI scans in migraine patients. The purpose of the present study was to analyze the relation between hs-CRP levels and WMHs in migraine patients.

Methods
Subjects
This case–control clinical study was performed with patients who had migraine newly diagnosed at the neurology outpatient clinics of Baskent Medical Faculty from October 2011 to December 2013 and who had brain MRI scans as a part of their evaluation. Inclusion criteria were duration of migraine symptoms ≥ 1 year, headache frequency ≥ 2 attacks/month, and absence of any known vascular risk factors, inflammatory disease, chronic illness, metabolic disease, or infections. Patients were excluded for (1) migraine duration < 1 year; (2) history of cerebrovascular or cardiovascular disease, arterial hypertension (blood pressure > 130/80 mm Hg), diabetes mellitus, or hyperlipidemia (low-density lipoprotein cholesterol ≥ 160 mg/dL); (3) body mass index < 18 kg/m^2 or > 35 kg/m^2; (4) abnormal plasma hs-CRP level (>10 mg/L); (5) smoking cigarettes > 1 pack/day; (6) current pregnancy, lactation, or hormonal contraceptive use; (7) alcohol or substance abuse; (8) drug use such as antiplatelet agents, anticoagulants, statins, or hormonal drugs; (9) renal, metabolic, psychiatric, inflammatory, infectious, or immune disease; (10) musculoskeletal disorders or fibromyalgia; or (11) possible "symptomatic migraine" in which the MRI showed arteriovenous malformations, ischemic infarcts, brain tumors, or other conditions that may be associated with migraine. In addition, patients who had high levels of hs-CRP (≥10 mg/L) were excluded from the study because high levels of hs-CRP (>10 mg/L) may represent nonspecific inflammation and lack positive predictive value [23,24]. There were 300 consecutive migraine patients considered for the study, and 84 patients were excluded (infection, 17 patients; thyroid disease, 12 patients, thyroid stimulating hormone, range 3.5 - 4.9 μIU/mL; no laboratory tests available, 11 patients; declined MRI scan, 10 patients; low-density lipoprotein cholesterol > 160 mg/dL, 9 patients; positive antinuclear antibody, 9 patients; hs-CRP > 10 mg/L, 8 patients; antidouble-stranded DNA autoantibody, 5 patients; silent lacunar infarct, 3 patients). The other 216 consecutive, newly diagnosed migraine patients were included in the study (165 women [76%] and 51 men [24%]; age range, 18–50 y [mean age, 31 ± 7 y]).

Healthy control subjects (216 subjects: 150 women [69.4%] and 66 men [30.6%]) aged between 18 and 50 years (mean age, 32.46 ± 7.54) were recruited consecutively from hospital staff, laboratory staff, relatives of patients, and the general population. Inclusion criteria for the control subjects were (1) absence of headaches such as migraine, tension-type headache, or cluster headache; (2) absence of other neurologic or systemic disease; and (3) presence of a match with migraine patients by age (±2 y), sex, body mass index, education level, and smoking habits. Exclusion criteria for control subjects were the same as for the migraine group. The study was approved by the local ethics committee of the Medical Faculty of Baskent University Hospital, and all migraine and control subjects gave informed consent to participate in the study and have MRI scans and laboratory tests.

Evaluation

Patients were diagnosed as having migraine according to the criteria of the International Classification of Headache Disorders II [1]. A detailed history of migraine was obtained including disease duration (y), age at onset, average duration of current headache (h), presence of aura, trigger factors, accompanying symptoms, frequency per month, and location and severity of pain. Severity of headache was evaluated with visual analog score (range, 1 [minimum pain] to 10 [maximum pain]). Migraine headache attack frequency was defined as the number of attacks per month. All patients and control subjects received a complete physical and neurologic examination. Comorbidities (coronary artery disease, stroke, diabetes mellitus, or thyroid disease) and intercurrent illnesses such as respiratory or urinary infections were determined from the patient history, physical examination, and laboratory tests (biochemical and hematologic tests). Blood pressure, body weight, height, smoking habits, and education level were recorded for all migraine patients and control subjects. No migraine patients took any medication within 3 days before blood sampling. Patients previously had used medications for acute pain such as acetaminophen, nonsteroidal anti-inflammatory drugs, triptans, or caffeine for headache, but patients who used analgesics daily were excluded from the study. Patients who were treated for migraine prophylaxis with drugs such as propranolol, topiramate, or valproic acid were excluded.

White matter hyperintensities

All 432 participants had cerebral MRI brain scanning (1.5 Tesla, Siemens Magnetom Vision Plus, Siemens, Munich, Germany) with the orbitomeatal line as reference. The scans included ≥ 3 sequences: sagittal T1-weighted, axial T2-weighted, and axial fluid attenuated inversion recovery (FLAIR) images. The slice thickness was 5 mm, the gap was 1 mm, and no intravenous contrast was used.

All MRI scans were reviewed and scored by a radiologist who was blinded to the clinical details. The scans were visually assessed for the presence and features of WMHs including appearance, number, size, distribution (infratentorial or supratentorial), and anatomic location. The number and size of the WMHs were determined on the FLAIR images and grouped according to location and distribution. Subgroups were delineated according to the distribution of the WMH following the methodology previously described in multiple sclerosis patients [31]. These subgroups were juxtacortical, subcortical, and periventricular. The locations of WMHs were defined as frontal, parietal, temporal, occipital, or infratentorial. Periventricular WMHs were defined as being anterior, posterior, or located at the lateral band. We included focal and punctate hyperintensities (size < 9 mm). Confluent and large hyperintensity lesions (>9 mm) were excluded. There were no WMHs at the corpus callosum. The McDonald and Barkhof MRI diagnostic criteria for dissemination in space in multiple sclerosis were applied to each patient to determine whether the criteria were satisfied [31,32].

Migraine and control subjects who had WMHs that were detected on brain MRI were evaluated with laboratory tests for vasculitis (anticardiolipin antibodies, antinuclear antibody, lupus anticoagulant, antidouble-stranded DNA autoantibody, and C3 and C4 levels). Migraine and control subjects who had WMHs underwent cardiac examination and transthoracic echocardiography to exclude patent foramen ovale and atrial septal defect; only 1 patient was excluded because of atrial septal defect on echocardiography.

High sensitivity C-reactive protein

Blood samples were obtained from the antecubital vein from control subjects and during a headache-free period from migraine patients. To exclude the potential effects of a recent attack, migraine patients had been free of migraine attack for ≥ 3 days before blood sampling. No subjects had taken anti-inflammatory drugs for ≥ 3 days before the study because these drugs may be associated with improved endothelial function and might have affected the results. Phlebotomy tubes contained no anticoagulant. Blood was centrifuged at $3000 \times g$ for 10 minutes and stored at $-20°C$ until analysis. Serum hs-CRP was measured by latex-enhanced immunoturbidimetry using monoclonal anti-CRP antibodies (Architect C 800, Abbott Diagnostic Systems, Abbott Park, IL, USA) (hs-CRP reference level, ≤ 5 mg/L).

Statistical analysis

Data analysis was performed with statistical software (IBM SPSS Statistics for Windows, Version 21.0, IBM Corp., Armonk, NY, USA). Statistical analysis of the numeric parameters that were normally distributed was performed with independent t test. Data that did not satisfy normal distribution approximation were analyzed with nonparametric Mann–Whitney test. Average values were reported as mean ± standard deviation (SD), and statistical analysis was performed with median values. Categorical and ordinal data were analyzed with Pearson chi-square and Fisher exact chi-square tests. Correlation analysis was performed with Spearman rank correlation. Factors affecting hs-CRP were investigated with regression analysis. However, to prove hypotheses of the regression analysis, transformation to the hs-CRP variable was applied to satisfy the normal distribution condition of the parameter. Factors affecting the presence of WMHs were analyzed with multiple logistic regression. In addition, descriptive statistics for categorical variables were specified as number (%), and median statistics for numeric variables were reported with range (minimum to maximum) and mean ± SD. In all analyses, statistical significance was defined by $P \le .05$ and decisions were at the 95% confidence level.

Results

In the 216 consecutive, newly diagnosed migraine patients who were included in the study, migraine without aura was diagnosed in 143 patients (66%) and migraine with aura was diagnosed in 73 patients (34%) (Table 1). The migraine and control groups were similar in mean age, body mass index, education, and frequency of smokers (Table 1). Frequency of family history of migraine and mean hs-CRP levels were similar between migraine patients with or without aura and were greater in migraine patients than control subjects (Table 1). Mean duration of migraine disease was statistically significantly greater in patients who had migraine with than without aura (Table 1). There was no statistically significant difference between the migraine groups in headache localization, headache duration, visual analog score, headache frequency, medication, education level, or smoking habits (Table 1).

The presence of WMHs and mean number of WMHs per subject were significantly higher in migraine patients (69 patients [31.9%]; 1.68 ± 3.12 mg/dL) than control subjects (21 subjects [9.7%]; 0.3 ± 1.3; $P \le .0001$) (Table 1). In the 69 migraine patients who had WMHs, 67 patients (97%) had supratentorial WMHs and 2 patients (3%) had infratentorial WMHs. In 15 of 69 (10.4%) migraine patients who had WMHs, the WMHs were present in > 1 anatomic location. In migraine patients, WMH diameter was ≤ 3 mm in 63 patients (91%) and 4 to 9 mm in 6 patients (9%). In all control subjects who had WMHs (21 patients [9.7%]), WMH diameter was ≤ 3 mm, and no infratentorial lesions were present.

The distribution of WMHs was significantly different between migraine and control subjects (Table 2). The presence and the number of WMHs per subject (juxtacortical, subcortical, and periventricular) were significantly higher in migraine patients than control subjects ($P \le .001$) (Table 2). The WMHs in the migraine and control groups were detected most frequently in the frontal lobe and least frequently in the occipital lobe (Table 2) ($P \le .05$). In the control group, the WMHs were detected only in the subcortical region (Table 2). Frequencies of juxtacortical and subcortical WMHs were similar between migraine patients with and without aura (not significant). Only migraine patients with aura had periventricular WMHs (Table 2), which were located in the anterior horn of the lateral ventricles; no patients had WMHs in the lateral ventricular bands or posterior horn of lateral ventricles (Table 2). In the 69 migraine patients, the WMHs were contiguous with the cortex in 18 patients (26%) and with the periventricular structure in 3 patients (4%) (Table 2). In 69 migraine patients who had WMHs, only 1 patient satisfied the 2010 McDonald criteria [32]. No patients satisfied the Barkhof criteria or radiologically isolated syndrome criteria [31,33].

There was no statistically significant correlation between hs-CRP level and WMHs in migraine and control subjects (r = 0.155; $P > .001$) (Table 3). In migraine patients, the hs-CRP levels were not significantly different between juxtacortical, subcortical, and periventricular WMHs (Table 4). There was no correlation between hs-CRP and headache characteristics (r < 0.042; not significant) (Table 4). The hs-CRP level was similar for females and males, and the presence and number of WMHs/subject were similar between females and males (Table 4). The WMHs (juxtacortical, subcortical, and periventricular) were not correlated with headache characteristics (migraine duration, visual analog score, or headache duration) (not significant).

Migraine disease was associated with a 4.35-fold increased risk of presence of WMHs (Table 5). In addition, age 1 year was associated with a 1.06-fold increased risk of the presence of the WMHs (Table 5).

Discussion

In the present study, serum hs-CRP levels were significantly higher in migraine patients than control subjects. Based on published Framingham coronary risk criteria, 57.9% migraine patients had moderate to high vascular risk [23,24]. The present data did not show associations between hs-CRP level and distribution of WMHs in migraine patients (Table 3). The prevalence of WMHs was 4.35-fold higher in migraine patients than control subjects (Table 5). The WMHs primarily involved the subcortical region and frontal lobe (Table 2). Only 1 migraine patient satisfied the revised 2010 McDonald criteria for multiple sclerosis [32].

A unique feature of the present study design was the simultaneous assessment of the associations of hs-CRP and WMHs in migraine patients. The participants had no known vascular risk factors or inflammatory disease. We included patients aged < 50 years to minimize the

Table 1 Characteristics of participants in study of migraine*

Characteristic		Control (n = 216)	Migraine without aura (n = 143)	Migraine with aura (n = 73)	P ≤[†]
Age (y)		32 ± 4.6	30.9 ± 7.6	32.6 ± 6.7	NS
Body mass index (kg/m²)		24.3 ± 3.3	24.4 ± 3.9	25 ± 4.1	NS
Sex					.002[‡]
	Female	150 (69.4)	105 (73.4)	60 (82.2)	
	Male	66 (30.6)	38 (26.6)	13 (17.8)	
hs-CRP (mg/L)	Mean ± SD	0.82 ± 0.58	1.76 ± 1.86	2.31 ± 2.30	.001[‡]
	Median (min-max)	0.69 (0.10-2.90)	1.09 (0.10-9.51)	1.48 (0.10-9.92)	
hs-CRP (no. of subjects [%])	<1 mg/L	147 (68.1)	65 (45.5)	28 (38.4)	.001[‡]
	1-3 mg/L	69 (31.9)	53 (37.1)	25 (34.2)	
	>3 mg/L	0 (0)	25 (17.5)	20 (27.4)	
WMHs present (no. of subjects [%])		21 (9.7)	44 (30.8)	25 (34.2)	.001[‡]
No. of WMHs per subject	Mean ± SD	0.34 ± 1.27	1.62 ± 3.07	1.66 ± 3	.001[‡]
	Median (min-max)	0 (0–10)	0 (0–16)	0 (0–15)	
No. of subjects with WMHs	0 WMH	195 (90.3)	99 (69.2)	48 (65.8)	.001[‡]
	1-2 WMHs	8 (3.7)	9 (6.3)	4 (6.5)	
	≥3 WMHs	13 (6.0)	35 (24.5)	21 (28.8)	
Migraine disease duration (y)	Mean ± SD	-	6.3 ± 5.2	10.1 ± 7	.001[§]
	Median (min-max)	-	5 (1 – 30)	10 (1 – 30)	
Headache localization	Half head	-	47 (32.9)	20 (27.4)	NS
	Entire head	-	96 (67.1)	53 (72.6)	
Visual analog score	Mean ± SD	-	7.3 ± 1.8	7.8 ± 1.8	NS
	Median (min-max)	-	7 (3–10)	8 (4–10)	
Headache frequency (no./mo)	Mean ± SD	-	7.6 ± 5.6	7.7 ± 5.6	NS
	Median (min- max)	-	6 (2–20)	5 (2–20)	
Headache duration (h)	Mean ± SD	-	25,46 ± 27,69	26,11 ± 27,62	NS
	Median (min - max)	-	18.0 (1–168)	18.0 (1–120)	
Medication	Acetaminophen	-	41 (28.7)	22 (30.1)	NS
	Nonsteroidal anti-inflammatory drug	-	86 (60.1)	41 (56.2)	
	Ergotamine	-	7 (4.9)	8 (11)	
	Triptan	-	9 (6.3)	2 (2.7)	
Education completed	Primary school	21 (25.6)	41 (28.9)	24 (32.9)	NS
	Secondary school	6 (7.3)	15 (10.6)	8 (11)	
	High school	29 (35.4)	41 (28.9)	22 (30.1)	
	University	26 (31.7)	45 (31.7)	19 (26)	
Family history of headache		23 (28)	110 (76.9)	58 (79.5)	.001[‡]
Smoking (≤1 pack/d)		20 (24.4)	35 (24.5)	18 (24.7)	NS
Thyroid stimulating hormone (µIU/mL)	Median ± SD	1.43 ± 0.73	1.42 ± 0.71	1.47 ± 0.77	NS
	Median (min - max)	1.26 (0.37-4.03)	1.25 (0.35-3.90)	1.41 (0.44-4.25)	
Ejection Fraction (%)	Median ± SD	65.67 ± 4.76	65.24 ± 3.61	64.44 ± 4.33	NS
	Median (min - max)	65 (60–75)	65 (60–74)	65 (60–75)	

*Data reported as mean ± SD, number of subjects (%), or median (range, minimum to maximum). *Abbreviations: hs-CRP* high sensitivity C-reactive protein, *WMH* white matter hyperintensity.
[†]NS, not significant (P > .05).
[‡]Significant difference between migraine patients and control subjects.
[§]Significant difference between migraine patients without or with aura.

Table 2 Anatomic location and distribution of juxtacortical, subcortical, and periventricular white matter hyperintensities in migraine and control subjects*

White matter hyperintensities		Control (n = 216)		Migraine without aura (n = 143)		Migraine with aura (n = 73)		$P \leq$[†]
Juxtacortical WMHs		0 (0)		12 (8.4)		6 (8.2)		.0001[‡]
Juxtacortical WMHs	Frontal	0 (0)		7 (4.9)		3 (4.1)		.0001[‡]
	Parietal	0 (0)		4 (2.8)		2 (2.7)		.03[‡]
	Temporal	0 (0)		1 (0.7)		1 (1.4)		NS
	Occipital	0 (0)		0 (0.5)		0 (0.5)		-
Juxtacortical WMHs		0.0 ± 0.0	0 (0–0)	0.1 ± 0.48	0 (0–3)	0.14 ± 0.53	0 (0–3)	0.0001[‡]
Juxtacortical WMHs	Frontal	0.0 ± 0.0	0 (0–0)	0.09 ± 0.41	0 (0–3)	0.05 ± 0.28	0 (0–2)	0.0001[‡]
	Parietal	0.0 ± 0.0	0 (0–0)	0.04 ± 0.26	0 (0–2)	0.07 ± 0.42	0 (0–3)	.02[‡]
	Temporal	0.0 ± 0.0	0 (0–0)	0.01 ± 0.08	0 (0–1)	0.01 ± 0.12	0 (0–1)	NS
	Occipital	0.0 ± 0.0	0 (0–0)	0.0 ± 0.0	0 (0–0)	0.0 ± 0.0	0 (0–0)	-
Subcortical WMHs		21 (9.7)		41 (28.7		24 (32.9)		.0001[‡]
Subcortical WMHs	Frontal	20 (9.3)		36 (25.2)		22 (30.1)		.0001[‡]
	Parietal	6 (2.8)		24 (16.8)		13 (17.8)		.0001[‡]
	Temporal	0 (0)		2 (1.4)		4 (5.5)		.03[‡]
	Occipital	0 (0)		1 (0.7)		0 (0)		-
Subcortical WMHs		0.34 ± 1.28	0 (0–10)	1.46 ± 2.9	0 (0–14)	1.60 ± 2.99	0 (0–13)	0.0001[‡]
Subcortical WMHs	Frontal	0.31 ± 1.19	0 (0–10)	0.94 ± 1.99	0 (0–11)	1.10 ± 2.12	0 (0–11)	.0001[‡]
	Parietal	0.03 ± 0.17	0 (0–1)	0.47 ± 1.32	0 (0–8)	0.42 ± 1.19	0 (0–8)	.0001[‡]
	Temporal	0.0 ± 0.0	0 (0–0)	0.08 ± 0.36	0 (0–2)	0.08 ± 0.36	0 (0–2)	0.014[‡]
	Occipital	0.0 ± 0.0	0 (0–0)	0.01 ± 0.17	0 (0–2)	0.0 ± 0.0	0 (0–0)	NS
Periventricular WMHs		0 (0)		0 (0)		3 (4.1)		.04[‖]
Periventricular WMH	Anterior	0 (0)		0 (0)		3 (4.1)		.04[‖]
	Posterior	0 (0)		0 (0)		0 (0)		-
	Lateral	0 (0)		0 (0)		0 (0)		-
Periventricular WMHs		0.0 ± 0.0	0 (0–0)	0.0 ± 0.0	0 (0–0)	0.04 ± 0.20	0 (0–1)	.02[‖]
Periventricular WMHs	Anterior	0.0 ± 0.0	0 (0–0)	0.0 ± 0.0	0 (0–0)	0.04 ± 0.20	0 (0–1)	.02[‖]
	Posterior	0.0 ± 0.0	0 (0–0)	0.0 ± 0.0	0 (0–0)	0.0 ± 0.0	0 (0–0)	-
	Lateral	0.0 ± 0.0	0 (0–0)	0.0 ± 0.0	0 (0–0)	0.0 ± 0.0	0 (0–0)	-

*Data reported as number of patients (%), mean ± SD, or median (range, minimum to maximum). *Abbreviation:* WMHs deep white matter hyperintensities.
[†]NS, not significant (*P* > .05).
[‡]Comparison between control subjects and migraine patients (with and without aura).
[‖]Comparison between migraine patients with and without aura.

effects of age-dependent WMHs. Limitations of the present study included the limited number of participants. In addition, an MRI scanner with a higher magnetic field than the scanner used may be more sensitive in detecting WMHs on FLAIR images. A more sensitive imaging protocol with thin slices (thickness, 3 mm) might have improved the detection of smaller lesions. Furthermore, some risk factors such as smoking and obesity were not strictly excluded; although we excluded heavy smokers (>1 pack/d), we did not exclude all cigarette smokers. There were no statistically significant differences between the migraine and control groups in smoking habits. Although all participants had body mass index ≤ 35 kg/m^2, some participants had body mass index > 30 kg/m^2, and

CRP level may increase with obesity [34]. Nevertheless, we observed no significant differences between the migraine and control groups in body mass index. In addition, it may be important to study other markers of endothelial dysfunction or inflammation such as tissue plasminogen activator antigen, von Willebrand factor activity, homocysteine level, or inflammatory cytokine levels to further evaluate the association of hs-CRP in the development of WMHs in migraine patients. We did not perform carotid Doppler studies to evaluate the possibility of microemboli.

The observed high hs-CRP levels in migraine patients were consistent with previous reports (Table 1) [15,25-27]. In contrast with the present study, the Reykjavik study reported that CRP levels were similar in migraine patients

Table 3 Relation between high sensitivity C-reactive protein and cerebral white matter hyperintensities on magnetic resonance imaging in migraine patients and control subjects*

Parameter		All participants (n = 432)		Control subjects (n = 216)		Migraine patients (n = 216)	
		r	$P \leq$[†]	r	$P \leq$[†]	R	$P \leq$[†]
WMHs		0.155	.001	0.165	0.015	0.024	NS
Juxtacortical WMHs		0.062	NS	-	-	−0.003	NS
Juxtacortical WMHs	Frontal	0.101	0.036	-	-	0.077	NS
	Parietal	−0.003	NS	-	-	−0.068	NS
	Temporal	−0.007	NS	-	-	−0.037	NS
Subcortical WMHs		0.148	0.002	0.165	.015	0.018	NS
Subcortical WMHs	Frontal	0.132	0.006	0.145	.033	0.008	NS
	Parietal	0.110	0.022	0.095	NS	0.031	NS
	Temporal	0.075	NS	-	-	0.041	NS
	Occipital	0.049	NS	-	-	0.036	NS
Periventricular WMHs		0.074	NS	-	-	0.054	NS
Periventricular WMHs Anterior		0.074	NS	-	-	0.054	NS

*Data reported as correlation coefficient r between hs-CRP and parameter. *Abbreviation: WMHs* white matter hyperintensities.
[†]NS, not significant ($P > .05$).

and control subjects; vascular risk factors and concomitant disease were not eliminated, and the mean age of participants was 55 years [35]. Furthermore, another study reported no association between hs-CRP levels and migraine, and patients had no vascular risk factors; however, the sample was small, mean age of participants was older than in the present study, and headache frequency and migraine disease duration were not reported [36]. In the present study, inclusion criteria ensured that headache frequency was ≥ 2 headaches/mo

and migraine disease duration was > 1 year. Elevated hs-CRP level is a sensitive marker of inflammation and arteriosclerosis [23]. The higher mean level of hs-CRP in migraine patients than control subjects is evidence that inflammation may contribute to migraine (Table 1). In migraine, elevation of CRP may be caused by oxidative stress, leukocyte activation, and inflammatory dilation of blood vessels, and inflammatory cytokines are increased during acute attacks of migraine and between attacks [13,14].

Table 4 Relation between high sensitivity C-reactive protein and location of cerebral white matter hyperintensities, headache characteristics, and sex differences in migraine patients*

Parameters		hs-CRP (mg/L)		$P \leq$[†]
Juxtacortical WMHs	Present	1.95 ± 2.22	1.13 (0.21 – 9.40)	NS
	Absent	1.94 ± 2.01	1.25 (0.10 – 9.92)	
Subcortical WMHs	Present	2.01 ± 2.20	1.35 (0.10 – 9.92)	NS
	Absent	1.91 ± 1.95	1.18 (0.19 – 9.80)	
Periventricular WMHs	Present	1.91 ± 0.83	2.04 (1.02 – 2.67)	NS
	Absent	1.94 ± 2.04	1.24 (0.10 – 9.92)	
Sex	Female	1.99 ± 2.14	1.21 (0.01 – 9.92)	NS
	Male	1.80 ± 1.62	1.35 (0.10 – 8.30)	
Migraine disease duration (y)	≤1	1.46 ± 2.04	0.75 (0.15 – 9.51)	NS
	2-6	1.92 ± 1.87	1.35 (0.10 – 9.40)	
	≥7	2.10 ± 2.18	1.31 (0.10 – 9.92)	
Headache duration (h)		r = −0.002		NS
Visual analog score		r = −0.028		NS
Headache frequency (no./mo)		r = 0.042		NS

*Data reported as mean ± SD, number of subjects (%), median (range, minimum to maximum), or correlation coefficient r between hs-CRP and parameters.
Abbreviations: hs-CRP high sensitivity C-reactive protein, *WMH* white matter hyperintensity.
[†]NS, not significant ($P > .05$).

Table 5 Factors affecting the presence of white matter hyperintensity*

Parameter	Odds ratio (95% confidence interval)	$P \leq$[†]
Migraine	4.35 (1.904 - 0.945)	.001[‡]
hs-CRP	1.05 (0.906 - 1.213)	NS
Age	1.06 (1.018 - 1.102)	.004[ll]
Body mass index	1.02 (0.942 - 1.100)	.NS

*Data reported as odds ration and 95% confidence interval.
Abbreviation: hs-CRP high sensitivity C-reactive protein.
[†]NS, not significant ($P > .05$).
[‡]Migraine increased the risk of the presence of WMH by 4.35-fold.
[ll]Age 1 y increased the risk of the presence of WMH by 1.06-fold.

Although migraine is a risk factor for WMHs, incidental findings on brain MRI scans are common, prevalence increases with age, and detection is more likely using high resolution MRI sequences than standard resolution sequences [16,17]. The prevalence of WMHs in adult migraine patients varies from 14% to 59% [16,20,21]. In the present study, WMHs were detected with 4.35-fold greater frequency on brain MRI scans in migraine patients than control subjects (Table 5). The reason for the association between headache and WMHs is unknown. The WMHs may be an indirect marker of focal cerebral hypoperfusion induced by migraine attacks. Repeated and prolonged oligemia during and after migraine attacks may affect the vulnerable small deep penetrating arteries, and the WMHs may represent minor brain injury caused by reduced local perfusion [22,37].

In the present study, hs-CRP levels were not associated with the presence and severity of WMHs on brain MRI scans in migraine patients (Tables 2 and 5), consistent with previous studies [30,38,39]. In contrast with our study, several previous studies reported a relation between hs-CRP levels and WMHs in elderly nondemented patients with unknown migraine history [28,29]. The Cardiovascular Health Study reported that CRP levels were associated with the presence of WMHs; participants were aged > 65 years, vascular risk factors were not eliminated, and patients had cerebral ischemic infarcts [29]. The Rotterdam Scan Study described a relation between CRP and WMHs (severity and 3-year progression of WMHs); the participants were aged 60 to 90 years and had cardiovascular risk factors [28]. Increased age and vascular risk factors have been associated with high levels of hs-CRP and the presence of WMHs [21,23,24]. Differences in the composition of study participants may have been important. In the present study, the participants were younger and apparently healthier than those of previous studies. The present participants had only migraine headache and no other health conditions, and possible confounding factors that could have affected hs-CRP levels and WMHs were avoided such as vascular risk factors, inflammatory disease, or chronic illness. We did

not include patients who had cerebral ischemic infarcts. Therefore, it is likely that we studied earlier stages of WMHs in migraine patients. The absence of an association between hs-CRP levels and WMHs may support the hypothesis that the hs-CRP level does not affect the brain pattern or severity of WMHs that are associated with migraine disease. The WMHs on MRI in migraine patients may be associated with migraine disease and may be determined genetically [18,40].

In the present study, the anatomic location of WMHs was different between patients who had different migraine subtypes and control subjects. Only migraine patients with aura had periventricular WMHs. The WMHs were located mostly in the subcortical region and frontal lobe (Table 2) The WMHs of the control subjects were located only in the subcortical region. The distribution of subcortical and juxtacortical WMHs was not different between migraine patients with or without aura (Table 2). A previous cross-sectional population study also showed a higher association between deep WMHs and migraine in patients who had migraine with than without aura [20]. In contrast with our study, there were no differences in the location of periventricular WMHs between migraine patients and control subjects. It was proposed that different mechanisms may affect the development of deep and periventricular WMHs in patients who have migraine with or without aura [18]. In addition, we did not find any differences between female and male migraine patients in the presence, number, or distribution of WMHs (Table 4). In contrast with the present study, the CAMERA 1 and 2 studies showed that women who had migraine, especially migraine without aura, had a higher incidence of deep WMHs and deep WMH progression than control subjects [18,19]. In the previous studies, migraine patients were older and had vascular risk factors, and the WMH classification was different than in the present study.

In the present study, we observed no associations between WMHs and migraine headache characteristics, similar to previous studies [19]. In contrast with the present findings, previous studies reported a positive correlation between WMHs and migraine headache characteristics, but in the previous studies, the patients were older and had more comorbid conditions than the present study participants [14,18,20].

Although revisions in 2010 simplified the McDonald criteria, allowing an earlier diagnosis of multiple sclerosis (enabling establishment of dissemination in space (DIS) and dissemination in time (DIT) even with a single scan), they imposed an importance to the issue of excluding alternative diagnoses. With the increasing use of brain MRI, the finding of asymptomatic intracranial abnormalities has increased, and there is increased awareness of MRI findings suggestive of multiple sclerosis in patients without typical multiple sclerosis symptoms [41]. The importance of this problem was highlighted by the definition of the entity termed *radiologically-isolated syndrome* (RIS) [33]. Half of the patients who have RIS had their initial MRI because of headache, and characteristic imaging features and clinical associations of WMHs in migraine should be determined [21]. Therefore, many studies have suggested new and different definitions of periventricular and juxtacortical lesions because they were not precisely defined previously [42]. However, newer definitions may cause confusion instead of enabling an accurate classification of WMHs that are observed incidently on brain MRI scans. In our study, we also tried to differentiate incidental MRI lesions from imaging characteritics and factors associated with migraine; we observed that the prevelance of WMHs was 4.35-times higher in migraine patients than control subjects. Although our cohort included few patients, only 1 of 69 patients with migraine (1.4%) satisfied the revised 2010 McDonald criteria for multiple sclerosis [32], consistent with another study that reported that the 2010 McDonald criteria were satisfied in 4 of 44 patients with migraine (9%) [21,32]. In another headache study, 2.4%-7.1% patients satisfied the Barkhof criteria and 24.4%-34.5% patients satisfied the McDonald criteria; in that study, the Barkhof and McDonald criteria were modified and included migraine patients with unknown medical history [42]. Therefore, these findings may have represented a false positive finding. Yet, it is important to be aware of WMHs because of the potential for diagnostic confusion. Aging, vascular risk factors, and inflammatory disease are associated with WMHs [21,20]. Nevertheless, none of our patients with migraine satisfied the Barkhof criteria. Therefore we suggest caution in interpreting asymptomatic MRI findings, especially in migraine patients, to avoid overdiagnosis. The Barkhof criteria may be more sensitive than McDonald 2010 multiple sclerosis criteria. The size of WMHs may be useful in differentiating migraine from demyelinating disease.

Conclusions

The present study showed that high levels of hs-CRP may be a marker of the proinflammatory state in migraine patients. However, the absence of correlation between hs-CRP and WMHs suggests that hs-CRP is not causally involved in the pathogenesis of WMHs in migraine patients. The WMHs were located mostly in the frontal lobe and subcortical area. The size and location of the WMHs may be important to differentiate WMHs from demyelination. Further prospective studies are justified to evaluate the relation between migraine and WMHs.

Abbreviations
CRP: C-reactive protein; WMHs: white matter hyperintensities; FLAIR: fluid attenuated inversion recovery; hs-CRP: high sensitivity C-reactive protein; MRI: magnetic resonance imaging.

Competing interests
The authors declare that they have no competing interests.

Authors' contributions
AYA, HL, and SA, conceived and designed the study and acquired and interpreted the data; AYA, USB, and MK revised the manuscript critically for important intellectual content. All authors read and approved the final manuscript.

Authors' information
A. Yilmaz Avci, assistant professor; H. Lakadamyali, associate professor; S. Arikan, assistant professor, U.S. Benli, professor; M. Kilinc, associate professor.

Acknowledgements
The authors thank Nagehan Kacar for statistical analysis.

Author details
[1]Department of Neurology, Baskent University, Saray Mah, Yunusemre cad, No. 1, Alanya-Antalya 07400 Ankara, Turkey. [2]Department of Radiology, Baskent University, Ankara, Turkey. [3]Department of Biochemistry, Baskent University, Ankara, Turkey.

References
1. Headache Classification Subcommittee of the International Headache Society (2004) The international classification of headache disorders: 2nd edition. Cephalalgia 24(suppl 1):9–160
2. Victor TW, Hu X, Campbell JC, Buse DC, Lipton RB (2010) Migraine prevalence by age and sex in the United States: a life-span study. Cephalalgia 30:1065–1072
3. Ertas M, Baykan B, Orhan EK, Zarifoglu M, Karli N, Saip S, Onal AE, Siva A (2012) One-year prevalance and the impact of migraine and tension-type headache in Turkey: a nationwide home-based study in adults. J Headache Pain 13:147–157
4. Schürks M, Rist PM, Bigal ME, Buring JE, Lipton RB, Kurth T (2009) Migraine and cardiovascular disease: systemic review and meta-analysis. BMJ 339:b3914, doi:10.1136/bmj.b3914
5. Bigal ME, Kurth T, Hu H, Santanello N, Lipton RB (2009) Migraine and cardiovascular disease: possible mechanisms of interaction. Neurology 72:1864–1871
6. Spector JT, Kahn SR, Jones MR, Jayakumar M, Dalal D, Nazarian S (2010) Migraine headache and ischemic stroke risk: an updated meta-analysis. Am J Med 123:612–624
7. Goldstein LB, Bushnell CD, Adams RJ, Appel LJ, Braun LT, Chaturvedi S, Creager MA, Culebras A, Eckel RH, Hart RG, Hinchey JA, Howard VJ, Jauch EC, Levine SR, Meschia JF, Moore WS, Nixon JV, Pearson TA, American Heart Association Stroke Council; Council on Cardiovascular Nursing; Council on Epidemiology and Prevention; Council for High Blood Pressure Research, Council on Peripheral Vascular Disease, and Interdisciplinary Council on Quality of Care and Outcomes Research (2011) Guidelines for the primary prevention of stroke: a guideline for healthcare professionals from the American Heart Association/American Stroke Association. Stroke 42:517–584
8. Kurth T, Schürks M, Logroscino G, Gaziano JM, Buring JE (2008) Migraine, vascular risk, and cardiovascular events in women: prospective cohort study. BMJ 337:a636, doi:10.1136/bmj.a636
9. MacClellan LR, Giles W, Cole J, Wozniak M, Stern B, Mitchell BD, Kittner SJ (2007) Probable migraine with visual aura and risk of ischemic stroke: the stroke prevention in young women study. Stroke 38:2438–2445
10. Henrich JB, Horwitz RI (1989) A controlled study of ischemic stroke risk in migraine patients. J Clin Epidemiol 42:773–780
11. Sacco S, Ornello R, Ripa P, Pistoia F, Carolei A (2013) Migraine and hemorrhagic stroke: a meta-analysis. Stroke 44:3032–3038
12. Bolay H, Reuter U, Dunn AK, Huang Z, Boas DA, Moskowitz MA (2002) Intrinsic brain activity triggers trigeminal meningeal afferents in migraine model. Nat Med 8:136–142
13. Waeber C, Moskowitz MA (2005) Migraine as an inflammatory disorder. Neurology 64(10 suppl 2):S9–S15
14. Sarchielli P, Alberti A, Baldi A, Coppola F, Rossi C, Pierguidi L, Floridi A, Calabresi P (2006) Proinflammatory cytokines, adhesion molecules, and

lymphocyte integrin expression in the internal jugular blood of migraine patients without aura assessed ictally. Headache 46:200–207

15. Tietjen GE, Herial NA, White L, Utley C, Kosmyna JM, Khuder SA (2009) Migraine and biomarkers of endothelial activation in young women. Stroke 40:2977–2982

16. Bashir A, Lipton RB, Ashina S, Ashina M (2013) Migraine and structural changes in the brain: a systematic review and meta-analysis. Neurology 81:1260–1268

17. Morris Z, Whiteley WN, Longstreth WT Jr, Weber F, Lee YC, Tsushima Y, Alphs H, Ladd SC, Warlow C, Wardlaw JM, Al-Shahi Salman R (2009) Incidental findings on brain magnetic resonance imaging: systemiic review and meta-analysis. BMJ 339:b3016, doi:10.1136/bmj.b3016

18. Kruit MC, van Buchem MA, Hofman PA, Bakkers JT, Terwindt GM, Ferrari MD, Launer LJ (2004) Migraine as a risk factor for subclinical brain lesions. JAMA 291:427–434

19. Palm-Meinders IH, Koppen H, Terwindt GM, Launer LJ, Konishi J, Moonen JM, Bakkers JT, Hofman PA, van Lew B, Middelkoop HA, van Buchem MA, Ferrari MD, Kruit MC (2012) Structural brain changes in migraine. JAMA 308:1889–1897

20. Kurth T, Mohamed S, Maillard P, Zhu YC, Chabriat H, Mazoyer B, Bousser MG, Dufouil C, Tzourio C (2011) Headache, migraine, and structural brain lesions and function: population based Epidemiology of Vascular Ageing-MRI study. BMJ 342:c7357, doi:10.1136/bmj.c7357

21. Seneviratne U, Chong W, Billimoria PH (2013) Brain white matter hyperintensities in migraine: clinical and radiological correlates. Clin Neurol Neurosurg 115:1040–1043

22. Bednarczyk EM, Remler B, Weikart C, Nelson AD, Reed RC (1998) Global cerebral blood flow, blood volume, and oxygen metabolism in patients with migraine headache. Neurology 50:1736–1740

23. Bassuk SS, Rifai N, Ridker PM (2004) High-sensitivity C-reactive protein: clinical importance. Curr Probl Cardiol 29:439–493

24. Ridker PM, Cook N (2004) Clinical usefulness of very high and very low levels of C-reactive protein across the full range of Framingham risk scores. Circulation 109:1955–1959

25. Kurth T, Ridker PM, Buring JE (2007) Mgraine and biomarkers of cardiovascular disease in women. Cephalalgia 28:49–56

26. Welch KM, Brandes AW, Salerno L, Brandes JL (2006) C-reactive protein may be increased in migraine patients who present with complex clinical features. Headache 46:197–199

27. Vanmolkot FH, de Hoon JN (2007) Increased C-reactive protein in young adult patients with migraine. Cephalalgia 27:843–846

28. van Dijk EJ, Prins ND, Vermeer SE, Vrooman HA, Hofman A, Koudstaal PJ, Breteler MM (2005) C-reactive protein and cerebral small-vessel disease: the Rotterdam Scan Study. Circulation 112:900–905

29. Fornage M, Chiang YA, O'Meara ES, Psaty BM, Reiner AP, Siscovick DS, Tracy RP, Longstreth WT Jr (2008) Biomarkers of inflammation and MRI-defined small vessel disease of the brain: the Cardiovascular Health Study. Stroke 39:1952–1959

30. Schmidt R, Schmidt H, Pichler M, Enzinger C, Petrovic K, Niederkorn K, Homer S, Ropele S, Watzinger N, Schumacher M, Berghold A, Kostner GM, Fazekas F (2006) C-reactive protein, carotid atherosclerosis, and cerebral small-vessel disease: results of the Austrian Stroke Prevention Study. Stroke 37:2910–2916

31. Barkhof F, Filippi M, Miller DH, Scheltens P, Campi A, Polman CH, Comi G, Adèr HJ, Losseff N, Valk J (1997) Comparison of MRI criteria at first presentation to predict conversion to clinically definite multiple sclerosis. Brain 120(pt 11):2059–2069

32. Polman CH, Reingold SC, Banwell B, Clanet M, Cohen JA, Filippi M, Fujihara K, Havrdova E, Hutchinson M, Kappos L, Lublin FD, Montalban X, O'Connor P, Sandberg-Wollheim M, Thompson AJ, Waubant E, Weinschenker B, Wolinsky JS (2011) Diagnostic criteria for multiple sclerosis: 2010 revisions to the McDonald criteria. Ann Neurol 69:292–302

33. Okuda DT, Mowry EM, Beheshtian A, Waubant E, Branzini SE, Goodin DS, Hauser SL, Pelletier D (2009) Incidental MRI anomalies suggestive of multiple sclerosis: the radiologically isolated syndrome. Neurology 72:800–805

34. Rexrode KM, Pradhan A, Manson JE, Buring JE, Ridker PM (2003) Relationship of total and abdominal adiposity with CRP and IL-6 in women. Ann Epidemiol 13:674–682

35. Gudmundsson LS, Aspelund T, Scher AI, Thorgeirsson G, Johannsson M, Launer LJ, Gudnason V (2009) C-reactive protein in migraine sufferers similar to that of non-migraineurs: the Reykjavik study. Cephalalgia 29:1301–1310

36. Guldiken B, Guldiken S, Demir M, Turgut N, Kabayel L, Ozkan H, Ozcelik E, Tugrul A (2008) Insulin resistance and high sensitivity C-reactive protein in migraine. Can J Neurol Sci 35:448–451

37. Cutrer FM, Sorensen AG, Weisskoff RM, Ostergaard L, Sanchez del Rio M, Lee EJ, Rosen BR, Moskowitz MA (1998) Perfusion-weighted imaging defects during spontaneous migrainous aura. Ann Neurol 43:25–31

38. Wada M, Nagasawa H, Kurita K, Koyama S, Arawaka S, Kawanami T, Tajima K, Daimon M, Kato T (2008) Cerebral small vessel disease and C-reactive protein: results of a cross-sectional study in community-based Japanese elderly. J Neurol Sci 264:43–49

39. Reitz C, Berger K, de Maat MP, Stoll M, Friedrichs F, Kardys I, Witteman JC, Breteler MM (2007) CRP gene haplotypes, serum CRP, and cerebral small-vessel disease: the Rotterdam Scan Study and the MEMO Study. Stroke 38:2356–2359

40. Atwood LD, Wolf PA, Heard-Costa NL, Massaro JM, Beiser A, D'Agostino RB, DeCarli C (2004) Genetic variation in white matter hyperintensity volume in the Framingham Study. Stroke 35:1609–1613

41. Granberg T, Martola J, Kristofferson-Wiberg M, Aspelin P, Fredrikson S (2013) Radiologically isolated syndrome - incidental magnetic resonance imaging findings suggestive of multiple sclerosis, a systematic review. Mult Scler 19:271–280

42. Liu S, Kullnat J, Bourdette D, Simon J, Kraemer DF, Murchison C, Hamilton BE (2013) Prevalence of brain magnetic resonance imaging meeting Barkhof and McDonald criteria for dissemination in space among headache patients. Mult Scler 19:1101–1105

9

Visual evoked potentials in subgroups of migraine with aura patients

Gianluca Coppola[1*], Martina Bracaglia[2], Davide Di Lenola[2], Cherubino Di Lorenzo[3], Mariano Serrao[2], Vincenzo Parisi[1], Antonio Di Renzo[1], Francesco Martelli[4], Antonello Fadda[4], Jean Schoenen[5] and Francesco Pierelli[2,6]

Abstract

Background: Patients suffering from migraine with aura can have either pure visual auras or complex auras with sensory disturbances and dysphasia, or both. Few studies have searched for possible pathophysiological differences between these two subgroups of patients.

Methods: Methods - Forty-seven migraine with aura patients were subdivided in a subgroup with exclusively visual auras (MA, $N = 27$) and another with complex neurological auras (MA+, $N = 20$). We recorded pattern-reversal visual evoked potentials (VEP: 15 min of arc cheques, 3.1 reversal per second, 600 sweeps) and measured amplitude and habituation (slope of the linear regression line of amplitude changes from the 1st to 6th block of 100 sweeps) for the N1-P1 and P1-N2 components in patients and, for comparison, in 30 healthy volunteers (HV) of similar age and gender distribution.

Results: VEP N1-P1 habituation, i.e. amplitude decrement between 1st and 6th block, which was obvious in most HV (mean slope −0.50), was deficient in both MA (slope +0.01, $p = 0.0001$) and MA+ (−0.0049, $p = 0.001$) patients. However, VEP N1-P1 amplitudes across blocks were normal in MA patients, while they were significantly greater in MA+ patients than in HVs.

Conclusions: Our findings suggest that in migraine with aura patients different aura phenotypes may be underpinned by different pathophysiological mechanisms. Pre-activation cortical excitability could be higher in patients with complex neurological auras than in those having pure visual auras or in healthy volunteers.

Keywords: Migraine with aura, Visual aura, Complex aura, Visual evoked potentials, Habituation, Cortical excitability

Background

Migraine with aura (MA) is defined as attacks of neurological symptoms that last no more than 60 min and may be followed or accompanied by headache (International Classification of Headache Disorders 3beta 2013). The most common aura symptoms are visual (e.g. scintillating scotoma), while sensory and aphasic auras are present in a smaller proportion of patients [1, 2]. According to Rasmussen and Olesen [3], 51 % of migraine auras are purely visual, while 4 % comprise sensory symptoms in addition to the visual ones and 6 % language disturbances in addition to visual and sensory disturbances.

The most likely cause of the migraine aura, Leão's cortical spreading depression (CSD), consists of a brief neuronal depolarisation followed by a long-lasting wave of neuronal depression that often spreads postero-anteriorly in the occipital cortex and can reach the parietal and/or temporal lobes [4, 5]. Indirect evidence for CSD occurrence in migraine patients stems from functional neuroimaging [6–8] and electrophysiological [9] studies. Although in animal models CSD is able to activate peripheral and central trigeminovascular neurons that underlie the migraine headache [10, 11], knowledge is lacking on the possible relation of CSD to interictal neural alterations that may predispose to migraine attacks.

During the last decade various research groups have demonstrated significant changes of bioelectrical activity in the visual cortex of migraine patients over the migraine cycle. In particular, cortical visual evoked potentials (VEPs)

* Correspondence: gianluca.coppola@gmail.com
[1]G.B. Bietti Foundation-IRCCS, Department of Neurophysiology of Vision and Neurophthalmology, Via Livenza 3, 00198 Rome, Italy
Full list of author information is available at the end of the article

are used to infer the mass activity of visual cortical neurons. Most, though not all [12], VEP, recordings have shown that the brain of migraineurs with and without aura is characterized by an interictal deficit of habituation during stimulus repetition, and by its ictal normalization [13–16].

It was suggested that migraine with aura is a condition with a spectrum of clinical subtypes that likely differ in pathophysiological mechanisms [17]. Distinct electrophysiological abnormalities were especially found at the neuromuscular junction in patients suffering from complex neurological auras characterized by visual symptoms followed by sensorimotor and dysphasic symptoms [18] or from prolonged auras [19]. Using 1H-MR-spectroscopy, migraine patients with visual symptoms and at least one of paraesthesia, paresis, or dysphasia had a significant lactate increase in the visual cortex during sustained visual stimulation, while this was not the case in controls and patients with exclusive visual aura. In the latter group, however, lactate levels were already elevated at baseline and remained consistently high during the visual stimulation [20]. Besides its role as energy substrate of the brain, lactate acts as a neuromodulator and interacts with glutamate [21], GABA [22], and monoamines [23], which suggest that it is important in regulating the activity of cortical neurons. Lactate may increase to attenuate the electrical activity of excessively active neurons as observed in experimental models [22, 24, 25] and in healthy humans during sustained visual stimulation [26]. Considering these data and those obtained by NMR spectroscopy showing altered metabolic homeostasis of the migraineur's brain [27, 28], it is of interest to verify whether activity of visual cortical neurons is increased in migraine patients suffering from complex auras respective to those experiencing pure visual symptoms. We decided therefore to compare amplitude and habituation of pattern reversal VEP in healthy volunteers, migraine patients with pure visual auras, and in patients with complex neurological auras including at least one of sensory and language symptoms in addition to visual disturbances. Considering the abovementioned NMR spectroscopy studies and our prior interictal VEP studies in migraine with aura [14, 15], we reasoned that subgroups of migraine with aura patients would show both common and specific neurophysiological abnormalities. We hypothesized that VEP amplitude would be higher in migraine with complex aura than in migraine with pure visual aura, while habituation would be equally deficient in both MA subgroups.

Methods

Subjects

We initially enrolled 58 consecutive migraine patients with typical aura (MAtot, ICHD-3beta code 1.2.1.1) who attended our headache clinic. We discarded recordings of 10 patients who did not fulfil our primary inclusion criteria (see below), and of one patient because he was an outlier. The final analysis set comprises therefore 47 patients (32 women, mean age 31.8 years). Patients were subdivided into those who experienced pure visual aura (MA, $N = 27$) and those who had in addition paraesthesia and/or dysphasia (i.e. complex neurological auras; MA+, $N = 20$). Auras usually developed gradually and were followed by headache. None had hemiplegic or brainstem auras or persistent aura without infarction. All patients had a varying combination of attacks with or without aura. We took information on various clinical characteristics by collecting up to two-month headache diaries at the time of the screening visit and the day of the recording session. Patients had to indicate duration of migraine history (years), attack frequency (n/month), attack duration (hours), and number of days elapsed since the last migraine attack (in 35 out of 47 patients) (Table 1).

A primary inclusion criterion was being attack-free for at least 3 days before and after the recording sessions, as checked by collecting headache diaries, and by telephone or e-mail interviews. Migraine patients were recorded in the interictal period. The time range of 3 days was chosen to avoid the accidental inclusion of patients recorded during an attack. In fact, according to the International classification of Headache Disorders, a migraine attack can last up to 3 days. Of the patients initially recorded, ten patients had an attack within 3 days after the recording session, and thus their VEP data were not included in the present analysis. We chose to focus on interictal recordings because some previous studies

Table 1 Clinical and demographic characteristics of healthy volunteers (HV), the total group of migraine with aura patients (MAtot) and its subgroups with pure visual aura (MA) or visual aura associated with paraesthesia and/or dysphasia (MA+). Data are expressed as means ± SD

Characteristics	HV (n = 30)	MAtot (n = 47)	MA (n = 27)	MA+ (n = 20)
Women (n)	18	32	17	15
Age (years)	33.4 ± 13.4	31.8 ± 9.3	31.7 ± 9.4	32.5 ± 9.5
Duration of migraine history (years)		16.1 ± 9.9	15.3 ± 9.5	17.0 ± 10.5
Attack frequency/month (n)		2.5 ± 2.6	2.1 ± 2.2	2.9 ± 3.0
Attack duration (hours)		28.8 ± 25.4	29.9 ± 27.2	27.4 ± 23.3
Days since the last migraine attack		17.5 ± 16.1	15.3 ± 16.4	20.6 ± 15.9

showed that habituation reflects the periodicity between 2 migraine attacks, i.e. is lacking between attacks and normalizes immediately before and during an attack [15, 29]. For comparison, we enrolled a group of 30 age-matched healthy volunteers (18 women, mean age 33.4 years) recruited among medical school students and healthcare professionals, randomly recorded between patients. Exclusion criteria were regular medication intake (i.e. antibiotics, corticosteroids, antidepressants, benzodiazepines, prophylactic migraine drugs) except for the contraceptive pill, failure to reach a best-corrected visual acuity of > 8/10, history of other neurological diseases, systemic hypertension, diabetes or other metabolic disorders, connective or autoimmune diseases, and any other type of primary or secondary headache. Female participants were always recorded at mid-cycle. All participants (HV and MwA) were naïve to the study procedure. We did not give any recommendation and/or information to HV or patients about potential clinical benefits or harms associated with the recordings.

All participants received a complete description of the study and granted written informed consent. The ethical review board "Sapienza" University of Rome, Polo Pontino, approved the project.

Visual evoked potentials

Subjects were sitting in an acoustically isolated room with dimmed lights in front of a TV monitor surrounded by a uniform luminance field of 5 cd/m^2. To obtain a stable pupillary diameter, each subject adapted to the ambient room light for 10 min before the VEP recordings. VEP were elicited by right monocular stimulation. Visual stimuli consisted of full-field checkerboard patterns (contrast 80 %, mean luminance 50 cd/m^2) generated on a TV monitor; the reversal rate was 1.55 Hz (3.1 reversal per second)). At the viewing distance of 114 cm, the single checks subtended a visual angle of 15 min, while the checkerboard subtended 23°. Recordings were

done with the best corrected visual acuity of > 8/10 at the viewing distance. Subjects were instructed to fixate with their right eye a red dot in the middle of the screen with the contralateral eye covered by a patch to maintain stable fixation. VEP were recorded from the scalp through silver cup electrodes positioned at Oz (active electrode) and at Fz (reference electrode, 10/20 system). A ground electrode was placed on the right forearm. Signals were amplified by Digitimer™ D360 pre-amplifiers (band-pass 0.05–2000 Hz, gain 1000) and recorded with a CED™ power 1401 device (Cambridge Electronic Design Ltd, Cambridge, UK). A total of 600 consecutive sweeps each lasting 200 ms were collected and sampled at 4000 Hz.

After applying off-line a 35 Hz low-pass digital filter, cortical responses were partitioned in 6 sequential blocks of 100, consisting of at least 95 artifact-free sweeps. Responses in each block were averaged off-line ("block averages") using the Signal™ software package version 4.10 (CED Ltd). Artefacts were automatically rejected using the Signal™ artefact rejection tool if the signal amplitude exceeded 90 % of analog-to-digital converter (ADC) range and was controlled by visual inspection. Through this approach, we made sure to exclude all severe artefacts but not to remove any signal systematically because background EEG amplitudes vary between subjects. The EP-signal was corrected off-line for DC-drifts, eye movements and blinks.

VEP components were identified according to their latencies: N1 was defined as the most negative peak between 60 and 90 ms, P1 as the most positive peak following N1 between 80 and 120 ms and N2 as the most negative peak following P1 at between 125 and 150 ms (Fig. 1). We measured the peak-to-peak amplitude of the N1–P1 and P1–N2 complexes. Habituation was defined as the slope of the linear regression line for the 6 blocks. All recordings were collected in the morning (between 09.00 and 11.00 a.m.) by the same investigators (D.D.L and C.D.L.), who did not meet the participants

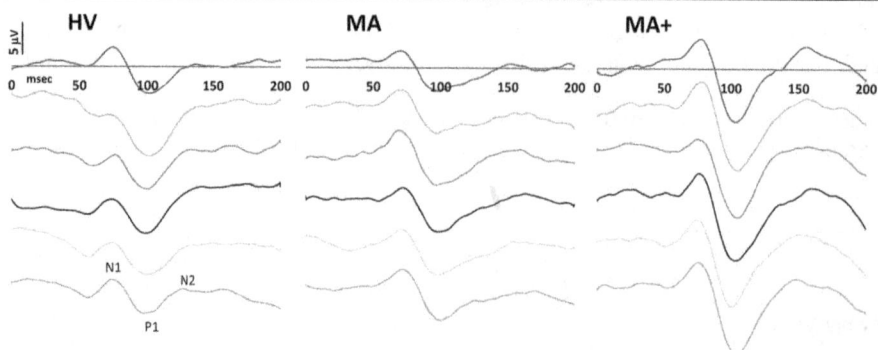

Fig. 1 Representative recordings (low pass filter 35 Hz) of visual evoked potentials in a healthy volunteer (HV), a migraine patient with pure visual aura (MA), and a migraine patient with complex aura (MA+) recorded between attacks. The 6 successive blocks of 100 averaged responses from top to bottom illustrate the difference between the 3 subjects in 1st block N1-P1 and P1-N2 amplitudes, and in amplitude change (habituation) over the 6 blocks

prior to the examination, since they were not involved in recruitment and inclusion of subjects. All recordings were numbered anonymously and analyzed blindly off-line by one investigator (M.B.), who was not blinded to the order of the blocks.

Statistical analysis

We used the Statistica for Windows (StatSoft Inc.), version 8.0 for all analyses. Preliminary descriptive analysis showed that the VEP N1–P1 and P1–N2 peak-to-peak amplitudes of the six blocks and the habituation slopes had a non-normal distribution. After log transformation, all data reached normal distribution (Kolmogorov-Smirnov test, $p > 0.2$).

A General Linear Model approach was used to analyze the "between-factor" × "within-factors" interaction effect. The between-subject factor was "group" (HV *vs.* MAtot or HV *vs.* MA subgroups); the within-subject factor was "blocks". Two models of repeated measures ANOVA (rm-ANOVA) followed by univariate ANOVAs were employed to investigate the interaction effect. Univariate results were analyzed only if Wilks' Lambda multivariate significance criterion was achieved. The sphericity of the covariance matrix was verified with the Mauchly Sphericity Test; in the case of violation of the sphericity assumption, Greenhouse-Geisser (G-G) epsilon (ε) adjustment was used. In rm-ANOVA and ANOVA models, partial eta^2 $\left(\eta_p^2\right)$ and observed power (op) were used as measures of effect size and power, respectively. To define which comparison(s) contributed to the major effects, post hoc tests were performed with Tukey Honest Significant Difference (HSD) test.

A regression analysis was used to disclose linear trends in VEP amplitude across blocks (slope) in each group. For slope, we employed ANOVA with group factor "group" (HV *vs.* MAtot or HV *vs.* MA subgroups), using Tukey test for post hoc analysis. Also for ANOVA partial eta^2 and op was used. Statistical significance was set at $p < 0.05$.

Pearson's correlation test was used to search for correlations among VEP amplitude slopes and clinical variables (duration of migraine history, attack frequency, attack duration, days since the last migraine attack).

Results

Recordings from 47 participants who fulfilled the inclusion criteria yielded analysable VEP data. The two patient subgroups MA and MA+ did not differ in other clinical features (Table 1).

Total group of migraine with aura patients (MAtot)

N1, P1 and N2 latencies were not significantly different between HV and MAtot ($p > 0.05$) (Table 2).

In the rm-ANOVA model with N1–P1 peak-peak amplitude as dependent variable, multivariate test was significant for the "*group*" × "*blocks*" interaction effect (Wilks' Lambda = 0.745, $F_{5,71} = 4.862$, $p = 0.0007$) (Table 3). After checking that the sphericity assumption was not violated (Mauchley Test: $p = 0.104$), univariate rm-ANOVAs for N1–P1 peak-peak amplitude confirmed the significant interaction factor effect ($F_{5,375} = 5.261$, $p = 0.0001$, partial $\eta^2 = 0.066$, op = 0.988) observed (see above) at the multivariate test. Post-hoc analysis showed that VEP amplitudes differed between groups only in the last block (5.97 µV in HV vs. 7.42 µV in MAtot, $p = 0.038$, raw data are shown in Fig. 2). In HV, N1–P1 amplitude was significantly lower in the 6th compared to the 1st block ($p = 0.0008$). This was not so in MAtot, where this comparison did not reach the significance level ($p = 0.994$).

In the rm-ANOVA model with P1-N2 peak-peak amplitude as dependent variable, multivariate test was not significant for the "*group*" × "*blocks*" interaction effect (Wilks' Lambda = 0.869, $F_{5,71} = 2.149$, $p = 0.069$) (Table 4).

The linear regression N1–P1 slope of VEP amplitudes over all blocks differed significantly between the two groups ($F_{1,75} = 24.493$, $p < 0.0001$, partial $\eta^2 = 0.246$, op = 0.998; raw data are shown in Fig. 3). The P1–N2 slope of the linear regression analysis was not different between groups ($F_{1,75} = 3.312$, $p = 0.073$, partial $\eta^2 = 0.042$, op = 0.435; Fig. 3).

In the MAtot group the N1–P1 amplitude slope correlated positively with the number of days elapsed since the last migraine attack (r = 0.351, $p = 0.045$). There were no other significant correlation between neurophysiological and clinical data.

Subgroups of migraine with aura patients

N1, P1 and N2 latencies were not significantly different between HV, MA or MA+ ($P > 0.05$) (Table 2).

Table 2 Latencies (in milliseconds) of VEPs in healthy volunteers (HV), the total group of migraine with aura patients (MAtot) and its subgroups with pure visual aura (MA) or visual aura associated with paraesthesia and/or dysphasia (MA+). Data are expressed as means ± SD.

Electrophysiological parameters (ms)	HV (n = 30)	MAtot (n = 47)	MA (n = 27)	MA+ (n = 20)
N1 (N75)	76.5 ± 6.4	75.7 ± 5.2	75.4 ± 5.8	75.9 ± 4.6
P1 (P100)	103.5 ± 5.9	103.1 ± 6.7	102.9 ± 5.7	103.4 ± 8.0
N2 (145)	144.2 ± 10.4	141.7 ± 11.9	140.6 ± 9.6	142.6 ± 11.4

Table 3 N1–P1 VEP component amplitude (μV) and habituation slope in healthy volunteers (HV), the total group of migraine with aura patients (MAtot) and its subgroups with pure visual aura (MA) or visual aura associated with paraesthesia and/or dysphasia (MA+). Data are expressed as means ± SD

N1-P1	HV (n = 30)	MAtot (n = 47)	MA (n = 27)	MA+ (n = 20)
1st amplitude block (μV)	6.97 ± 2.90	7.28 ± 3.23	6.53 ± 3.36	8.27 ± 2.83
2nd amplitude block (μV)	7.15 ± 3.02	7.39 ± 3.23	6.43 ± 3.29	8.69 ± 2.70
3rd amplitude block (μV)	6.87 ± 2.79	7.40 ± 2.96	6.49 ± 2.83	8.64 ± 2.74
4th amplitude block (μV)	6.55 ± 2.74	7.16 ± 3.17	6.12 ± 3.07	8.57 ± 2.81
5th amplitude block (μV)	6.25 ± 2.57	7.34 ± 3.00	6.49 ± 2.97	8.49 ± 2.70
6th amplitude block (μV)	5.97 ± 2.63	7.42 ± 3.02	6.65 ± 3.09	8.45 ± 2.64
Slope	−0.50 ± 0.36	+0.006 ± 0.40	+0.01 ± 0.30	+0.0049 ± 0.18

In the rm-ANOVA model with N1–P1 peak-peak amplitude as dependent variable, multivariate test was significant for the "group" × "blocks" interaction effect (Wilks' Lambda = 0.711, $F_{10,140}$ = 2.608, p = 0.006). After checking that the sphericity assumption was not violated (Mauchley Test: p = 0.126), univariate rm-ANOVAs for N1-P1 peak-peak amplitude confirmed the significant interaction factor effect ($F_{10,370}$ = 3.025, p = 0.001, partial η^2 = 0.076, op = 0.982) observed (see above) at the multivariate test. On post-hoc analysis there was a significant increase of N1-P1 VEP amplitude from the 2nd to the 6th block in MA+ compared with MA, and from the 4th to the 6th block in MA+ compared with HV (row data are shown in Fig. 2). In both MA and MA+, the comparison between the 6th and the 1st N1-P1 amplitude block did not reach the significance level (p > 0.05).

In the rm-ANOVA model with P1–N2 peak-peak amplitude as dependent variable, multivariate test was not significant for the "group" × "blocks" interaction effect (Wilks' Lambda = 0.834, $F_{10,140}$ = 1.335, p = 0.218).

The linear regression N1–P1 slope of VEP amplitudes over all blocks differed significantly between the three groups ($F_{2,74}$ = 12.219, p < 0.0001, partial η^2 = 0.248, op = 0.995; raw data are shown in Fig. 2). Post-hoc analysis showed that the slope of N1–P1 VEP amplitude changes over all 6 blocks was less steep in MA and in MA+ patients than in HV (p = 0.0001, p = 0.001 respectively, raw data are shown in Fig. 3), but it was equally steep between MA subgroups (p = 0.894).

The P1–N2 slope of the linear regression analysis was not different between groups ($F_{2,74}$ = 1.720, p = 0.186, partial η^2 = 0.044, op = 0.351; Fig. 3).

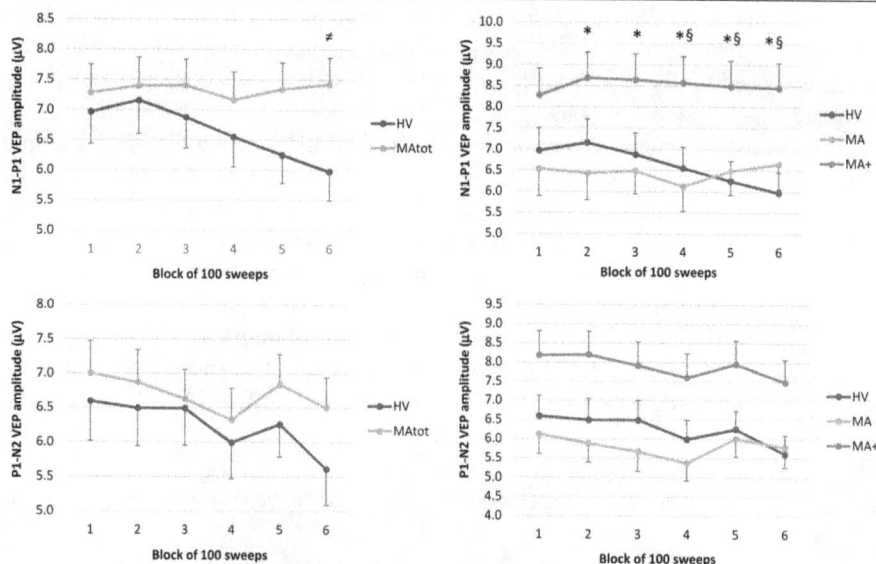

Fig. 2 Raw amplitudes (mean ± SEM) of N1-P1 (upper graphs) and P1-N2 (lower graphs) VEP components in 6 sequential blocks of 100 recordings. On the left healthy volunteers [HV, n = 30] are compared to the total group of migraine with aura patients [MAtot, n = 47]; on the right they are compared to the 2 subgroups of patients with pure visual aura [MA, n = 27] and patients with complex aura [MA+, n = 20]. ≠ p < 0.05 MAtot vs HV; *p < 0.05 MA+ vs MA; § p < 0.05 MA+ vs HV

Table 4 P1-N2 VEP component amplitude (μV) and habituation slope in healthy volunteers (HV), the total group of migraine with aura patients (MAtot) and its subgroups with pure visual aura (MA) or visual aura associated with paraesthesia and/or dysphasia (MA+). Data are expressed as means ± SD

P1-N2	HV (n = 30)	MAtot (n = 47)	MA (n = 27)	MA+ (n = 20)
1st amplitude block (μV)	6.59 ± 3.16	7.00 ± 3.07	6.12 ± 2.65	8.18 ± 3.26
2nd amplitude block (μV)	6.49 ± 3.03	6.87 ± 3.26	5.88 ± 2.55	8.20 ± 3.70
3rd amplitude block (μV)	6.49 ± 2.94	6.62 ± 3.10	5.67 ± 2.66	7.91 ± 3.25
4th amplitude block (μV)	5.99 ± 2.85	6.32 ± 2.88	5.37 ± 2.36	7.60 ± 3.08
5th amplitude block (μV)	6.26 ± 2.59	6.84 ± 2.93	6.01 ± 2.45	7.96 ± 3.19
6th amplitude block (μV)	5.61 ± 2.86	6.50 ± 2.78	5.78 ± 2.70	7.47 ± 2.64
Slope	−0.35 ± 0.73	−0.09 ± 0.42	−0.06 ± 0.47	−0.13 ± 0.35

In MA+, Pearson's test disclosed that the N1–P1 habituation slope correlated negatively with attack frequency ($r = -0.489$, $p = 0.034$) and positively with days elapsed since last attack ($r = 0.578$, $p = 0.019$), correlations that were not found in MA patients (Fig. 4).

Discussion

The purpose of the present study was to extend our electrophysiological investigations of visual cortex reactivity in migraine by searching for differences between two distinct phenotypes of migraine with aura.

First, we confirm the previous finding that during continuous stimulation amplitude of the VEP N1–P1 component, but not of P1–N2, does not habituate over sequential blocks of averaged responses in migraine with aura patients between attacks while it does so in healthy volunteers [15]. An additional novel finding is that, relative to HV, VEP N1–P1 habituation is deficient both in migraine with pure visual aura (MA) and in patients with complex aura (MA+).

A second striking result is that the amplitude of visual responses differs between patients having pure visual aura and those with complex auras. MA+ patients consistently have greater N1–P1 VEP amplitudes than MA patients. Contrary to MA+, MA patients do not differ from healthy volunteers in VEP N1–P1 and P1–N2 block amplitudes,

although they have reduced habituation over the 6 sequential blocks of 100 averaged VEP responses.

To the best of our knowledge, this is the first study of visual evoked responses in patients with different migraine aura phenotypes. It identifies within the migraine spectrum a subgroup of patients with complex neurological auras in whom excitability of the visual cortex appears genuinely increased, as evidenced by an increased VEP N1–P1 amplitude and decreased habituation. Previous VEP studies have yielded conflicting results in groups of migraine with aura (MwA) patients without phenotype distinction. In some reports the grand-average of VEP N1–P1 and/or P1–N2 amplitudes was found greater in MwA patients than in controls [30–35] and/or in migraine without aura (MO) patients [31, 36, 37]. The amplitude of steady-state VEP harmonics was also larger in MwA than in MO or HV [38]. In other studies, on the contrary, VEP amplitudes were found reduced in MwA [39], even when compared to MO [40]. Most often, VEP amplitudes in MwA were reported to be in the normal range [13–15, 41–44]. Our finding of low or normal visual cortex excitability in patients with pure visual auras, which is similar to migraine without aura patients [45] but contrasts with increased VEP amplitude and deficient habituation in patients with complex auras, may help to explain some of the abovementioned

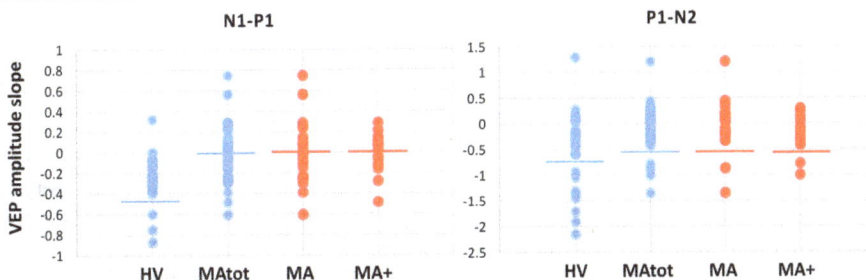

Fig. 3 Raw habituation slope of VEP N1-P1 and P1–N2 peak-to-peak amplitudes (mean ± SEM) over 6 sequential blocks of 100 averaged responses in healthy volunteers (HV, n = 30), patients with pure visual aura (MA, n = 27), patients with complex aura (MA+, n = 20) and the 2 latter groups combined (MAtot, n = 47)

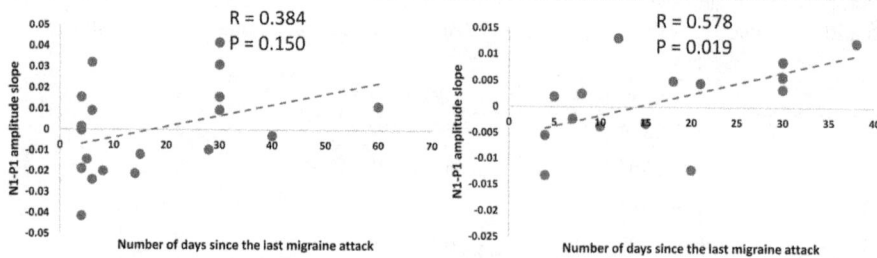

Fig. 4 Correlation between the days elapsed between the recordings and the last migraine attack and the slope of N1–P1 VEP amplitude changes over 6 sequential blocks of averaged responses (linear regression: dashed line). This correlation was significant in the group of patients with complex aura (MA+, right panel), but not in patients with pure visual aura (MA, left panel)

discrepant results. In fact, pooling patients with different migraine phenotypes (MO and MwA or different MA subgroups) in different proportions increases the variance of VEP results between studies. This probably fueled in part the controversy about the presence or not of interictal cortical hyperexcitability in migraine. In a previous review paper, we reasoned that in its strict physiological definition of a stimulus–response curve, the cortex would be hyperexcitable if it generates a response to a subliminal stimulus and/or if its response to a supraliminal stimulus is increased in amplitude. Because in most previous studies VEP amplitude in MO patients and, according to the present results, also in MA patients, increases during stimulus repetition, while remaining within a normal range (see Fig. 2), we proposed to abandon the general term "hyperexcitability" in favour of "hyperresponsivity" to characterise the response pattern of the migrainous brain to repeated stimulations [46]. As shown here, the functional abnormality is clearly different in MA+ patients in whom the initial VEP amplitude to a low number of stimuli is increased compared to both HV and MA, indicating that their visual cortex is genuinely hyperexcitable.

From a pathophysiological point of view, it is interesting to compare MA+ and chronic migraine that is also thought to be associated with true cortical hyperexcitability. The evidence in chronic migraine comes from studies of somatosensory evoked potentials [47] and magnetoencephalographic visual evoked responses [48]. The difference with MA+ is that in the latter VEP amplitude was increased in virtually all blocks of averagings and habituation was deficient over 6 blocks, while in chronic migraine only the 1st block of averaged visual or somatosensory responses was increased in amplitude, but not the subsequent blocks, leaving habituation normal. The electrophysiological pattern in migraine with complex neurological auras may therefore suggest that the visual cortex is locked in a state of persistent hyperexcitability.

The pathophysiological determinants of different aura phenotypes and related differences in interictal visual evoked potential profiles remain speculative. Cortical spreading depression (CSD) is thought to be the pathophysiological substrate of the migraine aura. CSD is an electrochemical wave that usually starts in the posterior regions of the brain and spreads anteriorly at approx. 3 mm/min, accompanied by biphasic cerebral blood flow changes [4]. In several brain imaging studies performed during attacks, though not in all, [49, 50] the vascular and metabolic changes accompanying the migraine aura spread more anteriorly in patients with complex neurological symptoms and hemiplegia than in those with only visual disturbances. The recovery from CSD depends largely on intact neurovascular coupling to match the increased energy demand and to restore ion gradients via the Na^+/K^+ ATPase pump [51]. The distance, to which CSD spreads during MwA attacks, and thus the clinical phenotype of the aura, depends on the balance between factors that predispose the brain to CSD and others that inhibit CSD and allow the parenchyma to recover.

The neurovascular tone is modulated by local factors such as oxygen availability or lactate concentrations, and by subcortical monoaminergic projections [52, 53]. During continuous visual stimulation neurovascular coupling is impaired in migraine patients between attacks, especially in migraine with aura [34, 54, 55]. There is also circumstantial evidence from biochemical and functional neuroimaging studies that monoaminergic, in particular serotonergic, transmission from the brainstem to the thalamus and cortex is altered in migraine [56]. Finally, convergent data from various laboratories have shown that the mitochondrial energy reserve and ATP levels are significantly reduced in the brain of migraineurs between attacks [27, 28]. Based on these biochemical and functional data, we have proposed that migraine is characterized interictally by a cycling dysregulation of the serotoninergic control of thalamo-cortical activity that causes varying degrees of cortical hyperresponsivity and thus increased energy demands, which, under the influence of triggering or aggravating factors, may disrupt homeostasis and lead to an attack [14, 57].

Several studies suggest that the abnormalities of energy metabolism could be more pronounced in migraine with complex neurological aura. The phosphocreatine/phosphate (PCr/Pi) ratio, a marker of the brain's energy reserve, differed significantly between patients with different aura phenotypes and was lowest in those with more complex auras [58]. In a 1H-MR-spectroscopy study [20] MA+ patients had a significant increase of lactate in the visual cortex during sustained visual stimulation, while this was not the case in HV and MA patients. Variants in the mitochondrial DNA, such as those that distinguish responders from non-responders to preventive antimigraine treatment with riboflavin [59], could play a role in the metabolic differences between aura phenotypes.

That genetic load can influence CSD patterns and severity is evidenced by the studies of the "knock-in" mice wearing CACNA1A [60] or ATP1A2 [61] mutations found respectively in familial hemiplegic migraine (FHM) type 1 and 2. In FHM1 mice having the S218L mutation that causes a more severe clinical phenotype in patients, CSD are more frequent and more spread out (up to the striatum) than in mice with the R192Q mutation. As mentioned, the common form of migraine with aura is not associated with the mutations found in FHM, but merely with common variants in a number of loci identified on genome-wide association studies (GWAS) that are seemingly not much different from those found in migraine without aura [62]. It remains to be determined whether the combination of such common genetic variants and their association with mitochondrial DNA variants may influence the clinical migraine phenotype, including that of the aura.

One can only speculate on the possible relation between the ictal phenomena, i.e. CSD and its spreading, and the VEP abnormalities found interictally. We know of only one study in photosensitive subjects with a photo-paroxysmal response to intermittent photic stimulation where increased VEP amplitude was correlated with spread of the paroxysmal EEG activity to more anterior brain areas [63]. In photo-paroxysmal responses and photically induced seizures, this could be the electrophysiological correlate of increased functional connectivity between occipital and parieto-temporo-frontal networks under the control of the thalamus [64–66]. A recent study showing in animals that CSD can activate the thalamic reticular nuclei that controls the flow of sensory information to the cortex, is therefore of major interest [67]. Translated to migraine pathophysiology, one may hypothesize that repeated thalamic activation by CSD could worsen the interictal impairment of thalamic/thalamocortical activity in migraine with complex auras [14, 68–71]. Studies correlating aura frequency and duration of the disorder with thalamic/thalamocortical activity in MwA are necessary to test this hypothesis.

Whatever the possible relation between ictal CSD and interictal VEP might be, the pathophysiological mechanisms underlying VEP habituation are not permanently influenced by the ictal phenomena, even in MA+ patients. In the latter, indeed, like in MwA patients overall and in migraine without aura [15], the VEP habituation deficit is obvious between attacks. Moreover, in MA+, but not in MA patients, it worsens progressively with time elapsed since the last migraine attack and decreases with increased attack frequency; in other words, VEP habituation increases with proximity to an attack. To explain this difference between MA+ and MA, we speculate that MA+ patients are carrying the most pronounced genetic load predisposing them to more prominent pathophysiological dysfunctions. For instance, we intend to explore the possibility that MA+ is the migraine with aura phenotype with the most pronounced deficit of short-range lateral inhibition within the visual cortex, an abnormality that we also found directly related to the distance from the last attack in a previous study of a mixed group of migraine with and without aura patients [15]. Taken together with our present results, this would indicate that the inhibitory performance and habituation with stimulus repetition decreases with the distance from the last migraine attack. A psychophysical study using visual metacontrast masking test, found a similar correlation between inhibitory processes and the number of days elapsed since the last attack [72]. The biochemical correlate of impaired inhibitory mechanisms could be lactate-induced downregulation of GABA activity in the visual cortex. As mentioned, in MA+ lactate levels increase in the occipital cortex during visual stimulation [20] there is emerging evidence that lactate, besides its role as energy substrate, has a concentration-dependent downregulating effect on GABAergic neurotransmission [22].

As other neurophysiological studies, ours has some methodological shortcomings. For instance, the investigators were blinded during off-line analyses of VEP data, as applied in previous studies by independent groups [15, 73], but not to diagnosis during the recording session, although this is probably only a minor risk for bias. As a matter of fact, in a clinical setting it is quasi impossible to totally blind a neurophysiological study. Even in VEP studies that found no abnormalities in migraineurs and were claimed to be blinded to diagnosis [12, 74, 75], blinding was not perfect for various reasons according to the reported methodology: 1) the neurophysiologist knew which set of responses belonged to each of the 6 blocks of averagings [74], which allows a selection bias in favour of low amplitude responses and thus normal habituation [76]; 2) the neurophysiologist was not blinded to check size [74], to which VEP amplitudes are quite sensitive [77]; 3) after each recording, the investigators guessed the correct diagnosis in more than half of subjects [12]; 4) although the investigators were blinded to diagnosis during the first examination, they were not during the 3 subsequent recording sessions [75].

Though we refer herein to habituation as the common feature of responses to any type of repeated sensory stimuli and to its classical definition of "a behavioral response decrement that results from repeated stimulation and that does not involve sensory adaptation/sensory fatigue or motor fatigue" [78, 79], we cannot totally exclude that changes in the level of attention and contrast pattern adaptation may have influenced our results. This is nonetheless unlikely for the following reasons. In previous studies VEP amplitudes after full field stimulation were not significantly influenced by attention and reaction time task conditions [80, 81]. Moreover, the effects of contrast adaptation on the P1 peak are small (peak time shift approx. 3 ms, amplitude unchanged) and require to take place stimulations lasting about 25 min [82, 83], contrasting with a 3 min 20 sec duration of a VEP recording session in our study.

We also are aware that our samples are relatively small and that clinical correlations are retrospective. Further studies are needed to repeat the analysis in a larger clinical sample with various migraine phenotypes and with a longitudinal, prospective follow-up of patients, allowing to record them during attacks as well as at different time points between attacks.

Conclusions

To summarize, this study shows that the clinical heterogeneity of migraine with aura is reflected in distinct visual evoked potential profiles. Patients with complex neurological auras differ from those with strictly visual auras by an interictal increase of VEP amplitudes suggestive of an underlying genuine persistent visual cortical hyperexcitability. Whether this is related to CSD features, their effect on cortex and thalamus or to a common neurobiological or genetic denominator between CSD and VEP profile determinants remains to be determined.

Abbreviations

CSD: cortical spreading depression; GWAS: genome-wide association studies; HV: Healthy Volunteer; MA: migraine with pure visual Aura; MA+: migraine with complex aura; MAtot: total group of migraine with aura patients; MO: migraine without aura; MwA: migraine with aura; VEP: visual evoked potential.

Competing interests

The authors declare that they have no competing interests.

Authors' contributions

GC made substantial contributions to interpretation of data as well as in drafting the manuscript. MS, VP, JS and FP were implied in the interpretation of data as well as in drafting the manuscript; ADR, FM, and AF gave critical revision of the manuscript for important intellectual content. CDL, DDL

and MB were implied in recording and analyzing data. All authors read and approved the final manuscript.

Acknowledgment
Italian Ministry of Health and Fondazione Roma financially supported the research for this paper.

Author details
[1]G.B. Bietti Foundation-IRCCS, Department of Neurophysiology of Vision and Neurophthalmology, Via Livenza 3, 00198 Rome, Italy. [2]Department of Medical and Surgical Sciences and Biotechnologies, "Sapienza" University of Rome Polo Pontino, Latina, Italy. [3]Fondazione Don Gnocchi, Milan, Italy. [4]Istituto Superiore di Sanità, Dipartimento Tecnologie e Salute, Rome, Italy. [5]Headache Research Unit, Department of Neurology-CHR Citadelle, University of Liège, Liège, Belgium. [6]IRCCS-Neuromed, Pozzilli, IS, Italy.

References
1. Russell M, Olesen J (1996) A nosographic analysis of the migraine aura in a general population. Brain 119:355–361
2. Eriksen M, Thomsen L, Andersen I, Nazim F, Olesen J (2004) Clinical characteristics of 362 patients with familial migraine with aura. Cephalalgia 24:564–575
3. Rasmussen B, Olesen J (1992) Migraine with aura and migraine without aura: an epidemiological study. Cephalalgia 12:221–228
4. Lauritzen M (2001) Cortical spreading depression in migraine. Cephalalgia 21:757–760
5. Charles A, Baca S (2013) Cortical spreading depression and migraine. Nat Rev Neurol 9:637–644
6. Olesen J, Friberg L, Olsen T, Iversen H, Lassen N, Andersen A, et al (1990) Timing and topography of cerebral blood flow, aura, and headache during migraine attacks. Ann Neurol 28:791–798
7. Cao Y, Welch K, Aurora S, Vikingstad E (1999) Functional MRI-BOLD of visually triggered headache in patients with migraine. Arch Neurol 56:548–554
8. Hadjikhani N, Sanchez D, Wu O, Schwartz D, Bakker D, Fischl B, et al (2001) Mechanisms of migraine aura revealed by functional MRI in human visual cortex. Proc Natl Acad Sci U S A 98:4687–4692
9. Bowyer SM, Aurora KS, Moran JE, Tepley N, Welch KM (2001) Magnetoencephalographic fields from patients with spontaneous and induced migraine aura. Ann Neurol 50:582–587
10. Zhang X, Levy D, Noseda R, Kainz V, Jakubowski M, Burstein R, et al (2010) Activation of meningeal nociceptors by cortical spreading depression: implications for migraine with aura. J Neurosci 30:8807–8814
11. Zhang X, Levy D, Kainz V, Noseda R, Jakubowski M, Burstein R, et al (2011) Activation of central trigeminovascular neurons by cortical spreading depression. Ann Neurol 69:855–865
12. Omland P, Nilsen K, Uglem M, Gravdahl G, Linde M, Hagen K, et al (2013) Visual Evoked Potentials in Interictal Migraine: No Confirmation of Abnormal Habituation. Headache 53:1071–1086
13. Afra J, Cecchini AP, De Pasqua V, Albert A, Schoenen J (1998) Visual evoked potentials during long periods of pattern-reversal stimulation in migraine. Brain 121(Pt 2):233–241
14. Coppola G, Ambrosini A, Di Clemente L, Magis D, Fumal A, Gérard P, et al (2007) Interictal abnormalities of gamma band activity in visual evoked responses in migraine: an indication of thalamocortical dysrhythmia? Cephalalgia 27:1360–1367
15. Coppola G, Parisi V, Di Lorenzo C, Serrao M, Magis D, Schoenen J, et al (2013) Lateral inhibition in visual cortex of migraine patients between attacks. J Headache Pain 14:20
16. Coppola G, Di Lorenzo C, Schoenen J, Pierelli F (2013) Habituation and sensitization in primary headaches. J Headache Pain 14:65
17. Eriksen M, Thomsen L, Olesen J (2006) Implications of clinical subtypes of migraine with aura. Headache 46:286–297
18. Ambrosini A, de Noordhout A, Alagona G, Dalpozzo F, Schoenen J (1999) Impairment of neuromuscular transmission in a subgroup of migraine patients. Neurosci Lett 276:201–203
19. Ambrosini A, de Noordhout A, Schoenen J (2001) Neuromuscular transmission in migraine patients with prolonged aura. Acta Neurol Belg 101:166–170
20. Sándor P, Dydak U, Schoenen J, Kollias S, Hess K, Boesiger P, et al (2005) MR-spectroscopic imaging during visual stimulation in subgroups of migraine with aura. Cephalalgia 25:507–518

21. Sickmann H, Walls A, Schousboe A, Bouman S, Waagepetersen H (2009) Functional significance of brain glycogen in sustaining glutamatergic neurotransmission. J Neurochem 1:80–86

22. Bozzo L, Puyal J, Chatton J (2013) Lactate modulates the activity of primary cortical neurons through a receptor-mediated pathway. PLoS One 8:10

23. Matsui T, Soya S, Kawanaka K, Soya H (2015) Brain Glycogen Decreases During Intense Exercise Without Hypoglycemia: The Possible Involvement of Serotonin. Neurochem Res 40:1333–1340

24. Gilbert E, Tang J, Ludvig N, Bergold P (2006) Elevated lactate suppresses neuronal firing in vivo and inhibits glucose metabolism in hippocampal slice cultures. Brain Res 1117:213–223

25. Shimizu H, Watanabe E, Hiyama T, Nagakura A, Fujikawa A, Okado H et al (2007) Glial Nax channels control lactate signaling to neurons for brain [Na+] sensing. Neuron 54:59–72

26. Sappey-Marinier D, Calabrese G, Fein G, Hugg J, Biggins C, Weiner M, et al (1992) Effect of photic stimulation on human visual cortex lactate and phosphates using 1H and 31P magnetic resonance spectroscopy. J Cereb Blood Flow Metab 12:584–592

27. Barbiroli B, Montagna P, Cortelli P, Funicello R, Iotti S, Monari L, et al (1992) Abnormal brain and muscle energy metabolism shown by 31P magnetic resonance spectroscopy in patients affected by migraine with aura. Neurology 42:1209–1214

28. Watanabe H, Kuwabara T, Ohkubo M, Tsuji S, Yuasa T (1996) Elevation of cerebral lactate detected by localized 1H-magnetic resonance spectroscopy in migraine during the interictal period. Neurology 47:1093–1095

29. Judit A, Sándor PS, Schoenen J (2000) Habituation of visual and intensity dependence of auditory evoked cortical potentials tends to normalize just before and during the migraine attack. Cephalalgia 20:714–719

30. Coutin-Churchman P, Padrón de Freytez A (2003) Vector analysis of visual evoked potentials in migraineurs with visual aura. Clin Neurophysiol 114:2132–2137

31. Shibata K, Osawa M, Iwata M (1997) Pattern reversal visual evoked potentials in classic and common migraine. J Neurol Sci 145:177–181

32. Shibata K, Osawa M, Iwata M (1998) Pattern reversal visual evoked potentials in migraine with aura and migraine aura without headache. Cephalalgia 18:319–323

33. Oelkers R, Grosser K, Lang E, Geisslinger G, Kobal G, Brune K, et al (1999) Visual evoked potentials in migraine patients: alterations depend on pattern spatial frequency. Brain 122(Pt 6):1147–1155

34. Zaletel M, Strucl M, Bajrović F, Pogacnik T (2005) Coupling between visual evoked cerebral blood flow velocity responses and visual evoked potentials in migraneurs. Cephalalgia 25:567–574

35. Shibata K, Yamane K, Iwata M, Ohkawa S (2005) Evaluating the effects of spatial frequency on migraines by using pattern-reversal visual evoked potentials. Clin Neurophysiol 116:2220–2227

36. Sand T, Zhitniy N, White LR, Stovner LJ (2008) Visual evoked potential latency, amplitude and habituation in migraine: a longitudinal study. Clin Neurophysiol 119:1020–1027

37. Sand T, White L, Hagen K, Stovner L (2009) Visual evoked potential and spatial frequency in migraine: a longitudinal study. Acta Neurol Scand Suppl 189:33–37

38. Shibata K, Yamane K, Otuka K, Iwata M (2008) Abnormal visual processing in migraine with aura: a study of steady-state visual evoked potentials. J Neurol Sci 271:119–126

39. Nguyen B, McKendrick A, Vingrys A (2012) Simultaneous retinal and cortical visually evoked electrophysiological responses in between migraine attacks. Cephalalgia 32:896–907

40. Khalil NM, Legg NJ, Anderson DJ (2000) Long term decline of P100 amplitude in migraine with aura. J Neurol Neurosurg Psychiatry 69:507–511

41. Schoenen J, Wang W, Albert A, Delwaide P (1995) Potentiation instead of habituation characterizes visual evoked potentials in migraine patients between attacks. Eur J Neurol 2:115–122

42. Afra J, Ambrosini A, Genicot R, Albert A, Schoenen J (2000) Influence of colors on habituation of visual evoked potentials in patients with migraine with aura and in healthy volunteers. Headache 40:36–40

43. Afra J, Proietti Cecchini A, Sándor PS, Schoenen J (2000) Comparison of visual and auditory evoked cortical potentials in migraine patients between attacks. Clin Neurophysiol 111:1124–1129

44. Ozkul Y, Bozlar S (2002) Effects of fluoxetine on habituation of pattern reversal visually evoked potentials in migraine prophylaxis. Headache 42:582–587

45. Coppola G, Currà A, Sava SL, Alibardi A, Parisi V, Pierelli F et al (2010) Changes in visual-evoked potential habituation induced by hyperventilation in migraine. J Headache Pain 11:497–503

46. Coppola G, Pierelli F, Schoenen J (2007) Is the cerebral cortex hyperexcitable or hyperresponsive in migraine? Cephalalgia 27:1427–1439

47. Coppola G, Iacovelli E, Bracaglia M, Serrao M, Di Lorenzo C, Pierelli F et al (2013) Electrophysiological correlates of episodic migraine chronification: evidence for thalamic involvement. J Headache Pain 14:76

48. Chen W, Wang S, Fuh J, Lin C, Ko Y, Lin Y et al (2011) Persistent ictal-like visual cortical excitability in chronic migraine. Pain 152:254–258

49. Floery D, Vosko M, Fellner F, Fellner C, Ginthoer C, Gruber F, et al (2012) Acute-onset migrainous aura mimicking acute stroke: MR perfusion imaging features. AJNR Am J Neuroradiol 33:1546–1552

50. Iizuka T, Tominaga N, Kaneko J, Sato M, Akutsu T, Hamada J et al (2015) Biphasic neurovascular changes in prolonged migraine aura in familial hemiplegic migraine type 2. J Neurol Neurosurg Psychiatry 86:344–353

51. Piilgaard H, Lauritzen M (2009) Persistent increase in oxygen consumption and impaired neurovascular coupling after spreading depression in rat neocortex. J Cereb Blood Flow Metab 29:1517–1527

52. Hamel E (1985) (1985) Perivascular nerves and the regulation of cerebrovascular tone. J Appl Physiol 100:1059–1064

53. Gordon G, Choi H, Rungta R, Ellis-Davies G, MacVicar B (2008) Brain metabolism dictates the polarity of astrocyte control over arterioles. Nature 456:745–749

54. Descamps B, Vandemaele P, Reyngoudt H, Deblaere K, Leybaert L, Paemeleire K, et al (2011) Absence of haemodynamic refractory effects in patients with migraine without aura: an interictal fMRI study. Cephalalgia 31:1220–1231

55. Griebe M, Flux F, Wolf M, Hennerici M, Szabo K (2014) Multimodal assessment of optokinetic visual stimulation response in migraine with aura. Headache 54:131–141

56. Hamel E (2007) Serotonin and migraine: biology and clinical implications. Cephalalgia 27:1293–1300

57. Schoenen J (1996) Deficient habituation of evoked cortical potentials in migraine: a link between brain biology, behavior and trigeminovascular activation? Biomed Pharmacother 50:71–78

58. Schulz U, Blamire A, Corkill R, Davies P, Styles P, Rothwell P, et al (2007) Association between cortical metabolite levels and clinical manifestations of migrainous aura: an MR-spectroscopy study. Brain 130:3102–3110

59. Di Lorenzo C, Pierelli F, Coppola G, Grieco GS, Rengo C, Ciccolella M, et al (2009) Mitochondrial DNA haplogroups influence the therapeutic response to riboflavin in migraineurs. Neurology 72:1588–1594

60. Eikermann-Haerter K, Dileköz E, Kudo C, Savitz SI, Waeber C, Baum MJ, et al (2009) Genetic and hormonal factors modulate spreading depression and transient hemiparesis in mouse models of familial hemiplegic migraine type 1. J Clin Invest 119:99–109

61. Leo L, Gherardini L, Barone V, De F, Pietrobon D, Pizzorusso T, et al (2011) Increased susceptibility to cortical spreading depression in the mouse model of familial hemiplegic migraine type 2. PLoS Genet 7:10

62. Nyholt D, Anttila V, Winsvold B, Kurth T, Stefansson H, Kallela M, et al (2015) Concordance of genetic risk across migraine subgroups: Impact on current and future genetic association studies. Cephalalgia 35:489–499

63. Siniatchkin M, Moeller F, Shepherd A, Siebner H, Stephani U (2007) Altered cortical visual processing in individuals with a spreading photoparoxysmal EEG response. Eur J Neurosci 26:529–536

64. Moeller F, Siebner H, Wolff S, Muhle H, Granert O, Jansen O et al (2009) Mapping brain activity on the verge of a photically induced generalized tonic-clonic seizure. Epilepsia 50:1632–1637

65. Moeller F, Muthuraman M, Stephani U, Deuschl G, Raethjen J, Siniatchkin M (2013) Representation and propagation of epileptic activity in absences and generalized photoparoxysmal responses. Hum Brain Mapp 34:1896–1909

66. Hanganu A, Groppa S, Deuschl G, Siebner H, Moeller F, Siniatchkin M et al (2015) Cortical Thickness Changes Associated with Photoparoxysmal Response. Brain Topogr 28:702–709

67. Tepe N, Filiz A, Dilekoz E, Akcali D, Sara Y, Charles A, et al (2015) The thalamic reticular nucleus is activated by cortical spreading depression in freely moving rats: prevention by acute valproate administration. Eur J Neurosci 41:120–128

68. Coppola G, Vandenheede M, Di Clemente L, Ambrosini A, Fumal A, De Pasqua V et al (2005) Somatosensory evoked high-frequency oscillations reflecting thalamo-cortical activity are decreased in migraine patients between attacks. Brain 128:98–103

69. DaSilva AFM, Granziera C, Tuch DS, Snyder J, Vincent M, Hadjikhani N (2007) Interictal alterations of the trigeminal somatosensory pathway and periaqueductal gray matter in migraine. Neuroreport 18:301–305

70. Rocca MA, Pagani E, Colombo B, Tortorella P, Falini A, Comi G, et al (2008) Selective diffusion changes of the visual pathways in patients with migraine: a 3-T tractography study. Cephalalgia 28:1061–1068

71. Datta R, Aguirre G, Hu S, Detre G, Cucchiara B (2013) Interictal cortical hyperresponsiveness in migraine is directly related to the presence of aura. Cephalalgia 33:365–374

72. Shepherd A, Wyatt G, Tibber M (2011) Visual metacontrast masking in migraine. Cephalalgia 31:346–356

73. Bednář M, Kubová Z, Kremláček J (2014) Lack of visual evoked potentials amplitude decrement during prolonged reversal and motion stimulation in migraineurs. Clin Neurophysiol 125:1223–1230

74. Omland P, Uglem M, Engstrøm M, Linde M, Hagen K, Sand T, et al. (2014) Modulation of visual evoked potentials by high-frequency repetitive transcranial magnetic stimulation in migraineurs. Clin Neurophysiol. doi:10.1016/j.clinph.2014.12.035

75. Omland P, Uglem M, Hagen K, Linde M, Tronvik E, Sand T (2015) Visual evoked potentials in migraine: Is the "neurophysiological hallmark" concept still valid? Clin Neurophysiol. doi:10.1016/j.clinph.2014.12.035.

76. Brighina F, Cosentino G, Fierro B (2015) Habituation or lack of habituation: What is really lacking in migraine? Clin Neurophysiol. doi:10.1016/j.clinph.2015.05.028.

77. Harter MR, White CT (1968) Effects of contour sharpness and check-size on visually evoked cortical potentials. Vision Res 8:701–711

78. Thompson RF, Spencer WA (1966) Habituation: a model phenomenon for the study of neuronal substrates of behavior. Psychol Rev 73:16–43

79. Rankin CH, Abrams T, Barry RJ, Bhatnagar S, Clayton DF, Colombo J, et al (2009) Habituation revisited: an updated and revised description of the behavioral characteristics of habituation. Neurobiol Learn Mem 92:135–138

80. Skuse N, Burke D (1992) Sequence-dependent deterioration in the visual evoked potential in the absence of drowsiness. Electroencephalogr Clin Neurophysiol 84:20–25

81. Hoshiyama M, Kakigi R (2001) Effects of attention on pattern-reversal visual evoked potentials: foveal field stimulation versus peripheral field stimulation. Brain Topogr 13:293–298

82. Heinrich T, Bach M (2002) Contrast adaptation in retinal and cortical evoked potentials: no adaptation to low spatial frequencies. Vis Neurosci 19:645–650

83. Heinrich S, Bach M (2001) Adaptation dynamics in pattern-reversal visual evoked potentials. Doc Ophthalmol 102:141–156

10

Subclinical vestibular dysfunction in migraine patients: a preliminary study of ocular and rectified cervical vestibular evoked myogenic potentials

Chul-Ho Kim, Min-Uk Jang, Hui-Chul Choi and Jong-Hee Sohn[*]

Abstract

Background: Many studies have identified various vestibular symptoms and laboratory abnormalities in migraineurs. Although the vestibular tests may be abnormal, the changes may exist without vestibular symptoms. To date, vestibular-evoked myogenic potential (VEMP) has been the easiest and simplest test for measuring vestibular function in clinical practice. Cervical VEMP (cVEMP) represents a vestibulo-collic reflex, whereas ocular VEMP (oVEMP) reflects a vestibulo-ocular pathway. Therefore, we determined whether ocular and rectified cervical VEMPs differed in patients with migraine or tension type headache (TTH) and compared the results to controls with no accompanying vestibular symptoms.

Methods: The present study included 38 females with migraine without aura, 30 with episodic TTH, and 50 healthy controls without vestibular symptoms. oVEMP and cVEMP using a blood pressure manometer were recorded during a headache-free period. From the VEMP graphs, latency and amplitude parameters were analyzed, especially following EMG rectification in cVEMP.

Results: With respect to oVEMP, the migraine group exhibited significantly longer mean latencies of bilateral n1 and left p1 than the other groups ($p < 0.05$). Amplitudes of n1-p1 were lower than in other groups, but the difference did not reach statistical significance. In regards to cVEMP, p13 and n23 latencies and amplitudes after rectification did not differ significantly among groups.

Conclusions: An abnormal interictal oVEMP profile was associated with subclinical vestibular dysfunction in migraineurs, suggesting pathology within the vestibulo-ocular reflex. oVEMP is a more reliable measure than cVEMP to evaluate vestibular function in migraineurs, although results from the two tests in patients with migraine are complementary.

Keywords: Vestibular evoked myogenic potential (VEMP), Ocular VEMP, Cervical VEMP, Migraine

Background

Dizziness and vertigo are frequent symptoms accompanying primary headache disorders, especially migraine [1]. Migraine has long been associated with various vestibular symptoms and several vestibular syndromes [2]. Additionally, several studies have identified several vestibular laboratory abnormalities in migraineurs [3].

* Correspondence: deepfoci@hallym.or.kr
Department of Neurology, Chuncheon Sacred Heart Hospital, Hallym University College of Medicine, 153 Gyo-dong, Chuncheon-si, Gangwon-do 200-704, Republic of Korea

Of the various methods used to evaluate the vestibular system, vestibular evoked myogenic potential (VEMP) is a non-invasive and simple clinical test. Cervical VEMP (cVEMP) represents an uncrossed vestibulo-collic reflex, which assesses saccular function, the inferior vestibular nerve and vestibular nuclei, and serves as a pathway through the lower brainstem to the motor neurons of the sternocleidomastoid muscle [4]. The more recently described ocular VEMP (oVEMP), a manifestation of a crossed vestibulo-ocular pathway, reflects predominantly utricular function and involves the medial longitudinal fasciculus, oculomotor nuclei and nerves, and extraocular muscles following activation of the vestibular nerve and nucleus [4, 5]. While cVEMP descends via the vestibulospinal tract through the lower brainstem, oVEMP ascends via the medial longitudinal fasciculus through the upper brainstem. Additionally, recent studies suggest that oVEMP is produced by otolith afferents in the superior vestibular nerve division, whereas cVEMP, evoked by sound, is believed to be an inferior vestibular nerve reflex [6]. Using oVEMP and cVEMP together allows for the evaluation of both ascending and descending vestibular pathways in the brainstem and identifies a higher percentage of abnormalities [4]. Thus, the combined measures of oVEMP and cVEMP provide complementary information.

VEMP presentation differs in individual patients according to the method used for assessment, diagnosis of migraine subtype, and the presence of vestibular symptoms, as reported in literature. Several authors have reported absent or delayed cVEMPs [7–10], whereas others have found cVEMPs of normal latency but reduced amplitude in migraineurs [11, 12]. In contrast with most previous studies, a normal interictal cVEMP profile was reported in patients with migraine with or without aura and vestibular migraine [13]. Recently, interest in oVEMP studies for migraine has increased. High rates of absent oVEMP and higher amplitude asymmetry ratios or reduced amplitudes have been shown in vestibular migraine (VM) [14, 15], whereas prolonged latency and lower amplitudes were found in migraineurs without vestibular symptoms [16].

Although previous VEMP reports have been inconsistent, VEMP remains the easiest and simplest method for measuring vestibular activity in clinical practice to date. Measurement of both ocular and cervical VEMPs provides more information because the results are complementary. Additionally, several studies on patients with migraine without vestibular symptoms have reported vestibular deficits in various vestibular function tests. In particular, findings such as defective oculomotor function, dysfunctional equilibrium, and peripheral and central vestibular deficits have been described [17–21]. Patients with tension-type headache (TTH) often report balance disorders or subjective imbalance [22, 23]. However, little is known about vestibular function in those with TTH without manifested vestibulopathy.

Thus, we hypothesized that migraineurs with no accompanying vestibular symptoms exhibit subclinical vestibular dysfunction. We investigated vestibular function using ocular and rectified cervical VEMP methods in patients with migraine without aura and those with episodic TTH during headache-free periods.

Methods

Subjects

This study collected data obtained from consecutive first-visit patients with migraine without aura and episodic TTH treated in the neurology outpatient department of a university hospital. All participants were between 20 and 60 years of age, and only females were included to eliminate age and gender bias [24–26]. Headache diagnoses were classified by a board-certified neurologist based on the criteria of the International Classification of Headache Disorders-3 beta version (ICHD-3β) using patient history, a neurological examination, and laboratory or neuroimaging studies. To exclude other primary headaches, patients were required to have at least a 1-year history of migraine or TTH headaches prior to enrollment. Patients who had auras or vestibular symptoms during headache attacks were excluded. In total, 38 patients with migraine without aura and 30 patients with episodic TTH based on the ICHD-3β were enrolled in the study. Subjects with episodic TTH were defined as those with headaches lasting from 1 to 15 days per month (frequent episodic TTH). The control group consisted of age-matched volunteers. We recruited the control group by inviting persons who accompanied the patients to join the study (e.g., friends) and also through advertisements (e.g., posted notices in the hospital). Controls were free of headaches for at least three months prior to the study, experienced no more than an occasional mild headache (<5 times per year) and had not sought medical treatment for headaches.

All participants were underwent physical and neurological examinations performed by an experienced neurologist. Participants were asked to complete a questionnaire regarding their headache symptoms, including frequency, duration, and intensity, during the previous 4 weeks. Headache frequency (days/week) was calculated by dividing the number of days with headaches by 4 weeks. Headache duration (hours/day) was calculated by dividing the sum of the total hours of headaches by the number of days with headaches and headache intensity (numeric rating scale [NRS]: 0 = no pain to 10 = unbearable pain) was calculated as the mean NRS for days with headaches. We also obtained a comprehensive neuro-otological history from all participants. The detailed interview for assessing vestibular symptoms in headache patients or diagnosing VM according to the ICHD-3β included questions about clinical features (e.g., main type of vertigo and duration, frequency, severity) and concomitant symptoms. Exclusion criteria included subjects with hearing loss, middle ear disease or surgery, history of vestibular disease, history of recurrent vertigo or vertigo that lasted more than one day or required hospitalization, a cervical disorder that affected head movement, the presence of neurological disorders (e.g. stroke, multiple sclerosis), pregnancy, daily medication to prevent headaches and/or antidepressant medication, medication-overuse headache, and patients with VM.

Written informed consent was obtained from all subjects prior to enrollment. The university hospital ethics committee approved this study.

VEMP recordings

VEMP tests were performed by an examiner blinded to group and patient clinical examination data. VEMP recordings were performed using a Nicolet EDX EMP/EP machine (Natus Neurology, Middleton, WI, USA). Patients with headache underwent VEMP testing on headache-free days. Specifically, recordings in migraine patients were obtained interictally at least 3 days after the last and before the next migraine attack.

oVEMP

For oVEMP testing, the active electrode was placed ~1 cm below the center of the inferior eyelid contralateral to the sound stimulation, with the reference electrode located 15 mm below the active electrode and the ground electrode on the forehead. Patients were tested in a seated position. During the test, patients were asked to look upward to a fixed point 2 m away and 25-30° above the horizontal line. Electromyography (EMG) signals were amplified and band pass-filtered between 30 and 3000 Hz. Sound stimuli were presented through headphones as short tone burst sounds (500 Hz) at a frequency of 5 Hz. In total, 100 stimuli were applied to each ear and repeated twice consecutively at 130 dB normal hearing level (nHL).

cVEMP

For cVEMP testing, the active electrode was placed on the upper one-third of the sternocleidomastoid (SCM) muscle, ipsilateral to the sound stimulation, with the reference electrode on the anterior margin of the clavicle and the ground electrode on the forehead. Patients were tested in a seated position. To contract the SCM, we used the blood pressure cuff method [27]. Subjects had to flex the head ~30° forward and rotate it ~30° to the opposite side. While holding the cuff between the right hand and jaw, the subject pushed with her head against the hand-held cuff to generate a cuff pressure of 40 mmHg. The obtained cuff pressures and background muscle activity based on visual feedback system of the VEMP machine were monitored by the subject and investigator during the recording period. EMG signals were amplified and band pass-filtered between 20 and 2000 Hz. Sound stimuli (500 Hz) were presented through headphones as rarefaction clicks 0.1 ms in

duration and at a frequency of 5 Hz. In total, 128 stimuli were applied to each ear and repeated twice consecutively at a 125 dB nHL.

VEMP analysis

From the oVEMP graphs, unrectified signals from 100 trials were averaged. The first negative and positive responses were designated as n1 and p1 waves, respectively. The oVEMP response was only considered reliable if the n1 and p1 peaks were reproducible in two consecutive trace runs. Additionally, the cVEMP response was only considered reliable if the p13 and n23 peaks were reproducible in two consecutive runs of the unrectified trace. The p13-n23 responses were observed best in the unrectified trace. Initial positive and negative polarities of the waveform with peaks were termed p13 and n23 on the basis of their respective latencies. Rectified values were used since the VEMP response amplitude is significantly affected by the force of muscular contraction or stimulus intensity. After rectification (Synergy Reader software, version 20.1), peak latencies of p13 and n23 and amplitude parameters p13 and n23 were measured. The results of both runs were averaged, providing the final response from which the peak-to-peak amplitude (n1-p1) and absolute latencies (n1, p1) in oVEMP and rectified amplitude and absolute latencies (p13, n23) in cVEMP were derived. Interside differences of n1 and p1 latencies in oVEMP and p13 and n23 latencies in cVEMP were calculated. Amplitude asymmetry ratio (AR) was calculated in oVEMP and cVEMP as follows: (larger response - smaller response) / (larger response + smaller response) × 100 [4].

Statistical analyses

Statistical analyses were performed using 'R' (version 3.01; R Foundation for Statistical Computing, Vienna, Austria) and P-values <0.05 were considered to indicate statistical significance. The planned sample of 38 migraineurs and 46 healthy subjects resulted in a power of 90 % for detecting a 40 % reduction in the bilateral oVEMP response at a significance level of 0.05 using a two-sided Fisher's exact test [16]. Additionally, the sample size calculation for the t-test to detect the difference in N1 latencies between the migraine and healthy control groups required 24 and 48 subjects, respectively. Data were expressed as the means ± standard deviation (SD) for continuous variables and as numbers (rates) for categorical variables. Continuous variables were compared using a two-sample t-test or Wilcoxon's rank sum test, whereas categorical variables were evaluated using the χ^2 test or Fisher's exact test. Results of oVEMP and cVEMP parameters were compared among three subgroups. Multiple group analyses were performed using one-way analysis of variance (ANOVA) or the

Kruskal-Wallis test. Pair-wise comparisons were assessed using the Wilcoxon's rank sum test with Bonferroni correction.

Results

Clinical characteristics

The present study included 38 females with migraine without aura, 30 episodic TTH and 50 healthy controls. Mean age in the migraine, TTH and control groups was 35.5, 33.3 and 35.1 years, respectively. The mean age did not differ significantly among groups. Clinical and headache characteristics are shown in Table 1.

oVEMP abnormalities

Eight patients in the migraine group (7, 18.4 % unilateral; 1, 2.6 % bilateral) demonstrated absent oVEMP responses, while responses could not be obtained for three patients in the TTH group (2, 6.7 % unilateral; 1, 3.3 % bilateral) and five patients in the control group (3, 6.0 % unilateral; 2, 4.0 % bilateral). A low response rate was observed in migraineurs, but no statistical difference was detected in the response rate of oVEMP among groups (Table 2). In oVEMP, the migraine group had mean latencies of bilateral n1 and left p1 significantly longer than the other groups ($p < 0.05$). Mean amplitudes of n1-p1 were lower than in the other groups, but the difference did not reach statistical significance (Table 3). No significant difference was observed in the AR amplitude or interaural latency differences of oVEMP. Illustrated examples of oVEMP tracings in controls and patients with migraine are shown in Fig. 1. Box plots of statistically significant oVEMP parameters are shown in Fig. 2.

cVEMP abnormalities

Four patients in the migraine group (4, 10.5 % unilateral; 0, 0 % bilateral), seven patients in the TTH group (7, 23.3 % unilateral; 0, 0 % bilateral) and four patients (3, 6.0 % unilateral; 1, 2.0 % bilateral) in the control group showed absent cVEMP responses. There was no statistically significant difference among the groups with respect to cVEMP response rate (Table 2). Illustrated examples of rectified cVEMP tracings in

controls and patients with migraine are shown in Fig. 1. Additionally, p13 and n23 latencies and rectified amplitudes of cVEMP in migraine without aura and TTH patients did not differ significantly from those of healthy controls (Table 4). Moreover, no significant difference was observed in the amplitude AR or interaural latency differences of cVEMP.

Discussion

In our study, significantly prolonged latency in oVEMP was detected in migraine without aura versus TTH and

Table 2 VEMP response rates in headache patients and healthy controls

	TTH (n = 30)	Migraine (n = 38)	Controls (n = 50)
oVEMP			
Bilateral response, n (%)	27 (90.0 %)	30 (78.9 %)	45 (90.0 %)
Unilateral response, n (%)	2 (6.7 %)	7 (18.4 %)	3 (6.0 %)
No response, n (%)	1 (3.3 %)	1 (2.6 %)	2 (4.0 %)
cVEMP			
Bilateral response, n (%)	23 (76.7 %)	34 (89.5 %)	46 (92.0 %)
Unilateral response, n (%)	7 (23.3 %)	4 (10.5 %)	3 (6.0 %)
No response, n (%)	0 (0 %)	0 (0 %)	1 (2.0 %)

TTH tension-type headache, *oVEMP* ocular vestibular evoked myogenic potential, *cVEMP* cervical vestibular evoked myogenic potential

Table 3 oVEMP results of headache patients and healthy controls

Parameters	TTH	Migraine	Controls
Left side			
latency n1 (ms)	11.29 ± 0.78**	12.34 ± 1.43*,**	11.29 ± 0.73*
latency p1 (ms)	16.09 ± 0.83	17.05 ± 1.95*	16.11 ± 0.82*
n1-p1 interpeak latency (ms)	4.79 ± 0.87	4.75 ± 1.22	4.82 ± 0.92
n1-p1 amplitude	11.64 ± 6.73	8.00 ± 5.21+	11.66 ± 9.14
Right side			
latency n1 (ms)	11.42 ± 0.86**	12.41 ± 1.41*,**	11.58 ± 0.90*
latency p1 (ms)	16.41 ± 0.89	16.99 ± 2.02	16.20 ± 1.04
n1-p1 interpeak latency (ms)	4.99 ± 1.02	4.58 ± 1.24	4.62 ± 1.00
n1-p1 amplitude	11.29 ± 6.77	7.51 ± 4.47+	11.76 ± 10.79
Interside difference			
interaural latency diff., n1	0.64 ± 0.86	0.91 ± 0.97	0.74 ± 0.72
interaural latency diff., p1	0.64 ± 0.55	0.84 ± 0.95	0.78 ± 0.62
amp. asymmetry ratio, n1	0.23 ± 0.17	0.28 ± 0.17	0.23 ± 0.16
amp. asymmetry ratio, n1	0.22 ± 0.19	0.28 ± 0.21	0.24 ± 0.15

*$p < 0.05$, statistically significant between patients with migraine and controls; **$p < 0.05$, statistically significant between patients with migraine and patients with TTH; values are expressed as the means ± standard deviation

TTH tension-type headache, *oVEMP* ocular vestibular-evoked myogenic potential, *amp* amplitude

Table 1 Clinical and headache characteristics of the study groups

	TTH (n = 30)	Migraine (n = 38)	Control (n = 50)	P-value
Age (years)	33.37 ± 13.70	35.58 ± 12.26	35.14 ± 13.47	NS
Frequency (day/week)	1.52 ± 0.93	2.14 ± 2.05	-	
Duration (hours/day)	5.35 ± 6.01	9.51 ± 8.83	-	
Intensity (NRS)	4.13 ± 1.61	6.29 ± 2.10	-	

Values are expressed as mean ± standard deviation

TTH tension-type headache, *NRS* numeric rating scale, *NS* non-significant

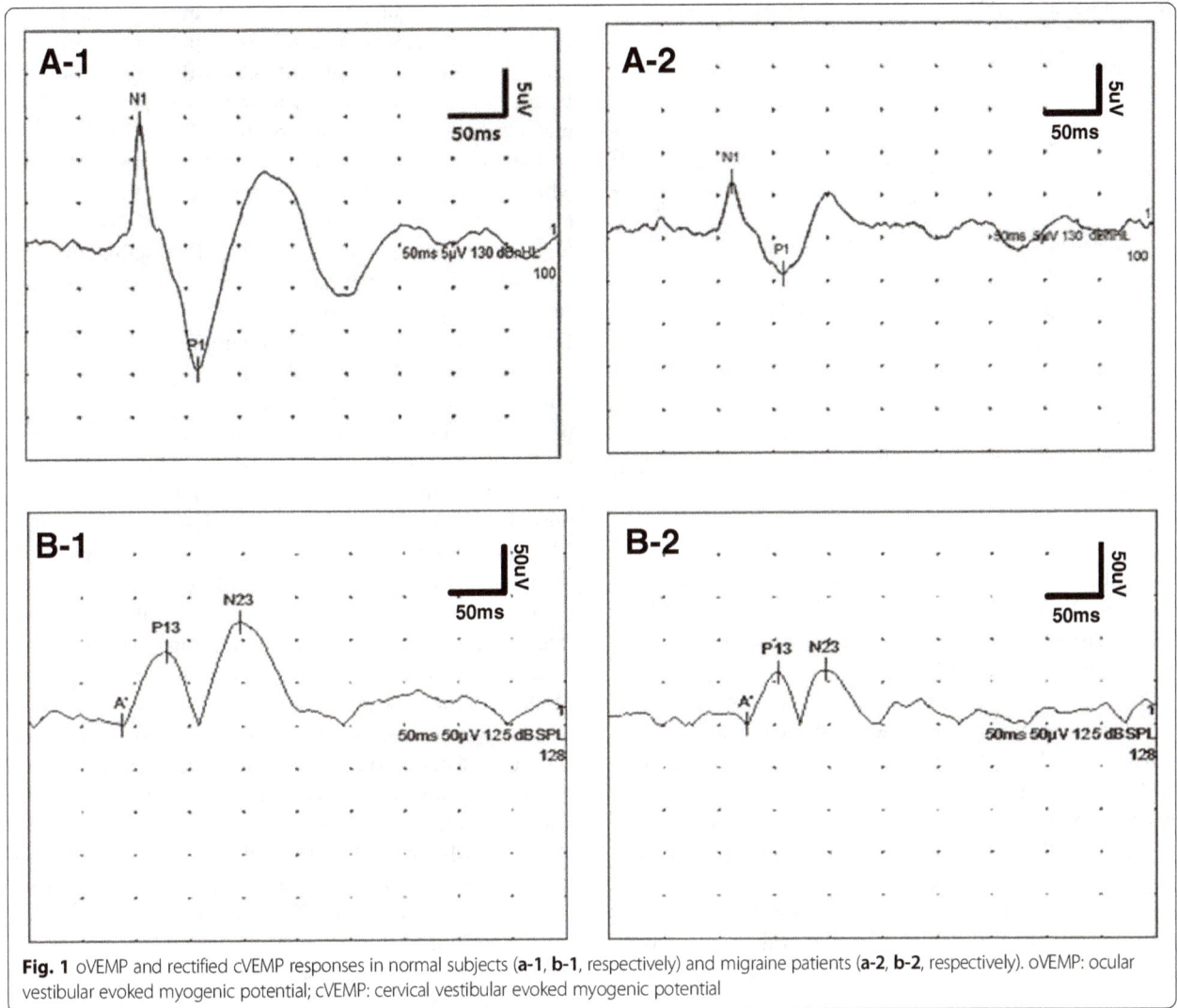

Fig. 1 oVEMP and rectified cVEMP responses in normal subjects (**a-1**, **b-1**, respectively) and migraine patients (**a-2**, **b-2**, respectively). oVEMP: ocular vestibular evoked myogenic potential; cVEMP: cervical vestibular evoked myogenic potential

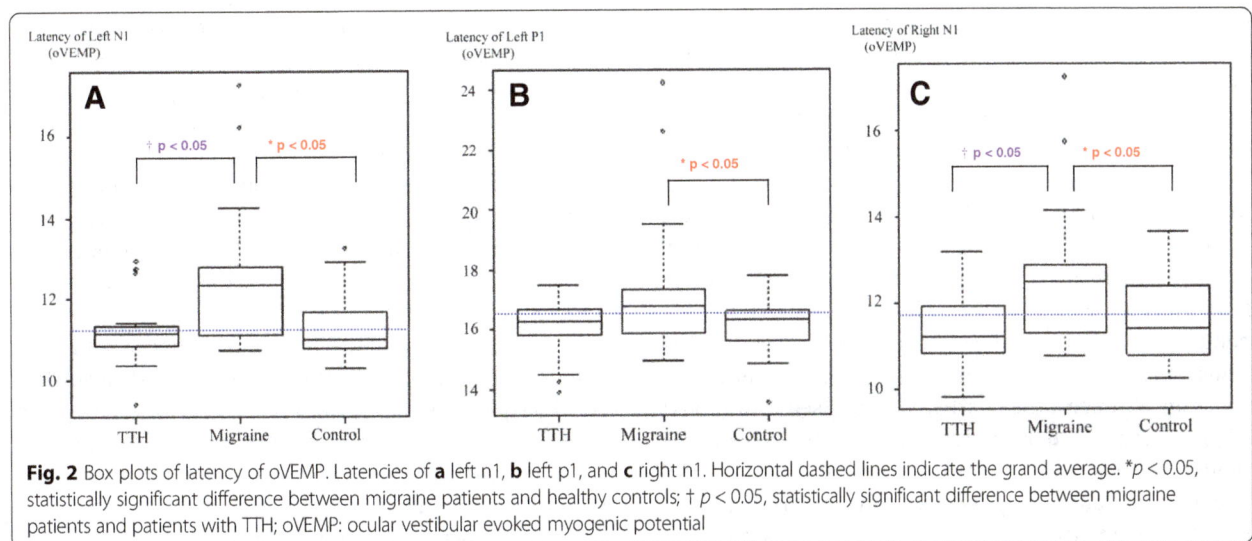

Fig. 2 Box plots of latency of oVEMP. Latencies of **a** left n1, **b** left p1, and **c** right n1. Horizontal dashed lines indicate the grand average. *$p < 0.05$, statistically significant difference between migraine patients and healthy controls; † $p < 0.05$, statistically significant difference between migraine patients and patients with TTH; oVEMP: ocular vestibular evoked myogenic potential

Table 4 Rectified cVEMP results of headache patients and controls

Parameters	TTH	Migraine	Controls	P value
Left side				
latency p13 (ms)	12.78 ± 1.37	13.57 ± 2.37	12.84 ± 1.81	NS
latency n23 (ms)	20.82 ± 2.01	21.98 ± 3.01	21.32 ± 2.06	NS
p13 rectified amp (μV)	42.43 ± 19.10	38.61 ± 24.95	39.41 ± 21.81	NS
n23 rectified amp (μV)	53.22 ± 13.90	58.52 ± 37.73	50.95 ± 34.25	NS
Right side				
latency p13 (ms)	12.89 ± 2.45	13.68 ± 2.16	13.01 ± 2.00	NS
latency n23 (ms)	21.06 ± 2.17	22.09 ± 3.10	21.56 ± 2.29	NS
p13 rectified amp (μV)	38.97 ± 21.05	34.49 ± 23.40	41.79 ± 25.55	NS
n23 rectified amp (μV)	49.98 ± 15.70	46.38 ± 28.37	57.79 ± 39.72	NS

Values are expressed as the means ± standard deviation

TTH tension-type headache, *cVEMP* cervical vestibular evoked myogenic potential, *amp* amplitude, *NS* non-significant

control groups. However, there was no significant difference in cVEMP parameters among the migraine, TTH and control groups. These results suggest pathology within the oVEMP pathway or the ascending utriculo-ocular reflex in migraineurs. Thus, migraineurs showed subclinical vestibulopathies with oVEMP abnormalities during a headache-free period.

cVEMP and oVEMP provide valuable information regarding the location and nature of the lesion(s) affecting central vestibular pathways because the vestibulo-collic and vestibulo-ocular reflex pathways diverge beyond the nerve root entry zone [4, 28]. Using oVEMP and cVEMP together allows for the evaluation of both ascending and descending vestibular pathways, resulting in the identification of a higher percentage of abnormalities [4, 28–30]. Patients who have brainstem involvement in multiple sclerosis or internuclear ophthalmoplegia show higher abnormality rates in oVEMP than in cVEMP [29, 31]. Additionally, oVEMP is more sensitive than cVEMP for detecting silent brainstem lesions in multiple sclerosis patients and vestibular dysfunction in VM patients [14, 29]. Furthermore, because oVEMP latencies are dependent primarily on afferent and efferent reflex limbs and central transmission, prolonged latencies are likely due to the degradation of central vestibular processing of otolith signals rather than a decline in peripheral vestibular function [26]. VEMP amplitudes can be used as independent quantitative measures of otolith function [4]. Thus, peripheral vestibular disorders frequently involve an absence of oVEMPs or decreased amplitudes, whereas prolonged latencies may indicate central vestibular lesions [32]. Significantly prolonged oVEMP latencies in our study suggest an underlying functional abnormality in the central vestibular system.

Herein, bilaterally or unilaterally absent oVEMP responses were observed in 21 % of patients in the migraine group, while absent cVEMP responses were found in 10.5 % of patients in the migraine group. Several previous reports showed absent oVEMP responses in the migraine group (53.3 %) and VM group (28 %), whereas absent cVEMP responses were detected in 8 % of VM patients [14, 16]. Similar to previous studies, a high unresponsive rate of oVEMP in migraineurs was observed in our study, although the difference did not reach statistical significance. These findings also suggest defective oVEMP pathways in migraineurs.

Various vestibular function test studies have been conducted on patients with migraines during the interictal period. Several works reported vestibular abnormalities in the form of involvement of peripheral or central vestibular pathways or both [18, 19, 33]. One study reported dysfunction in the vestibulo-ocular reflex, whereas another indicated underlying dysfunction in the vestibulospinal system [21, 34]. Other reports showed interictal dysfunction of vestibulocerebellar origin in migraineurs [20, 35]. These findings suggest that migraineurs without vestibular symptoms exhibit vestibular abnormalities, generally indicating subclinical vestibulopathies in patients with migraines. Additionally, the distribution between central and peripheral vestibular findings did not differ between VM and migraine patients [18]. More recently, in a report evaluating cVEMP and oVEMP pathways in patients with VM, the rates of abnormal oVEMPs were significantly higher without cVEMP abnormalities, similar to our study, although the subjects suffered symptoms on the same day of testing [14]. Thus, subclinical vestibular dysfunction may be an integral part of migraine pathophysiology and could be related to fundamental pathophysiological similarities between migraine and VM. Recently, positron emission tomography (PET) studies have demonstrated thalamo-cortical involvement or increased thalamic activation in VM patients [36, 37]. Additionally, voxel-based morphometry studies have identified gray matter volume reductions in patients with VM [38]. These functional and structural alterations in patients with VM resemble those previously described in patients with migraine. VM likely represents the pathophysiological paradigm of a connection between migraine and the vestibular system [39].

Subclinical vestibulopathy in migraineurs may be related to multiple potential interactions between the trigeminal and vestibular systems at various levels. In migraine patients, stimulation of the trigeminal nuclei has produced spontaneous nystagmus [40]. Conversely, vestibular nuclei receive both serotonergic inputs from the dorsal raphe nucleus and noradrenergic inputs from the locus coeruleus, and activation of these pain structures during migraine can affect central vestibular processing [3]. These reciprocal connections between the vestibular nuclei and trigeminal nucleus caudalis may provide a mechanism whereby vestibular signals influence trigeminovascular pathways and trigeminal information processing during migraine attacks [41]. Additionally, studies using functional MRI showed that the vestibular system is represented at a cortical level [42]. The presence of descending cortical projections on vestibular nuclei has been demonstrated in cats. Researchers concluded that neurons in cortical areas were able to modulate vestibular reflexes [43]. Minor cerebellar abnormalities related to eye and arm movements have also been described in asymptomatic migraine patients [20, 35]. Although semicircular canal and otolith afferents terminate in the vestibular nuclei region, both inputs project to the caudal vermis of the cerebellum and Purkinje cells in the cortex of the nodulus/uvula inhibit the vestibular nuclei [44]. These various potential interconnections between migraine and the vestibular system can cause abnormalities in vestibular function tests in migraineurs during the interictal period. A recent blood oxygen level-dependent (BOLD) functional MRI study conducted in patients with VM, patients with migraine without aura, and healthy controls during the interictal period, revealed that caloric vestibular stimulation elicited statistically significant activation in the bilateral insular cortex, thalamus, cerebellum, and brainstem of all subjects [36]. In particular, discrete activation in the periaqueductal gray matter was observed in migraine patients, suggesting a peculiar relationship between vestibular stimulation and the activation of brain areas that play key roles in pain processing [45]. This reciprocal connection between brainstem vestibular nuclei and structures involved in modulation of trigeminal nociceptive inputs may explain the VEMP abnormalities in migraineurs.

Due to the measurement method and/or technical factors, oVEMP is more valuable in assessing vestibular function in patients with headache compared to cVEMP. During cVEMP recordings, amplitude-related parameters change according to the degree of tonic contraction of the SCM showing a direct correlation; the more tonic the muscle tension, the larger the cVEMP amplitude response [4]. Decreased response rate and amplitude or prolonged latencies on cVEMP and oVEMP occur with age increase over 60 years [24, 26]. Regarding the influence of gender on oVEMPs, one study found oVEMPs to be independent of gender [31], whereas another study reported that the mean oVEMP amplitude in males was significantly larger than in females [25]. Thus, in our study, we only included females 20–60 years of age based on these known age and gender effects. To control the amount of muscle tension between right and left

muscles, we used a feedback method with a blood pressure manometer and analyzed VEMP parameters following EMG rectification in cVEMP [27, 46]. Many patients with primary headache disorders, such as TTH and migraine, also have accompanying pericranial, neck and shoulder muscle tenderness and/or associated myofascial pain syndrome. These conditions can affect muscle tension or posture during cVEMP measurements. Thus, the cVEMP method may provide inaccurate information in patients with migraine and TTH because the degree of muscle contraction affects the cVEMP result and its interpretation. Consequently, oVEMP may be the more sensitive method for evaluating the vestibular system in primary headache disorders.

Our study had several limitations. First, highly selected patients from a neurology clinic at a regional university hospital were recruited. The sample size was small, and the study used a cross-sectional design that provided limited causal information. Second, the present data did not identify statistically significant correlations between VEMP parameters and headache clinical parameters such as frequency, duration, and intensity (data not shown). Additionally, this study was based on outpatient subjects and only administered the headache questionnaire at the first visit; therefore, detailed headache characteristics recorded using a headache diary should be considered in future studies to more accurately identify the correlations between electrophysiological data and headache parameters. Furthermore, prospective longitudinal studies including information regarding impact or disabilities due to headache may be warranted. Third, sound stimulation was applied at 500 Hz, which showed a 100 % response rate in both oVEMP and cVEMP of healthy subjects [47]. However, VEMPs were not obtained in approximately 8-10 % of subjects in the control group, as previous studies showed similar results [14, 16]. oVEMP and cVEMP predominantly represent saccular stimulation, and bone vibration activates both utricular and saccular afferents [4]. Thus, we should consider the use of a bone vibrator in future studies.

Conclusions

In conclusion, this study provides electrophysiological evidence that abnormalities of the oVEMP pathway can be observed in patients with migraine without aura who are not experiencing vestibular symptoms during a headache-free period. These findings appear to be related to subclinical vestibulopathy in migraineurs. Thus, oVEMP may be useful in evaluating alterations in the vestibular system in patients with migraine as well as other types of primary headaches.

Abbreviations

oVEMP: Ocular vestibular-evoked myogenic potential; cVEMP: Cervical vestibular-evoked myogenic potential; ICHD-3β: The International Classification of Headache Disorders-3 beta version; VM: Vestibular migraine; EMG: Electromyography; nHL: Normal hearing level; AR: Amplitude asymmetry ratio; PET: Positron emission tomography; BOLD: Blood oxygen level-dependent imaging.

Competing interests

The authors declare that they have no competing interests.

Authors' contributions

Conception and design of the experiments: JHS. Performance of experiments: CHK, MUJ, HCC, and JHS. Data analysis: CHK and JHS. Writing of the manuscript: JHS. All authors read and approved the final manuscript.

References

1. Bisdorff A, Andree C, Vaillant M, Sandor PS (2010) Headache-associated dizziness in a headache population: prevalence and impact. Cephalalgia 30(7):815–820
2. Neuhauser HK, Radtke A, von Brevern M, Feldmann M, Lezius F, Ziese T, Lempert T (2006) Migrainous vertigo: prevalence and impact on quality of life. Neurology 67:1028–1033
3. Furman JM, Marcus DA, Balaban CD (2003) Migrainous vertigo: development of a pathogenetic model and structured diagnostic interview. Curr Opin Neurol 16:5–13
4. Rosengren SM, Welgampola MS, Colebatch JG (2010) Vestibular evoked myogenic potentials: Past, present and future. Clin Neurophysiol 121(5):636–651
5. Rosengren SM, McAngus Todd NP, Colebatch JG (2005) Vestibular-evoked extraocular potentials produced by stimulation with bone-conducted sound. Clin Neurophysiol 116(8):1938–1948
6. Rosengren SM, Kingma H (2013) New perspectives on vestibular evoked myogenic potentials. Curr Opin Neurol 26(1):74–80
7. Liao LJ, Young YH (2004) Vestibular evoked myogenic potentials in basilar artery migraine. Laryngoscope 114(7):1305–1309
8. Hong SM, Kim SK, Park CH, Lee JH (2011) Vestibular-evoked myogenic potentials in migrainous vertigo. Otolaryngol Head Neck Surg 144(2):284–287
9. Boldingh MI, Ljostad U, Mygland A, Monstad P (2011) Vestibular sensitivity in vestibular migraine: VEMPs and motion sickness susceptibility. Cephalalgia 31(11):1211–1219
10. Baier B, Stieber N, Dieterich M (2009) Vestibular-evoked myogenic potentials in vestibular migraine. J Neurol 256(9):1447–1454
11. Allena M, Magis D, De Pasqua V, Schoenen J, Bisdorff AR (2007) The vestibulo-collic reflex is abnormal in migraine. Cephalalgia 27(10):1150–1155
12. Roceanu A, Allena M, De Pasqua V, Bisdorff A, Schoenen J (2008) Abnormalities of the vestibulo-collic reflex are similar in migraineurs with and without vertigo. Cephalalgia 28(9):988–990
13. Kandemir A, Celebisoy N, Kose T (2013) Cervical vestibular evoked myogenic potentials in primary headache disorders. Clin Neurophysiol 124(4):779–784
14. Zaleski A, Bogle J, Starling A, Zapala DA, Davis L, Wester M, Cevette M (2015) Vestibular evoked myogenic potentials in patients with vestibular migraine. Otol Neurotol 36(2):295–302
15. Zuniga MG, Janky KL, Schubert MC, Carey JP (2012) Can vestibular-evoked myogenic potentials help differentiate Meniere disease from vestibular migraine? Otolaryngol Head Neck Surg 146(5):788–796
16. Gozke E, Erdal N, Ozkarakas H (2010) Ocular vestibular evoked myogenic potentials in patients with migraine. Acta Neurol Belg 110(4):321–324
17. Bir LS, Ardic FN, Kara CO, Akalin O, Pinar HS, Celiker A (2003) Migraine patients with or without vertigo: comparison of clinical and electronystagmographic findings. J Otolaryngol 32(4):234–238
18. Boldingh MI, Ljostad U, Mygland A, Monstad P (2013) Comparison of interictal vestibular function in vestibular migraine vs. migraine without vertigo. Headache 53(7):1123–1133
19. Casani AP, Sellari-Franceschini S, Napolitano A, Muscatello L, Dallan I (2009) Otoneurologic dysfunctions in migraine patients with or without vertigo. Otol Neurotol 30(7):961–967

20. Harno H, Hirvonen T, Kaunisto MA, Aalto H, Levo H, Isotalo E, Kallela M, Kaprio J, Palotie A, Wessman M, Farkkila M (2003) Subclinical vestibulocerebellar dysfunction in migraine with and without aura. Neurology 61(12):1748–1752
21. Ishizaki K, Mori N, Takeshima T, Fukuhara Y, Ijiri T, Kusumi M, Yasui K, Kowa H, Nakashima K (2002) Static stabilometry in patients with migraine and tension-type headache during a headache-free period. Psychiatry Clin Neurosci 56(1):85–90
22. Ashina M, Bendtsen L, Jensen R, Lassen LH, Sakai F, Olsen J (1999) Muscle hardness in patients with chronic tension-type headache: human model of muscle pain. Pain 79:201–205
23. Asai M, Aoki M, Hayashi H, Yamada N, Mizuta K, Ito Y (2009) Subclinical deviation of the subjective visual vertical in patients affected by a primary headache. Acta Otolaryngol 129:30–35
24. Su HCHT, Young YH, Cheng PW (2004) Aging effect on vestibular evoked myogenic potential. Oto Neurotol 25(6):977–980
25. Sung PH, Cheng PW, Young YH (2011) Effect of gender on ocular vestibular-evoked myogenic potentials via various stimulation modes. Clin Neurophysiol 122(1):183–187
26. Tseng CL, Chou CH, Young YH (2010) Aging effect on the ocular vestibular-evoked myogenic potentials. Otol Neurotol 31(6):959–963
27. Vanspauwen R, Wuyts FL, Van de Heyning PH (2006) Improving vestibular evoked myogenic potential reliability by using a blood pressure manometer. Laryngoscope 116(1):131–135
28. Rosengren SM, Nogajski JH, Cremer PD, Colebatch JG (2007) Delayed vestibular evoked responses to the eyes and neck in a patient with an isolated brainstem lesion. Clin Neurophysiol 118(9):2112–2116
29. Gazioglu SBC (2012) Ocular and cervical vestibular evoked myogenic potentials in multiple sclerosis patients. Clin Neurophysiol 123(9):1872–1879
30. Lin KY, Hsu YS, Young YH (2010) Brainstem lesion in benign paroxysmal vertigo children: evaluated by a combined ocular and cervical vestibular-evoked myogenic potential test. Int J Pediatr Otorhinolaryngol 74(5):523–527
31. Rosengren SM, Colebatch JG (2011) Ocular vestibular evoked myogenic potentials are abnormal in internuclear ophthalmoplegia. Clin Neurophysiol 122(6):1264–1267
32. Kantner C, Gurkov R (2012) Characteristics and clinical applications of ocular vestibular evoked myogenic potentials. Hear Res 294(1–2):55–63
33. Marcelli V, Furia T, Marciano E (2010) Vestibular pathways involvement in children with migraine: a neuro-otological study. Headache 50(1):71–76
34. Baker BJ, Curtis A, Trueblood P, Vangsnes E (2013) Vestibular functioning and migraine: comparing those with and without vertigo to a normal population. J Laryngol Otol 127(12):1169–1176
35. Sandor PS, Mascia A, Seidel L, de Pasqua V, Schoenen J (2001) Subclinical cerebellar impairment in the common types of migraine: a three-dimensional analysis of reaching movements. Ann Neurol 49(5):668–672
36. Russo A, Marcelli V, Esposito F, Corvino V, Marcuccio L, Giannone A, Cnforti R, Marciano E, Tedeschi G, Tessitore A (2014) Abnormal thalamic function in patients with vestibular migraine. Neurology 82(23):2120–2126
37. Shin JH, Kim YK, Kim HJ, Kim JS (2014) Altered brain metabolism in vestibular migraine: comparison of interictal and ictal findings. Cephalalgia 34(1):58–67
38. Obermann M, Wurthmann S, Steinberg BS, Theysohn N, Diener HC, Naegel S (2014) Central vestibular system modulation in vestibular migraine. Cephalalgia 34(13):1053–1061
39. Tedeschi G, Russo A, Conte F, Laura M, Tessitor A (2015) Vestibular migraine pathophysiology: insights from structural and functional neuroimaging. Neurol Sci 36(Suppl1):S37–S40
40. Marano E, Marcelli V, Di Stasio E, Bonuso S, Vacca G, Manganelli F, Marciano E, Perretti A (2005) Trigeminal stimulation elicits a peripheral vestibular imbalance in migraine patients. Headache 45(4):325–331
41. Buisseret-Delmas C, Compoint C, Delfini C, Buisseret P (1999) Organisation of reciprocal connections between trigeminal and vestibular nuclei in the rat. J Comp Neurol 409(1):153–168
42. Fasold O, von Brevern M, Kuhberg M, Ploner CJ, Villringer A, Lempert T, Wenzel R (2002) Human vestibular cortex as identified with caloric stimulation in functional magnetic resonance imaging. Neuroimage 17(3):1384–1393
43. Wilson VJ, Zarzecki P, Schor RH, Isu N, Rose PK, Sato H, Thomson DB, Umezaki T (1999) Cortical influences on the vestibular nuclei of the cat. Exp Brain Res 125(1):1–13

44. King S, Wang J, Priesol AJ, Lewis RF (2014) Central integration of canal and otolith signals is abnormal in vestibular migraine. Front Neurol 10(5):233. doi:10.3389/fneur.2014.00233
45. Borsook D, Burstein R (2012) The enigma of the dorsolateral pons as a migraine generator. Cephalalgia 32(11):803–812
46. Lee KJ, Kim MS, Son EJ, Lim HJ, Bang JH, Kang JG (2008) The usefulness of rectified VEMP. Clin Exp Otorhinolaryngol 1(3):143–147
47. Park HJ, Lee IS, Shin JE, Lee YJ, Park MS (2010) Frequency-tuning characteristics of cervical and ocular vestibular evoked myogenic potentials induced by air-conducted tone bursts. Clin Neurophysiol 121(1):85–89

11

Cervical non-invasive vagus nerve stimulation (nVNS) for preventive and acute treatment of episodic and chronic migraine and migraine-associated sleep disturbance: preliminary findings from a prospective observational cohort study

Thomas M. Kinfe[1,2]*, Bogdan Pintea[2], Sajjad Muhammad[2], Sebastian Zaremba[3,4], Sandra Roeske[4], Bruce J. Simon[5] and Hartmut Vatter[2]

Abstract

Background: The debilitating nature of migraine and challenges associated with treatment-refractory migraine have a profound impact on patients. With the need for alternatives to pharmacologic agents, vagus nerve stimulation has demonstrated efficacy in treatment-refractory primary headache disorders. We investigated the use of cervical non-invasive vagus nerve stimulation (nVNS) for the acute treatment and prevention of migraine attacks in treatment-refractory episodic and chronic migraine (EM and CM) and evaluated the impact of nVNS on migraine-associated sleep disturbance, disability, and depressive symptoms.

Methods: Twenty patients with treatment-refractory migraine were enrolled in this 3-month, open-label, prospective observational study. Patients administered nVNS prophylactically twice daily at prespecified times and acutely as adjunctive therapy for migraine attacks. The following parameters were evaluated: pain intensity (visual analogue scale [VAS]); number of headache days per month and number of migraine attacks per month; number of acutely treated attacks; sleep quality (Pittsburgh Sleep Quality Index [PSQI]); migraine disability assessment (MIDAS); depressive symptoms (Beck Depression Inventory® [BDI]); and adverse events (AEs).

Results: Of the 20 enrolled patients, 10 patients each had been diagnosed with EM and CM. Prophylaxis with nVNS was associated with significant overall reductions in patient-perceived pain intensity; median (interquartile range) VAS scores at baseline versus 3 months were 8.0 (7.5, 8.0) versus 4.0 (3.5, 5.0) points ($p < 0.001$). Baseline versus 3-month values (mean ± standard error of the mean) were 14.7 ± 0.9 versus 8.9 ± 0.8 ($p < 0.001$) for the number of headache days per month and 7.3 ± 0.9 versus 4.5 ± 0.6 ($p < 0.001$) for the number of attacks per month. Significant improvements were also noted in MIDAS ($p < 0.001$), BDI ($p < 0.001$), and PSQI global ($p < 0.001$) scores. No severe or serious AEs occurred.

(Continued on next page)

* Correspondence: thomas.kinfe@ukb.uni-bonn.de
This article was updated on December 22, 2015.
[1]Division of Functional Neurosurgery and Neuromodulation, Department of Neurosurgery, Rheinische Friedrich-Wilhelms University, Regina-Pacis-Weg 3, 53113 Bonn, Germany
[2]Department of Neurosurgery, Rheinische Friedrich-Wilhelms University, Regina-Pacis-Weg 3, 53113 Bonn, Germany
Full list of author information is available at the end of the article

(Continued from previous page)

Conclusion: In this study, treatment with nVNS was safe and provided clinically meaningful decreases in the frequency and intensity of migraine attacks in patients with treatment-refractory migraine. Improvements in migraine-associated disability, depression, and sleep quality were also noted.

Keywords: Neuromodulation, Headache, Acute therapy, Prophylactic therapy, Sleep impairment

Background

As a highly prevalent neurologic disorder, migraine headache exerts a considerable burden on individuals and society [1, 2], including substantial economic costs [3]. Recent findings from the Global Burden of Disease Study 2013 suggest that migraine ranks sixth among the top worldwide causes of disability [4, 5]. Along with premonitory (i.e. aura) and attack-associated symptoms (i.e. phonophobia, photophobia, nausea, and vomiting) [2], patients with migraine are likely to experience sleep disturbances [6, 7] and other comorbidities such as depression and anxiety [8, 9]. Sleep disturbances may trigger a migraine attack in the preictal state [6]. Patients with non-sleep migraine (NSM) demonstrate low thermal pain thresholds, whereas insufficient rest may evoke migraine attacks in patients with sleep migraine (SM) [6, 10].

Although there is no clear consensus on precisely how to define refractory migraine, a key parameter among commonly used clinical definitions is unresponsiveness to medications from multiple pharmacologic classes [11]. Thus, individuals with treatment-refractory migraine require alternatives to standard pharmacologic therapies. Neuromodulation therapy using implanted vagus nerve stimulation (VNS) devices has been successfully used to treat drug-resistant epilepsy [12] and depression [13], and numerous other methods of neuromodulation (e.g. occipital nerve stimulation, non-invasive VNS, transcranial direct current stimulation, repetitive transcranial magnetic stimulation, transcutaneous electrical nerve stimulation, transcutaneous supraorbital nerve stimulation, spinal cord stimulation) have been investigated for treating patients with migraine, with varying degrees of success [14]. Small studies and case reports have shown that implanted VNS may also alleviate migraine and cluster headache [15–18]. Data suggest that attenuation of pain by VNS occurs via inhibition of signalling through afferent vagus nerve fibres to the trigeminal nucleus caudalis (TNC) [19] and via modulation of inhibitory neurotransmitter release, resulting in decreased glutamate levels in the TNC [20, 21].

The use of implanted VNS devices for the treatment of headache disorders is hampered by inherent procedural risks (i.e. infection, lead migration, lead fracture, and battery replacement), health complications (i.e. voice disturbance, cough, headache, and paraesthesia), surgery cost, and the need for postoperative monitoring [22, 23]. Thus, a non-invasive vagus nerve stimulation (nVNS) device (gammaCore®; electroCore, LLC) has been developed and is CE-marked for the treatment of primary headache disorders [24]. Recent evidence suggests that nVNS is effective in the acute treatment of migraine [25, 26] and in the acute or prophylactic treatment of cluster headache [27–29]. An open-label pilot study that evaluated nVNS for the acute treatment of episodic migraine (EM) attacks reported that the efficacy of nVNS at 2 h after initiation of therapy was comparable to that of first-line pharmacologic interventions [25]. Barbanti and colleagues evaluated the use of nVNS for the acute treatment of migraine attacks in patients with chronic migraine (CM) and high-frequency EM [26]. The majority of patients with mild or moderate migraine attacks achieved pain relief or pain-free status at both 1 and 2 h after nVNS treatment [26].

No published studies to date have examined the effect of nVNS on sleep quality and depression in patients with migraine. We therefore conducted a 3-month, open-label, prospective, observational cohort study to investigate the safety and efficacy of acute and prophylactic nVNS treatment in patients with EM and CM and assess the effects of nVNS on sleep quality in these patients.

Methods

Study design

This was a 3-month, single-centre, open-label, prospective, observational cohort study to evaluate the impact of preventive and acute treatment with nVNS in patients with treatment-refractory EM and CM and migraine-associated sleep disturbances, disability, and depressive symptoms. Patients were referred to our department by a headache specialist (neurologist), and their diagnoses were confirmed by a multidisciplinary pain board consisting of neurologists, anaesthesiologists, neurosurgeons, psychiatrists, and pain nurses.

Ethics, consent, and permissions

Approval for this study was obtained from the institutional ethics committee. All patients provided written informed consent.

Study population

Patients who were diagnosed with EM (headaches occurring <15 days per month) or CM (headaches occurring ≥15 days per month) according to the *International Classification of Headache Disorders* criteria (3rd edition; beta version) [2] and who fulfilled all of the inclusion criteria and none of the exclusion criteria (Table 1) were enrolled. All patients enrolled in the study were considered refractory to prophylactic treatment having previously failed 4 or more classes of medications (i.e. beta [β]-blocker, anticonvulsant, tricyclic antidepressant, and calcium channel blocker) and behavioural therapy.

Stimulation paradigm

The nVNS device (provided by electroCore, LLC, Basking Ridge, NJ, USA) is a handheld, portable appliance that employs a constant voltage-driven signal consisting of a 1-millisecond burst of 5-kHz sine waves repeated at a frequency of 25 Hz, with stimulation intensity ranging from 0 to 24 V. The device is positioned against the side of the neck below the mandibular angle, medial to the sternocleidomastoid muscle and lateral to the larynx. Stimulations are delivered transcutaneously in the region of the cervical branch of the vagus nerve through 2 stainless steel disc electrodes that are manually coated with a conductive gel.

For prophylactic therapy, patients were instructed to administer two 2-min stimulations of nVNS (1 stimulation on each side of the neck in the regions of the right and left cervical vagus nerves) twice daily (morning and late afternoon; total of 4 doses per day) (Fig. 1). For acute therapy, patients were advised to administer two 2-min stimulations (1 stimulation on each side of the neck) at the time of acute medication intake. Before study commencement, all patients received training from the same instructor regarding how to use the device.

Assessments and end points

Data for all efficacy and safety outcomes were obtained from patient-completed headache diaries and by physician questioning during outpatient visits. Efficacy related to prophylactic therapy was assessed by evaluating the change from baseline in patient-reported pain intensity, number of headache days per month, and number of migraine attacks per month. Baseline values for the number of headache days per month and number of migraine attacks per month were determined on the basis of patient reporting and medical history. The efficacy of acute nVNS treatment on individual attacks was assessed using subjective patient reports of overall pain relief or pain freedom as self-reported at baseline and after 3 months of therapy. Data for all reported and treated attacks were pooled and analysed. The onset, severity, and frequency of treatment-related adverse events (AEs) were evaluated. Furthermore, impaired sleep quality (Pittsburgh Sleep Quality Index [PSQI] score) [30], depressive symptoms (Beck Depression Inventory® [BDI; Psychological Corporation of San Antonio, San Antonio, TX, USA] score) [31], and migraine disability (Migraine Disability Assessment [MIDAS]) scores and grades [32] were evaluated at baseline and after 3 months of nVNS treatment. Sleep disturbances were classified according to the onset of the migraine attack (SM vs NSM) and in relation to the time of sleep evaluation (interictal: 48 h from last attack; or preictal or postictal: <48 h from last attack) (Table 3).

Statistical analysis

Univariate analyses of data obtained at baseline and after 3 months of nVNS treatment were performed to determine changes in pain intensity (visual analogue scale [VAS] score), headache days/month, MIDAS score/grade, number of migraine attacks per month, and depressive (BDI) and sleep (PSQI) comorbidities. Comparisons of the outcomes at baseline and 3 months' follow-up were performed using the McNemar test for binominal variables

Table 1 Inclusion and exclusion criteria

Inclusion criteria	Exclusion criteria
• Chronic refractory headache disorder according to *ICHD-3* beta criteria • Age ≥18 years • Migraine attacks that are refractory to medical or behavioural therapy • Eligible for nVNS therapy • Willingness to comply with a defined follow-up interval • Intracranial and cervical pathologies ruled out by an MRI scan • Stable pain medication for 4 weeks prior to nVNS	• Other concomitant neuropsychiatric comorbidity that is not adequately classified or requires a specific diagnosis or treatment • Pregnancy • Previous invasive or non-invasive neuromodulation therapy or ablative procedure • Unwillingness to complete pain diary and provide information on pain intensity and migraine attack frequency (i.e. number of migraine attacks per month) • Cerebrovascular or cardiovascular disease

Abbreviations: *ICHD-3 International Classification of Headache Disorders (3rd edition)*, *MRI* magnetic resonance imaging, *nVNS* non-invasive vagus nerve stimulation

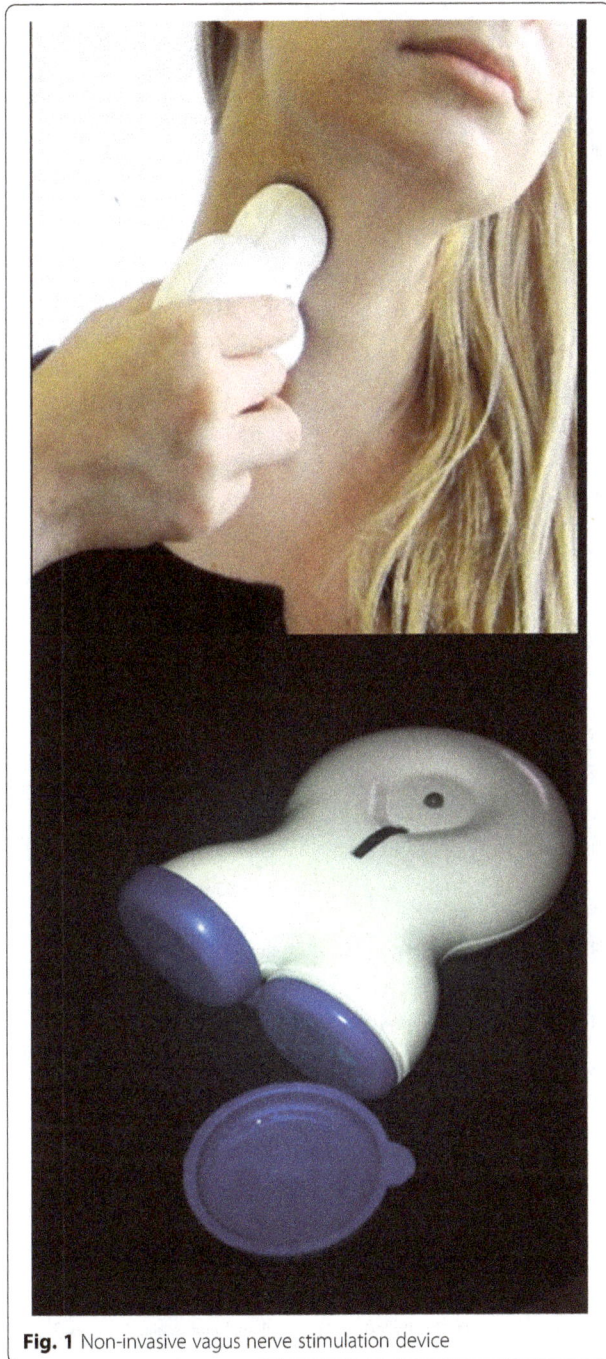

Fig. 1 Non-invasive vagus nerve stimulation device

and the Student *t* test or the Wilcoxon signed rank test, as appropriate, for continuous data. *P*-values <0.05 were considered significant. All patients were included in the analyses; subgroup analyses were performed for patients with EM and CM. Statistical analyses were performed independently by North American Science Associates Inc. (Minneapolis, MN, USA) using SAS® 9.2 (SAS Institute Inc., Cary, NC, USA).

Results

Demographic and baseline characteristics

Of the 20 participants, 16 were female and 4 were male, with an average age of 53.1 years (range, 35–72 years). Ten patients each had been diagnosed with EM (9 without aura/1 with aura) and CM (8 without aura/2 with aura). All patients were classified as MIDAS grade III/IV, with most having clinical signs of sleep disturbance (average PSQI score, 8.3 points; range, 2–17 points) and depressive symptoms (average BDI score, 17.3 points; range, 5–34 points) (Table 2). Evaluation of sleep patterns at baseline revealed that of 20 patients, 15 (6 EM/9 CM) had a disturbed sleep architecture (i.e. global PSQI score of >5 points), and most patients (18/20) had NSM (Table 3). The majority of patients (18/20) had body mass index (BMI) values ≤30 kg/m^2; 2 patients (1 EM/1 CM) had BMI values >30 kg/m^2.

Preventive use of nVNS

Median (interquartile range [IQR]) pain intensity (VAS score) in the total study population was 8 (7.5, 8.0) points at baseline and significantly declined to 4 (3.5, 5) points after 3 months of nVNS use ($p < 0.001$) (Fig. 2). Reductions in pain intensity were observed in both EM (baseline vs 3 months of nVNS treatment: 8 [7, 8] vs 3.5 [3, 4] points; $p = 0.002$) and CM (8 [8, 8] vs 5 [4, 5] points; $p = 0.002$) subgroups (Fig. 2). The overall mean ± standard error of the mean (SEM) number of headache days per month declined from 14.7 ± 0.9 to 8.9 ± 0.8 days ($p < 0.001$) (Fig. 3). Similarly, the number of headache days declined in both the EM (11.3 ± 0.6 vs 5.7 ± 0.5 days; $p < 0.001$) and CM (18.1 ± 0.8 vs 12.1 ± 0.6 days; $p < 0.001$) subgroups (Fig. 3). The number of migraine attacks per month declined significantly in the total population (7.3 ± 0.9 vs 4.5 ± 0.6 attacks; $p < 0.001$), the EM subgroup (4.9 ± 0.6 vs 3.0 ± 0.4 attacks; $p = 0.02$), and the CM subgroup (9.7 ± 1.2 vs 5.9 ± 0.8 attacks; $p < 0.001$) (Fig. 4).

Acute treatment with nVNS

All patients reported that they had treated each of their migraine attacks with adjunctive nVNS during the 3-month treatment phase. Overall, patients with EM treated 90 migraine attacks with nVNS, and patients with CM treated 177 migraine attacks with the device. All patients self-reported at least some overall pain relief with their pre-existing acute treatment at baseline and with adjunctive acute nVNS use at follow-up. Of the 9 patients who reported a maximum benefit of pain relief at baseline, 5 (2 EM/3 CM) were able to achieve pain freedom within 2 h after initiating adjunctive nVNS treatment as reported at 3 months ($p = 0.03$).

Table 2 Demographic and baseline characteristics

Patient No.	Sex	Age, years	Migraine Type	Number of Attacks per Month	Pain Intensity (VAS) Score	Number of Headache Days per Month	MIDAS Grade (score)	BDI Score	Prophylactic Medications	Acute Medications + Time to Achieve Pain Relief	BMI, kg/m²	Global PSQI Score
1	f	36	EM+	6	6	10	III (18)	18	4 Classes + Mg + Botox®	Triptan + 60 min	24	5
2	f	66	CM-	6	8	20	IV (45)	19	4 Classes + Botox	NSAID + 90 min	23	12
3	f	41	CM-	7	8	20	IV (39)	34	4 Classes	Triptan + 60 min	31	12
4	m	70	CM-	7	7	15	IV (39)	15	Calcium channel blocker	NSAID + 45 min	25	2
5	f	56	CM+	17	8	18	IV (51)	17	N/A	Triptan + 60 min	25	17
6	f	60	CM-	8	8	22	IV (44)	16	4 Classes + Botox	Triptan + 60 min	24	7
7	f	35	EM-	4	8	9	III (19)	8	4 Classes + Botox	Triptan + 60 min	17	8
8	m	50	EM-	5	7	9	IV (37)	23	4 Classes + Botox	NSAID + 160 min	40	6
9	f	50	EM-	3	9	9	IV (45)	5	4 Classes + Botox	Triptan + 30 min	22	7
10	f	35	CM-	12	8	15	IV (36)	11	4 Classes + Botox	Triptan + 60 min	22	12
11	m	39	EM-	4	8	12	III (19)	21	Calcium channel blocker + Mg + Ca++	NSAID + 150 min	29	7
12	f	52	EM-	4	8	12	III (19)	21	4 Classes + Mg	Triptan + 150 min	23	3
13	f	45	CM-	15	8	18	IV (33)	25	4 Classes + Botox	NSAID + 45 min	23	17
14	f	54	EM-	4	8	12	III (18)	17	4 Classes + Mg	Triptan + 120 min	25	4
15	f	60	EM-	10	8	14	III (19)	18	4 Classes + Mg	Triptan + 60 min	18	5
16	f	60	EM-	5	7	14	III (16)	16	4 Classes + Botox	Triptan + 120 min	20	11
17	f	59	CM+	10	8	15	III (18)	16	4 Classes + Botox	Triptan + 90 min	22	6
18	m	72	CM-	9	8	18	III (17)	15	4 Classes	NSAID + 90 min	22	8
19	f	60	CM-	6	8	20	IV (44)	16	4 Classes + Botox	Triptan + 60 min	24	6
20	f	62	EM-	4	7	12	III (16)	15	4 Classes + Botox	Triptan + 120 min	20	10

Abbreviations: *BDI* Beck Depression Inventory, *BMI* body mass index, *Ca++* calcium, *CM* chronic migraine, *EM* episodic migraine, *f/m* female/male, *Mg* magnesium, *MIDAS* Migraine Disability Assessment, *NSAID* nonsteroidal anti-inflammatory drug, *PSQI* Pittsburgh Sleep Quality Index, *VAS* visual analogue scale, *4 Classes* β-blocker, anticonvulsant, tricyclic antidepressant, calcium channel blocker, −/+ without aura/with aura

Migraine-associated comorbidities

In the total population, significant reductions were observed in the median (IQR) MIDAS score (baseline vs 3 months of nVNS treatment: 26 [18, 41.5] vs 15 [9, 34.5] points; $p < 0.001$) and MIDAS grade (3.5 [3, 4] vs 3 [2, 4]; $p = 0.008$) (Fig. 5a). A significant decrease in the MIDAS score was also observed in the CM subgroup (39 [33, 44] vs 16 [9, 36] points; $p = 0.002$) but not in the EM subgroup (Fig. 5a).

A significant reduction from baseline to 3 months in the mean ± SEM BDI score was noted in the total population (17.3 ± 1.4 vs 10.8 ± 1.1 points; $p < 0.001$), the EM subgroup (16.2 ± 1.8 vs 8.4 ± 0.9 points; $p < 0.001$), and the CM subgroup (18.4 ± 2.1 vs 13.2 ± 1.6 points; $p < 0.001$) (Fig. 5b).

Similarly, significant reductions in the global PSQI score were observed in the total population (7 [5.5, 11.5] vs 5 [5, 8.5] points; $p < 0.001$), the EM subgroup (6.5 [5, 8] vs 5 [5, 5] points; $p = 0.03$), and the

Table 3 Distribution of sleep patterns

Patient No.	Sex	Age, years	Migraine Type	Migraine Attack Onset	Sleep Evaluation	BMI, kg/m^2	Global PSQI Score
1	f	36	EM+	NSM	IC	24	5
2	f	66	CM-	NSM	IC	23	12
3	f	41	CM-	NSM	IC	31	12
4	m	70	CM-	NSM	IC	25	2
5	f	56	CM+	NSM	PC	25	17
6	f	60	CM-	NSM	PC	24	7
7	f	35	EM-	NSM	IC	17	8
8	m	50	EM-	NSM	IC	40	6
9	f	50	EM-	NSM	IC	22	7
10	f	35	CM-	NSM	IC	22	12
11	m	39	EM-	NSM	IC	29	7
12	f	52	EM-	SM	IC	23	3
13	f	45	CM-	NSM	IC	23	17
14	f	54	EM-	NSM	IC	25	4
15	f	60	EM-	NSM	IC	18	5
16	f	60	EM-	NSM	IC	20	11
17	f	59	CM+	NSM	IC	22	6
18	m	72	CM-	NSM	IC	22	8
19	f	60	CM-	SM	IC	24	6
20	f	62	EM-	NSM	PC	20	10

Abbreviations: *BMI* body mass index, *CM* chronic migraine, *EM* episodic migraine, *f/m* female/male, *IC* interictal, *NSM* non-sleep migraine, *PC* preictal or postictal, *PSQI* Pittsburgh Sleep Quality Index, *SM* sleep migraine, *–/+* without aura/with aura

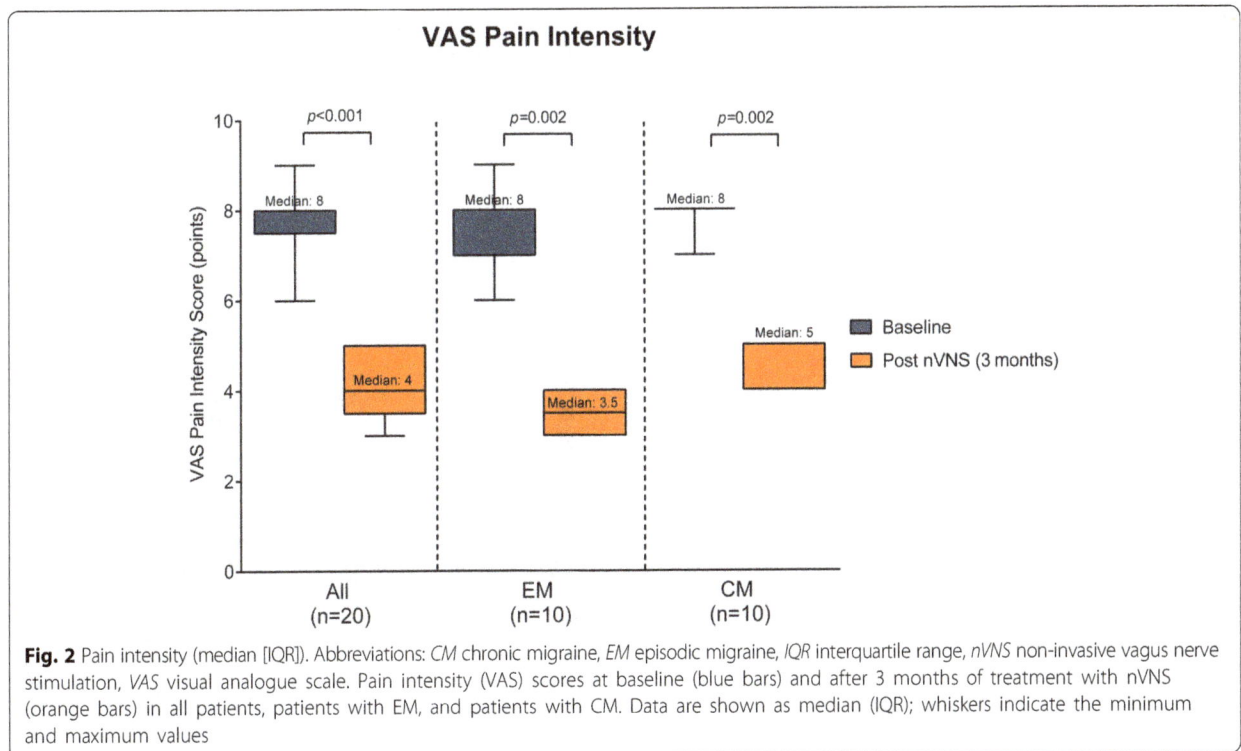

Fig. 2 Pain intensity (median [IQR]). Abbreviations: *CM* chronic migraine, *EM* episodic migraine, *IQR* interquartile range, *nVNS* non-invasive vagus nerve stimulation, *VAS* visual analogue scale. Pain intensity (VAS) scores at baseline (blue bars) and after 3 months of treatment with nVNS (orange bars) in all patients, patients with EM, and patients with CM. Data are shown as median (IQR); whiskers indicate the minimum and maximum values

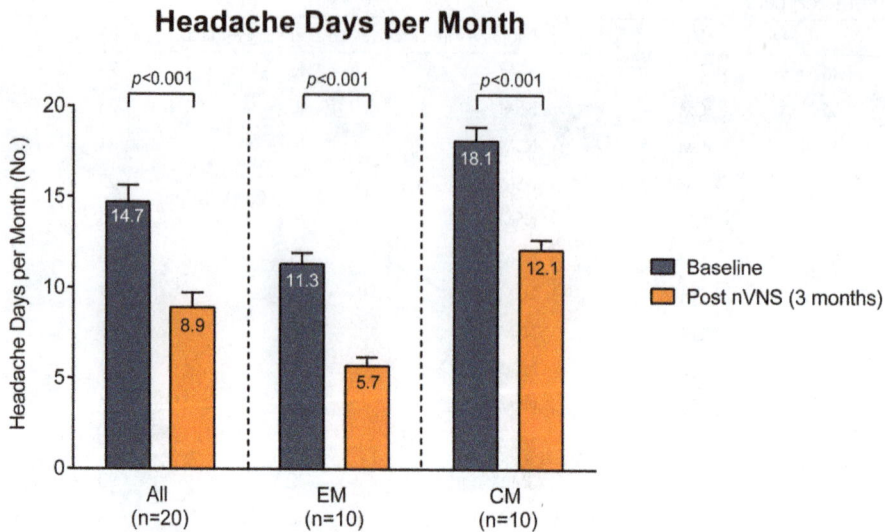

Fig. 3 Number of headache days per month (mean ± SEM). Abbreviations: *CM* chronic migraine, *EM* episodic migraine, *nVNS* non-invasive vagus nerve stimulation, *SEM* standard error of the mean. Number of headache days per month at baseline (blue bars) and after 3 months of treatment with nVNS (orange bars) in all patients, patients with EM, and patients with CM. Baseline measures were determined on the basis of patient reporting and medical history. Data are shown as mean ± SEM

CM subgroup (10 [6, 12] vs 8.5 [6, 10] points; $p = 0.02$) (Fig. 5c and Table 4). Reductions in PSQI subscores were significant in the total population for latency (1 [0.5, 3.5] vs 1 [0.5, 2] point; $p = 0.03$) and daytime dysfunction (2.5 [2, 4] vs 2 [1, 2] points; $p = 0.004$) (Table 4). Trends toward lower PSQI subscores after treatment were observed for daytime dysfunction in the EM subgroup (2.5 [2, 4] vs 2 [1, 2] points; $p = 0.06$) and for latency in the CM subgroup (2.5 [1, 5] vs 2 [1, 3] points; $p = 0.06$).

Incidence of AEs

Four patients reported mild treatment-related AEs, most commonly neck twitching and skin irritation. These AEs were transient, coincided with the period of stimulation, and resolved during the course of treatment. No severe or serious AEs occurred.

Discussion

In this study, a clinically meaningful response to 3 months of prophylactic nVNS therapy was observed

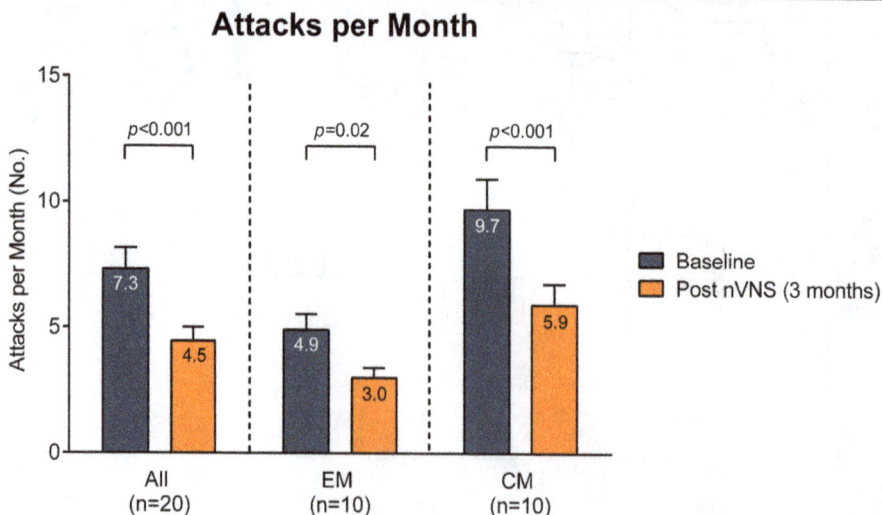

Fig. 4 Number of migraine attacks per month (mean ± SEM). Abbreviations: *CM* chronic migraine, *EM* episodic migraine, *nVNS* non-invasive vagus nerve stimulation, *SEM* standard error of the mean. The number of migraine attacks per month at baseline (blue bars) and after 3 months of treatment with nVNS (orange bars) in all patients, patients with EM, and patients with CM. Baseline measures were determined on the basis of patient reporting and medical history. Data are shown as mean ± SEM

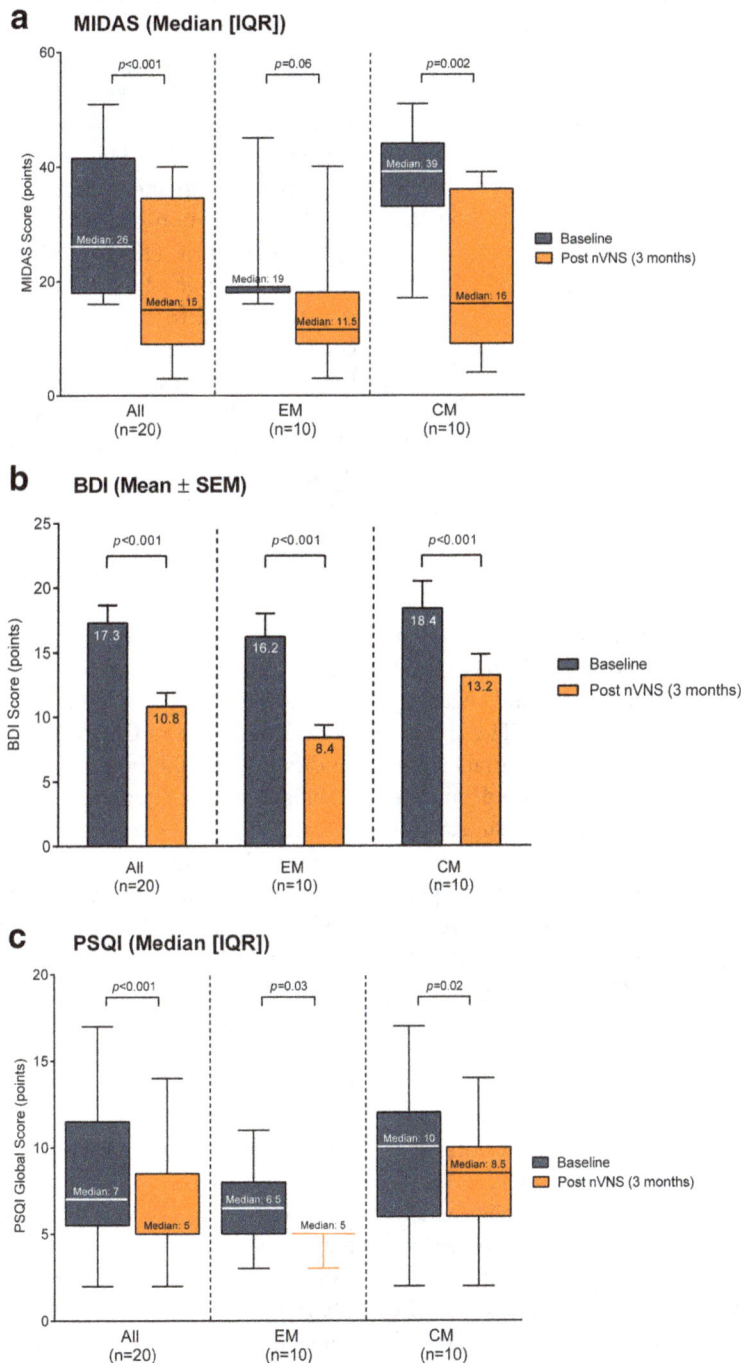

Fig. 5 Migraine disability and migraine-associated comorbidities. Abbreviations: *BDI* Beck Depression Inventory, *CM* chronic migraine, *EM* episodic migraine, *IQR* interquartile range, *MIDAS* Migraine Disability Assessment, *nVNS* non-invasive vagus nerve stimulation, *PSQI* Pittsburgh Sleep Quality Index, *SEM* standard error of the mean. MIDAS (**a**), BDI (**b**), and PSQI (**c**) scores at baseline (blue bars) and after 3 months of nVNS treatment (orange bars) in all patients, patients with EM, and patients with CM. Data are shown as median (IQR) for MIDAS and PSQI (whiskers indicate the minimum and maximum values) and as mean ± SEM for BDI

in the overall population as well as in the migraine subgroups (EM and CM), and nVNS was associated with significant reductions in pain intensity and number of headache days per month. A significant decrease in the number of migraine attacks per month was noted in the total population and in both subgroups. After 3 months, MIDAS scores and MIDAS grades significantly decreased in the total population. Significant improvements in BDI and PSQI scores were observed for the total population and for both

Table 4 Pittsburgh Sleep Quality Index (PSQI) scores

	Baseline	Post nVNS	P-value
PSQI global score	7 (5.5, 11.5)	5 (5, 8.5)	<0.001
PSQI subscores			
Subjective sleep quality	1 (1, 1)	1 (1, 1)	0.25
Sleep latency	1 (0.5, 3.5)	1 (0.5, 2)	0.03
Sleep duration	0 (0, 0)	0 (0, 0)	N/A
Sleep efficacy	0 (0, 0.5)	0 (0, 0.5)	N/A
Sleep disturbance	2 (1, 2)	1 (1, 2)	0.13
Sleep medication	0 (0, 1)	0 (0, 0.5)	0.13
Daytime dysfunction	2.5 (2, 4)	2 (1, 2)	0.004

Abbreviations: *IQR* interquartile range, *N/A* not applicable, *nVNS* non-invasive vagus nerve stimulation
Data are presented as median (IQR)

subgroups. Treatment with nVNS was well tolerated with no serious or severe treatment-related AEs.

Migraine is associated with a considerable economic burden [3], and findings from the International Burden of Migraine Study [33] suggest that therapies aimed at decreasing headache frequency and/or headache-related disability are important in containing costs and reducing the clinical and economic strain of migraine. The significant decreases in the number of headache attacks per month and MIDAS scores that were noted in the current study suggest that nVNS may have substantial utility in this regard.

The limitations of the current study include its open-label design, lack of control arm and prospective run-in period, self-recollected reporting of acute pain relief and pain freedom findings, and its small patient population. The lack of a control arm did not allow for examination of the placebo effect, which has been noted consistently in studies of migraine interventions [25, 34]. The method used for reporting acute pain relief and pain freedom was based on patients' general impressions and did not involve the use of a validated pain scale.

To date, 2 studies have investigated prophylactic therapy for migraine using non-invasive neuromodulation devices [35, 36]. Findings from the current study are consistent with those reported in a study of prophylactic therapy for CM using non-invasive transcutaneous auricular VNS [35] and those reported in a study of prophylactic therapy for migraine using non-invasive transcutaneous supraorbital stimulation [36]. However, unlike the current study, the aforementioned studies did not evaluate the effect of prophylactic nVNS therapy in both EM and CM subgroups.

This study was the first to examine the effect of nVNS on sleep quality in patients with migraine. Significant improvements in sleep quality after 3 months of treatment with nVNS were observed; however, further studies are required to validate these findings. Results from the current study also confirmed the favourable safety

profile of nVNS that was reported in previous studies of nVNS in the treatment of migraine [25, 26]. As first-line pharmacologic therapy for the acute treatment of migraine, triptans (i.e. serotonin 5-HT$_{1B/1D}$ agonists) are associated with a risk for cardiovascular/cerebrovascular side effects [37–39]. Thus, nVNS may serve as a safe alternative to triptans, which may potentially lower the risk for medication-overuse headache [40].

The therapeutic effects of nVNS reported in the current study are supported by findings from human neuroimaging studies and from animal studies of migraine pain and cortical spreading depression (CSD) [21, 41–43]. Functional magnetic resonance imaging studies in patients with migraine reflect heightened sensory facilitation, decreased inhibition in response to sensory stimuli, and lack of or decreased adaptation to interictal stimuli [44]. Neuroimaging studies of VNS demonstrate thalamic involvement, which is responsible for processing somatosensory information and regulating cortical activity [41]. Thus, in patients with migraine, nVNS therapy may help to counteract the decline in thalamocortical activity that is responsible for the decreased habituation to interictal stimuli [45]. The potential role of nVNS in migraine-associated pain and CSD has been investigated in animal studies [21, 42, 43]. In a rat model of trigeminal allodynia, Oshinsky and colleagues demonstrated that nVNS decreased trigeminal nociceptive stimulation by inhibiting nitric oxide–induced increases in glutamate levels in the TNC [21]. Further evaluation of the analgesic effect of VNS suggests that VNS inhibits the increase in *c-fos* expression in the TNC that occurs in response to painful stimuli [43]. With regard to migraine aura, which is believed to result from CSD [46], Chen and colleagues compared the effect of direct VNS using implanted VNS with the effect of nVNS in a rat model of CSD [42]. Compared with control treatment, both modes of VNS suppressed CSD susceptibility, with nVNS being more effective than direct VNS [42].

Evidence suggests that the degree of response to nVNS may vary depending on the side of stimulation [47]. Examination of cervical vagus nerve morphology at the site of electrode implantation shows that the right vagus nerve has a considerably larger surface area and more tyrosine hydroxylase–positive nerve fibres than the left vagus nerve, which may be relevant with respect to the side of stimulation [47]. Stimulation-mediated sympathetic- and catecholamine-driven effects and variations in the amount of epineurial connective tissue may modulate treatment response [47]. In the current study, patients administered treatment to both the right and left vagus nerves. However, in 3 recently published studies of nVNS for migraine and cluster headache, stimulation in the region of the right vagus nerve was implemented [25, 26, 29].

Conclusion

In conclusion, this study demonstrated that administration of nVNS therapy in patients with treatment-refractory migraine was associated with significant reductions in the monthly number of headache days, a preferred outcome measure in migraine studies, and pain intensity. In addition, there were clinically meaningful improvements in migraine-associated disability, depression, and sleep quality. The role of nVNS in migraine therapy is being further explored in ongoing large-scale, randomised, sham-controlled trials with long-term follow-up.

Abbreviations

AE: Adverse event; BDI: Beck Depression Inventory; BMI: Body mass index; CM: Chronic migraine; CSD: Cortical spreading depression; EM: Episodic migraine; IQR: Interquartile range; MIDAS: Migraine Disability Assessment; NSM: Non-sleep migraine; nVNS: Non-invasive vagus nerve stimulation; PSQI: Pittsburgh Sleep Quality Index; SEM: Standard error of the mean; SM: Sleep migraine; TNC: Trigeminal nucleus caudalis; VAS: Visual analogue scale; VNS: Vagus nerve stimulation.

Competing interests

Thomas M. Kinfe, MD, has received training support from St. Jude Medical, Inc. He also serves as a consultant for St. Jude Medical, Inc., and Medtronic Inc. Bogdan Pintea, MD, has received training support from St. Jude Medical, Inc. Bruce J. Simon, PhD, is an employee of electroCore, LLC.

Authors' contributions

All authors were involved in the development of the study design and participated in data collection and data analyses. All authors contributed to the development of this manuscript and provided their critique and their approval of the final draft for submission to *The Journal of Headache and Pain*.

Updates

This article was updated on December 22, 2015. A global calculation error has been corrected that affected a significant amount of data reported in the paper, resulting in a substantial change to the text, tables and figures.

Acknowledgements

The authors express their appreciation for the efforts and contributions of all investigators involved in this study. We acknowledge Günther Halfar (employee of electroCore, LLC, Basking Ridge, NJ, USA) for patient training and instruction and the contributions of Carolina Link, MD, Katharina Fassbender (study nurse), and Ute Wegener-Höpfner, MD. Gratitude is expressed to all patients who participated in the study.

Funding

This study was performed without any external funding. The nVNS devices were provided by electroCore, LLC (Basking Ridge, NJ, USA). Statistical analyses for the study were conducted by Candace McClure, PhD, of North American Science Associates Inc. (Minneapolis, MN, USA) and were supported by electroCore, LLC. Editorial support for this manuscript was provided by MedLogix Communications, LLC (Schaumburg, IL, USA) and was paid for by electroCore, LLC.

Author details

[1]Division of Functional Neurosurgery and Neuromodulation, Department of Neurosurgery, Rheinische Friedrich-Wilhelms University, Regina-Pacis-Weg 3, 53113 Bonn, Germany. [2]Department of Neurosurgery, Rheinische Friedrich-Wilhelms University, Regina-Pacis-Weg 3, 53113 Bonn, Germany. [3]Sleep Medicine, Department of Neurology, Rheinische Friedrich-Wilhelms University, Sigmund-Freud-Str. 25, D-53105 Bonn, Germany. [4]German Centre for Neurodegenerative Diseases (DZNE), Ernst-Robert-Curtius-Str. 12, 53117 Bonn, Germany. [5]electroCore, LLC, 150 Allen Road, Suite 201, Basking Ridge, NJ 07920, USA.

References

1. Hamelsky SW, Stewart WF, Lipton RB (2001) Epidemiology of migraine. Curr Pain Headache Rep 5(2):189–194
2. Headache Classification Committee of the International Headache Society (2013) The International Classification of Headache Disorders, 3rd edition (beta version). Cephalalgia 33(9):629–808. doi:10.1177/0333102413485658
3. Lanteri-Minet M (2014) Economic burden and costs of chronic migraine. Curr Pain Headache Rep 18(1):385. doi:10.1007/s11916-013-0385-0
4. Global Burden of Disease Study Collaborators (2015) Global, regional, and national incidence, prevalence, and years lived with disability for 301 acute and chronic diseases and injuries in 188 countries, 1990–2013: a systematic analysis for the Global Burden of Disease Study 2013. Lancet 386(9995): 743–800. doi:10.1016/S0140-6736(15)60692-4
5. Steiner TJ, Birbeck GL, Jensen RH, Katsarava Z, Stovner LJ, Martelletti P (2015) Headache disorders are third cause of disability worldwide. J Headache Pain 16:58. doi:10.1186/s10194-015-0544-2
6. Engstrøm M, Hagen K, Bjørk MH, Stovner LJ, Gravdahl GB, Stjern M, Sand T (2013) Sleep quality, arousal and pain thresholds in migraineurs: a blinded controlled polysomnographic study. J Headache Pain 14:12. doi:10.1186/1129-2377-14-12
7. de Tommaso M, Delussi M, Vecchio E, Sciruicchio V, Invitto S, Livrea P (2014) Sleep features and central sensitization symptoms in primary headache patients. J Headache Pain 15:64. doi:10.1186/1129-2377-15-64
8. Malone CD, Bhowmick A, Wachholtz AB (2015) Migraine: treatments, comorbidities, and quality of life, in the USA. J Pain Res 8:537–547. doi:10.2147/JPR.S88207
9. Pompili M, Serafini G, Di Cosimo D, Dominici G, Innamorati M, Lester D, Forte A, Girardi N, De Filippis S, Tatarelli R, Martelletti P (2010) Psychiatric comorbidity and suicide risk in patients with chronic migraine. Neuropsychiatr Dis Treat 6:81–91
10. Engstrøm M, Hagen K, Bjørk MH, Stovner LJ, Sand T (2014) Sleep quality and arousal in migraine and tension-type headache: the headache-sleep study. Acta Neurol Scand Suppl 198:47–54. doi:10.1111/ane.12237
11. Martelletti P, Katsarava Z, Lampl C, Magis D, Bendtsen L, Negro A, Russell MB, Mitsikostas DD, Jensen RH (2014) Refractory chronic migraine: a consensus statement on clinical definition from the European Headache Federation. J Headache Pain 15:47. doi:10.1186/1129-2377-15-47
12. Ryvlin P, Gilliam FG, Nguyen DK, Colicchio G, Iudice A, Tinuper P, Zamponi N, Aguglia U, Wagner L, Minotti L, Stefan H, Boon P, Sadler M, Benna P, Raman P, Perucca E (2014) The long-term effect of vagus nerve stimulation on quality of life in patients with pharmacoresistant focal epilepsy: the PuLsE (Open Prospective Randomized Long-term Effectiveness) trial. Epilepsia 55(6):893–900. doi:10.1111/epi.12611
13. Aaronson ST, Carpenter LL, Conway CR, Reimherr FW, Lisanby SH, Schwartz TL, Moreno FA, Dunner DL, Lesem MD, Thompson PM, Husain M, Vine CJ, Banov MD, Bernstein LP, Lehman RB, Brannon GE, Keepers GA, O'Reardon JP, Rudolph RL, Bunker M (2013) Vagus nerve stimulation therapy randomized to different amounts of electrical charge for treatment-resistant depression: acute and chronic effects. Brain Stimul 6(4):631–640. doi:10.1016/j.brs.2012.09.013
14. Martelletti P, Jensen RH, Antal A, Arcioni R, Brighina F, de Tommaso M, Franzini A, Fontaine D, Heiland M, Jurgens TP, Leone M, Magis D, Paemeleire K, Palmisani S, Paulus W, May A, European Headache Foundation (2013) Neuromodulation of chronic headaches: position statement from the European Headache Federation. J Headache Pain 14:86. doi:10.1186/1129-2377-14-86
15. Sadler RM, Purdy RA, Rahey S (2002) Vagal nerve stimulation aborts migraine in patient with intractable epilepsy. Cephalalgia 22(6):482–484
16. Hord ED, Evans MS, Mueed S, Adamolekun B, Naritoku DK (2003) The effect of vagus nerve stimulation on migraines. J Pain 4(9):530–534
17. Lenaerts ME, Oommen KJ, Couch JR, Skaggs V (2008) Can vagus nerve stimulation help migraine? Cephalalgia 28(4):392–395. doi:10.1111/j.1468-2982.2008.01538.x
18. Mauskop A (2005) Vagus nerve stimulation relieves chronic refractory migraine and cluster headaches. Cephalalgia 25(2):82–86. doi:10.1111/j.1468-2982.2005.00611.x
19. Bossut DF, Maixner W (1996) Effects of cardiac vagal afferent electrostimulation on the responses of trigeminal and trigeminothalamic neurons to noxious orofacial stimulation. Pain 65(1):101–109
20. Beekwilder JP, Beems T (2010) Overview of the clinical applications of vagus nerve stimulation. J Clin Neurophysiol 27(2):130–138. doi:10.1097/WNP.0b013e3181d64d8a

21. Oshinsky ML, Murphy AL, Hekierski H Jr, Cooper M, Simon BJ (2014) Noninvasive vagus nerve stimulation as treatment for trigeminal allodynia. Pain 155(5):1037–1042. doi:10.1016/j.pain.2014.02.009

22. Ben-Menachem E, Revesz D, Simon BJ, Silberstein S (2015) Surgically implanted and non-invasive vagus nerve stimulation: a review of efficacy, safety and tolerability. Eur J Neurol 22(9):1260–1268. doi:10.1111/ene.12629

23. Kotagal P (2011) Neurostimulation: vagus nerve stimulation and beyond. Semin Pediatr Neurol 18(3):186–194. doi:10.1016/j.spen.2011.06.005

24. electroCore. News. Electrocore receives FDA approval for chronic migraine study. http://www.electrocore.com/electrocore-receives-fda-approval-for-chronic-migraine-study. Accessed September 14, 2014.

25. Goadsby PJ, Grosberg BM, Mauskop A, Cady R, Simmons KA (2014) Effect of noninvasive vagus nerve stimulation on acute migraine: an open-label pilot study. Cephalalgia 34(12):986–993. doi:10.1177/0333102414524494

26. Barbanti P, Grazzi L, Egeo G, Padovan AM, Liebler E, Bussone G (2015) Non-invasive vagus nerve stimulation for acute treatment of high-frequency and chronic migraine: an open-label study. J Headache Pain 16:61. doi:10.1186/s10194-015-0542-4

27. Kinfe TM, Pintea B, Guresir E, Vatter H (2015) Partial response of intractable cluster-tic syndrome treated by cervical non-invasive vagal nerve stimulation (nVNS). Brain Stimul 8(3):669–671. doi:10.1016/j.brs.2015.01.002

28. Nesbitt AD, Marin JC, Tompkins E, Ruttledge MH, Goadsby PJ (2015) Initial use of a novel noninvasive vagus nerve stimulator for cluster headache treatment. Neurology 84(12):1249–1253. doi:10.1212/WNL.0000000000001394

29. Gaul C, Diener HC, Silver N, Magis D, Reuter U, Andersson A, Liebler E, Straube A (2015) Non-invasive vagus nerve stimulation for PREVention and Acute treatment of chronic cluster headache (PREVA): a randomised controlled study. Published online September 21, 2015. http://cep.sagepub.com/content/early/2015/09/21/0333102415607070.full.pdf+html. Cephalalgia. doi:10.1177/0333102415607070

30. Buysse DJ, Reynolds CF 3rd, Monk TH, Berman SR, Kupfer DJ (1989) The Pittsburgh Sleep Quality Index: a new instrument for psychiatric practice and research. Psychiatry Res 28(2):193–213

31. Beck AT, Ward CH, Mendelson M, Mock J, Erbaugh J (1961) An inventory for measuring depression. Arch Gen Psychiatry 4:561–571

32. Midas Questionnaire. http://www.migraines.org/disability/pdfs/midas.pdf. Accessed October 2, 2015.

33. Bloudek LM, Stokes M, Buse DC, Wilcox TK, Lipton RB, Goadsby PJ, Varon SF, Blumenfeld AM, Katsarava Z, Pascual J, Lanteri-Minet M, Cortelli P, Martelletti P (2012) Cost of healthcare for patients with migraine in five European countries: results from the International Burden of Migraine Study (IBMS). J Headache Pain 13(5):361–378. doi:10.1007/s10194-012-0460-7

34. Meissner K, Fassler M, Rucker G, Kleijnen J, Hrobjartsson A, Schneider A, Antes G, Linde K (2013) Differential effectiveness of placebo treatments: a systematic review of migraine prophylaxis. JAMA Intern Med 173(21):1941–1951. doi:10.1001/jamainternmed.2013.10391

35. Straube A, Ellrich J, Eren O, Blum B, Ruscheweyh R (2015) Treatment of chronic migraine with transcutaneous stimulation of the auricular branch of the vagal nerve (auricular t-VNS): a randomized, monocentric clinical trial. J Headache Pain 16(1):543. doi:10.1186/s10194-015-0543-3

36. Schoenen J, Vandersmissen B, Jeangette S, Herroelen L, Vandenheede M, Gerard P, Magis D (2013) Migraine prevention with a supraorbital transcutaneous stimulator: a randomized controlled trial. Neurology 80(8):697–704. doi:10.1212/WNL.0b013e3182825055

37. Goadsby PJ (2000) The pharmacology of headache. Prog Neurobiol 62(5):509–525

38. Ferrari MD, Roon KI, Lipton RB, Goadsby PJ (2001) Oral triptans (serotonin 5-HT(1B/1D) agonists) in acute migraine treatment: a meta-analysis of 53 trials. Lancet 358(9294):1668–1675. doi:10.1016/S0140-6736(01)06711-3

39. Dodick D, Lipton RB, Martin V, Papademetriou V, Rosamond W, MaassenVanDenBrink A, Loutfi H, Welch KM, Goadsby PJ, Hahn S, Hutchinson S, Matchar D, Silberstein S, Smith TR, Purdy RA, Saiers J, Triptan Cardiovascular Safety Expert Panel (2004) Consensus statement: cardiovascular safety profile of triptans (5-HT agonists) in the acute treatment of migraine. Headache 44(5):414–425. doi:10.1111/j.1526-4610.2004.04078.x

40. Saper JR, Da Silva AN (2013) Medication overuse headache: history, features, prevention and management strategies. CNS Drugs 27(11):867–877. doi:10.1007/s40263-013-0081-y

41. Chae JH, Nahas Z, Lomarev M, Denslow S, Lorberbaum JP, Bohning DE, George MS (2003) A review of functional neuroimaging studies of vagus nerve stimulation (VNS). J Psychiatr Res 37(6):443–455

42. Chen SP, Ay I, Lopes de Morais A, Qin T, Zheng Y, Sadhegian H, Oka F, Simon B, Elkermann-Haerter K, Ayata C (2015) Vagus nerve stimulation inhibits cortical spreading depression. Pain. [published online November 25, 2015].

43. Multon S, Schoenen J (2005) Pain control by vagus nerve stimulation: from animal to man…and back. Acta Neurol Belg 105(2):62–67

44. Schwedt TJ, Chiang CC, Chong CD, Dodick DW (2015) Functional MRI of migraine. Lancet Neurol 14(1):81–91. doi:10.1016/S1474-4422(14)70193-0

45. Coppola G, Vandenheede M, Di Clemente L, Ambrosini A, Fumal A, De Pasqua V, Schoenen J (2005) Somatosensory evoked high-frequency oscillations reflecting thalamo-cortical activity are decreased in migraine patients between attacks. Brain 128(Pt 1):98–103. doi:10.1093/brain/awh334

46. Cui Y, Kataoka Y, Watanabe Y (2014) Role of cortical spreading depression in the pathophysiology of migraine. Neurosci Bull 30(5):812–822. doi:10.1007/s12264-014-1471-y

47. Verlinden TJ, Rijkers K, Hoogland G, Herrler A (2015) Morphology of the human cervical vagus nerve: implications for vagus nerve stimulation treatment. Acta Neurol Scand. doi:10.1111/ane.12462

12

Altered functional connectivity of the marginal division in migraine: a resting-state fMRI study

Zhiye Chen[1,2], Xiaoyan Chen[2], Mengqi Liu[1], Shuangfeng Liu[1], Siyun Shu[3], Lin Ma[1] and Shengyuan Yu[2*]

Abstract

Background: The marginal division of neostriatum (MrD) is a flat, pan-shaped zone between the neostriatum and the globus pallidus, and previous documents demonstrated that it was involved in the modulation of pain. The aim of this study is to investigate the roles of the MrD of the human brain in the chronicization migraine using resting state functional magnetic resonance imaging (rs-fMRI).

Methods: Conventional MRI, 3D structure images, and rs-fMRI were performed in 18 patients with episodic migraines (EM), 16 patients with chronic migraine (CM), 44 patients with medication overuse headache plus chronic migraine (MOH + CM), and 32 normal controls (NC). MrD was defined using manual delineation on structural images, and was selected as the seed to calculate the functional connectivity (FC).

Results: Compared with the NC group, the decreased FC of MrD was observed in the EM and CM groups, and increased FC of MrD was demonstrated in all patient groups. Compared with the EM group, the decreased FC of MrD was revealed in the CM and MOH + CM groups, and the increased FC occurred only in the CM group. Increased FC of MrD alone was observed in the MOH + CM group compared with that in the CM group.

Conclusion: This study confirmed the double neuromodulation network of MrD in pain modulation and migraine chronicization; however, the mechanism requires further investigation.

Keywords: Migraine, Marginal division of the neostriatum, fMRI, Functional connectivity

Background

The marginal division of neostriatum (MrD) is a flat, pan-shaped zone between the neostriatum and the globus pallidus, consisting of spindle-shaped neurons and some special connections [1, 2]. This area was first discovered at the caudal border of the striatum and the surrounding areas on the rostral edge of the globus pallidus in rat brains using histochemical techniques in 1988 [1]. Gradually more relevant papers were published, some of which demonstrated that this region was rich in neurotransmitters [3–5] and might also play an important role in learning and memory [2, 6–8].

In addition, neurophysiological studies showed that MrD was involved in the modulation of pain due to

nociceptive neurons localized exclusively in rat striatums [9, 10]. Substance P, an important neuropeptide in the MrD, plays a key role in learning and memory [11], which is also related to headache [12]. The rats with lesions of the MrD induced by kainic acid experienced altered perception of neuropathic pain behaviors. This may also be associated with the evident increased substance P in the ipsilateral spinal cord dorsal horn [13]. Mu opioid receptors (MORs) are localized in the MrD, and it is one member of the seven transmembrane family of G-protein coupled receptors, which may underlie pain and analgesia in the MrD of rat striatum [14]. To date, however, it has remained unknown whether and how MrD participates in pain modulation in the human brain in vivo.

Brain imaging and imaging analysis techniques can provide a possibility to explore and evaluate MrD in vivo in the human brain. A current study demonstrated that

* Correspondence: yusy1963@126.com
[2]Department of Neurology, Chinese PLA General Hospital, Beijing 100853, China
Full list of author information is available at the end of the article

altered functional connectivity of MrD was shown in Alzheimer's disease by using resting state functional MRI (rs-fMRI) [15]. In our previous studies, this method was used to investigate the age and gender effects of functional connectivity of MrD for the normal subjects [16, 17]. In clinical practice, the decreased functional connectivity of MrD was demonstrated in a patient with right extremity pain caused by a malacia lesion in the left putamen using rs-fMRI, which suggested that the MrD may contribute to the pain modulation [18].

The aim of this study is to investigate the roles of MrD in the chronicization of migraine using rs-fMRI. We hypothesized that MrD was involved in the pain modulation in headache, and that the decreased functional connectivity of MrD would generate the pain and might be the cause of migraine, while the increased functional connectivity of MrD would be complementary for pain and might compensate the dysfunction of MrD neuromodulation. To address this hypothesis, we obtained functional MR images for normal controls (NC), episodic migraine (EM) patients, chronic migraine (CM) patients, and medication overuse headache plus with chronic migraine (MOH + CM) patients. Firstly, the functional connectivity of MrD was performed with within-group analysis to explore the functional connectivity pattern of different subtypes of headache. Secondly, the between-group analysis was performed between the headache groups and the NC group to explore the varying functional connectivity in the different subtypes of headache. Lastly, between-groups analysis was performed among the different subtypes of headache to explore the altered pattern of functional connectivity.

Method
Subjects
One hundred and ten subjects were recruited, including 18 EM patients, 16 CM patients, 44 MOH + CM patients, and 32 NCs. Patients were recruited from the International Headache Center, Department of Neurology, Chinese PLA General Hospital. All the following inclusion criteria should be fulfilled: 1) diagnosis of 1.3 CM, 8.2 MOH, and 1.1 and 1.2 migraine based on the International Classification of Headache Disorders, third Edition (beta version) (ICHD-III beta) [19]; 2) no migraine preventive medication used in the past 3 months; 3) age between 20 and 60 years; 4) right-handed; 5) absence of any chronic disorders, including hypertension, hypercholesterolemia, diabetes mellitus, cardiovascular diseases, cerebrovascular disorders, neoplastic diseases, infectious diseases, connective tissue diseases, other subtypes of headache, chronic pain other than headache, severe anxiety or depression preceding the onset of headache, psychiatric diseases, etc.; 6) absence of alcohol, nicotine, or other substance abuse; and 7) patient's willingness to engage in the study. NCs were recruited from the hospital's staff and their relatives. Inclusion criteria were similar to those of patients, except for the first two items. NCs should never have had any primary headache disorders or other types of headache in the past year. General demographic and headache information were registered and evaluated in our headache database. Additionally, we evaluated anxiety, depression, and cognitive function of all the participants by using the Hamilton Anxiety Scale (HAMA) [20], the Hamilton Depression Scale (HAMD) [21], the Chinese version of Mini-Mental State Examination (MMSE), and the Montreal Cognitive Assessment (MoCA) Beijing Version (www.mocatest.org). The exclusion criteria were the following: cranium trauma, illness interfering with central nervous system function, psychotic disorder, and regular use of a psychoactive or hormone medication. The study protocol was approved by the Ethical Committee of Chinese PLA General Hospital and complied with the Declaration of Helsinki. Informed consent was obtained from all participants before the study. MRI scans were taken in the interictal stage at least 3 days after a migraine attack for EM patients. All the subjects were right-handed and underwent conventional MRI examination to exclude the subjects with cerebral infarction, malacia, or occupying lesions. Alcohol, nicotine, caffeine, and other substances were avoided for at least 12 h before MRI examination.

MRI acquisition
Images were acquired on a GE 3.0T MR system (DISCOVERY MR750, GE Healthcare, Milwaukee, WI, USA) and a conventional eight-channel quadrature head coil was used. All subjects were instructed to lie in a supine position, and formed padding was used to limit head movement. Conventional T2-weighted image (TR = 5000 ms, TE = 113.4 ms, FOV = 24 cm × 24 cm, Matrix = 384 × 384) and T1-FLAIR (TR = 2040 ms, TE = 6.9 ms, FOV = 24 cm × 24 cm, Matrix = 384 × 256) were obtained first. Then, the rs-fMRI was performed, during which subjects were instructed to relax, keep their eyes closed, stay awake, remain still, and clear their heads of all thoughts. Functional images were obtained using a gradient echo-planar imaging (EPI) sequence (TR = 2000 ms, TE = 30 ms, flip angle = 90, slice thickness = 3 mm, slice gap = 1 mm, FOV = 24 cm × 24 cm, Matrix = 64 × 64), and 180 continuous EPI functional volumes were acquired axially over 6 min. Finally, a high resolution three-dimensional T1-weighted fast spoiled gradient recalled echo (3D T1-FSPGR) sequence was performed, which generated 360 contiguous axial slices [TR (repetition time) = 6.3 ms, TE (echo time) = 2.8 ms, flip angle = 15°, FOV (field of view) = 25.6 cm × 25.6 cm, Matrix = 256 × 256, slice thickness = 1 mm]. None of the subjects complained of any discomfort or fell

asleep during scanning. No obvious structural damage was observed based on the conventional MR images.

Data processing

All MR structural and functional images were processed using Statistical Parametric Mapping 8 (SPM8) (http://www.fil.ion.ucl.ac.uk/spm) and the rs-fMRI data analysis toolkit (REST v1.8) [22] running under MATLAB 7.6 (The Mathworks, Natick, MA, USA).

The data preprocessing was carried out as follows: (1) The first ten volumes of each functional time course was discarded to allow for T1 equilibrium and the participants to adapt; (2) Slice timing; (3) Head motion correction; (4) Spatial normalization. These steps were performed by SPM8. No subjects had head motion with more than 1.5 mm displacement in X, Y, and Z direction or 1.5^0 of any angular motion throughout the course of the scanning. The linear trend removal and temporal band-pass filtering (0.01–0.08 Hz) was performed by REST [22].

The functional connectivity analysis was performed as follows: (1) Spatial smooth (full width at half maximum (FWHM) = 6 mm) using SPM8; (2) MrD was defined using manual delineation on a *ch2bet* template in MRIcron software (v6.6, www.mricro.com) (Fig. 1); (3) Functional connectivity computation of the left and right MrD were performed using REST (v1.8). The time courses of bilateral MrD were extracted, and Pearson's correlations were used to calculate the functional connectivity between the extracted time courses and the averaged time courses of the whole brain in a voxel-wise manner. The white matter, cerebrospinal fluid (CSF), and the six head motion parameters were used as covariates. (4) The individual r-maps were normalized to Z-maps using Fisher's Z-transformation.

Statistical analysis

One-way analysis of variance (ANOVA) was applied to the comparison of the age, BMI, education, migraine duration, headache frequency, pain intensity, medication intake, HAMA, HAMD, MMSE, and MoCA score. An independent sample t-test was applied to the comparison of the duration of headache chronicity/medication between the CM and MOH + CM groups. Significant difference was set at a P value of < 0.05. The statistical analysis was performed using SPSS 19.0.

One-sample t-tests were performed using the functional connectivity Z-maps to detect the regions with significant functional connectivity of MrD. Analysis of covariance (ANCOVA) tests were performed to identify the regions with significant differences in connectivity to MrD among groups, covarying for age, gender, and education. Significance was set at a P value of <0.001 without correction. The minimal number of contiguous voxels was set at 10. The statistical analysis was performed by SPM 8 software.

Results

Demography and neuropsychological test

Demographic and clinical data are summarized in Table 1. One hundred and ten subjects were included in our study, comprising 44 patients with MOH + CM (35 females, nine males, mean age 42.3 ± 9.6 years), 16 patients with CM (12 females, four males, mean age 42.4 ± 8.7 years), 18 patients with EM (14 females, four males, mean age 37.8 ± 7.9 years), and 32 NCs (24 females, eight males, mean age 41.3 ± 10.8 years). Although the age of the EM group tended to be lower than that of the other three groups, there was no significant difference for gender and age among groups. Body mass index (BMI) was significantly higher in the CM group than that of the EM and NC groups, and it was also higher in the MOH + CM group than in the EM group, using ANCOVA analysis with age as the covariance. The education level of the MOH + CM and CM groups was significantly lower than that of the EM and NC groups. We defined education in 6 levels from illiterate to master or higher as grades 1 to 6.

The mean years of migraine was significantly higher in the MOH + CM group (mean 17.8 ± 9.1 years) than that in the CM (11.3 ± 9.3 years) and EM (12.4 ± 8.1 years) groups. Headache frequency was significantly higher in

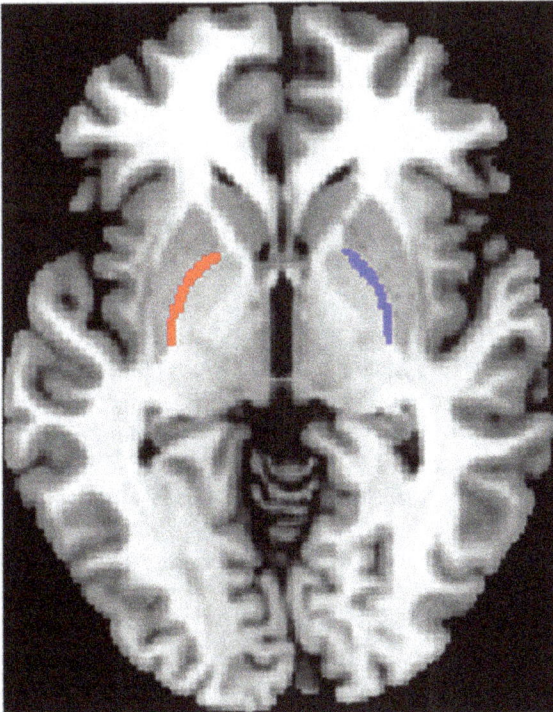

Fig. 1 Bilateral marginal divison was created by manual drawing based on ch2bet template in MRIcron software

Table 1 Demographic information of the subjects (mean ± SD)

	EM	CM	MOH + CM	NC	p value
N (F/M)	18 (14/4)	16 (12/4)	44 (35/9)	32 (24/8)	0.97
Age (years)	33.4 ± 11.0**	42.4 ± 8.7	42.3 ± 9.6	41.3 ± 10.8	0.01
Body mass index	21.3 ± 0.7	24.4 ± 0.7*	23.1 ± 0.4	22.5 ± 0.5	0.01
Education	4.4 ± 1.1	3.4 ± 1.3**	3.1 ± 1.2**	4.7 ± 1.0	0.00
Migraine duration (years)	12.4 ± 8.1	11.3 ± 9.3	17.8 ± 9.1*	-	0.02
Headache frequency (days/month)	3.5 ± 2.7	25.1 ± 5.9**	26.5 ± 5.0**	-	0.00
Pain intensity (VAS)	8.3 ± 1.5	7.9 ± 1.5	8.0 ± 1.4	-	0.46
Duration of headache chronicity/medication overuse (years)	-	3.0 ± 3.3	4.7 ± 4.8	-	0.20
Medication intake	4.9 ± 3.7	4.3 ± 3.8	119.7 ± 111.6**	-	0.00
HAMA	15.7 ± 9.9**	21.6 ± 10.9**	18.5 ± 8.7**	2.4 ± 1.5	0.00
HAMD	10.9 ± 7.3**	16.3 ± 10.5**	19.9 ± 11.9**	1.1 ± 0.9	0.00
MMSE (adjusted by education)	28.5 ± 0.7	26.9 ± 0.7	27.1 ± 0.5	28.3 ± 0.6	0.22
MoCA (adjusted by education)	26.1 ± 0.8	23.5 ± 0.9**	24.8 ± 0.6*	26.9 ± 0.7	0.02

* *VAS* visual anologue score, *HAMA* Hamilton anxiety scale, *HAMD* Hamilton depression scale, *MMSE* mini-mental state examination, *MoCA* the Montreal cognitive assessment, *EM* episodic migraine, *CM* chronic migraine, *MOH + CM* medication overuse headache plus with chronic migraine *:compared to NCs $P < 0.05$;**:-compared to NCs $P < 0.01$

the MOH + CM (mean headache days per month 26.5 ± 5.0) and CM (25.1 ± 5.9) groups than that in the EM group (3.5 ± 2.7). There was no significant difference in chronic headache duration between the MOH + CM group and the CM group or in pain intensity between the patient groups. The MOH + CM group took much more medication (mean number of pills per month 119.7 ± 111.6) than the CM (4.3 ± 3.8) and EM (4.9 ± 3.7) groups. The types of overused medication by MOH + CM patients included simple analgesics (3/44), triptan (1/44), opioids (1/44), combination analgesics (33/44), and multiple drug classes (6/44). CM patients and EM patients most frequently took combination analgesics as painkiller. None of the migraine patients regularly took preventive medication during the past 3 months.

Anxiety and depression scores were significantly higher in the three headache groups than that in NC group. The MOH + CM group showed a higher depression score, and the CM group showed a higher anxiety score than the EM group ($P < 0.05$). Cognitive function showed no significant difference among groups evaluated by MMSE but declined in the MOH + CM (mean score 24.8 ± 0.6) and CM (23.5 ± 0.9) groups compared with the NC group when evaluated by MoCA.

Functional connectivity of MrD - within-group analysis
Within-group analysis was performed, and a false discovery rate (FDR) was used with a p value set at < 0.05 with an extended threshold of 10 voxels. Regions with connectivity to MrD in each of the groups were acquired, and the functional connectivity maps were marked on the SPM8 T1 template.

Regions with positive functional connectivity of MrD were mainly in the bilateral basal ganglion regions, thalamus, insula, hippocampus, and right medial frontal orbital cortex, and the regions of negative functional connectivity of MrD were in the bilateral temporal lobes and middle frontal lobes in the NC group (Fig. 2).

In the EM group, regions with positive functional connectivity were mainly located in bilateral basal ganglion regions, and no evident negative functional connectivity was observed (Fig. 2).

In the CM and MOH + CM groups, regions with positive functional connectivity were located in bilateral basal ganglion regions. The regions with negative functional connectivity in the MOH + CM group were larger compared with the CM group, which were located in the bilateral middle frontal gyrus, cingulum, and right temporal lobes (Fig. 2).

Comparison of functional connectivity of MrD between the migraine groups and NC group
Table 2 shows the altered functional connectivity of MrD in migraineurs compared with NCs. In the EM group, the brain regions with decreased functional connectivity were mainly located in the right insula, and the brain regions with increased functional connectivity were mainly located in the right precentral gyrus and anterior cingulate cortex (ACC) (Fig. 3). In the CM group, the decreased functional connectivity of MrD was observed in the right cuneus and left middle cingulum cortex (MCC), and the increased functional connectivity was detected in the bilateral middle frontal gyrus, left hippocampus, and middle temporal gyrus (Fig. 3).

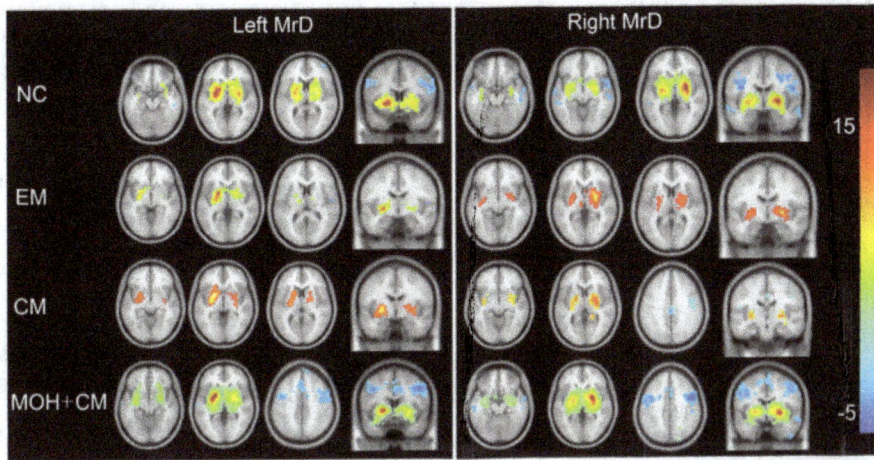

Fig. 2 MrD functional connectivity averaged over subject in the brain. Warm and cool colors represent positive and negative correlations. NC, normal control; EM, episodic migraine; CM, chronic migraine; MOH+CM, medication overuse headache plus chronic migraine;L, *left* MrD; R, *right* MrD

Interestingly, the decreased functional connectivity of MrD could not be observed in the MOH + CM group, while the increased functional connectivity was demonstrated in the left parahippocampus, right middle frontal gyrus, and inferior temporal gyrus (Fig. 3).

Comparison of functional connectivity of MrD among the CM, MOH + CM, and EM groups

Table 3 presents the altered functional connectivity of MrD among the CM, MOH + CM, and EM groups. Decreased functional connectivity of MrD was detected

Table 2 Comparison of functional connectivity of MrD between headache group and HC group

Group	Brain region	k value	P value	T value	x	y	z
EM vs. NC							
EM<NC							
Left	Insula_R	27	0.000	4.2	36	21	6
Right	Insula_R	23	0.000	4.3	33	18	6
EM>NC							
Left	Precentral_R	13	0.000	4.5	42	−15	36
Right	Cingulum_Ant_R	17	0.000	4.4	12	45	21
CM vs. NC							
CM<NC							
Left	Cuneus_R	10	0.000	4.7	9	−90	30
Right	Cingulum_Mid_L	66	0.000	5.7	0	−27	39
CM>NC							
Left	Frontal_Mid_L	21	0.000	4.52	−45	15	45
	Hippocampus_L	12	0.000	4.06	−30	−39	0
	Frontal_Mid_R	51	0.000	4.05	48	24	42
Right	Temporal_Mid_L	15	0.000	4.35	−54	3	−21
MOH + CMvs. NC							
MOH + CM>NC							
Left	Frontal_Mid_R	10	0.000	3.87	48	30	39
Right	Temporal_inf_R	12	0.000	4.56	48	−39	−21
	ParaHippocampa_L	18	0.000	4.42	−18	−21	−24

R right hemisphere, *L* left hemisphere, *Ant* anterior, *Mid* middle

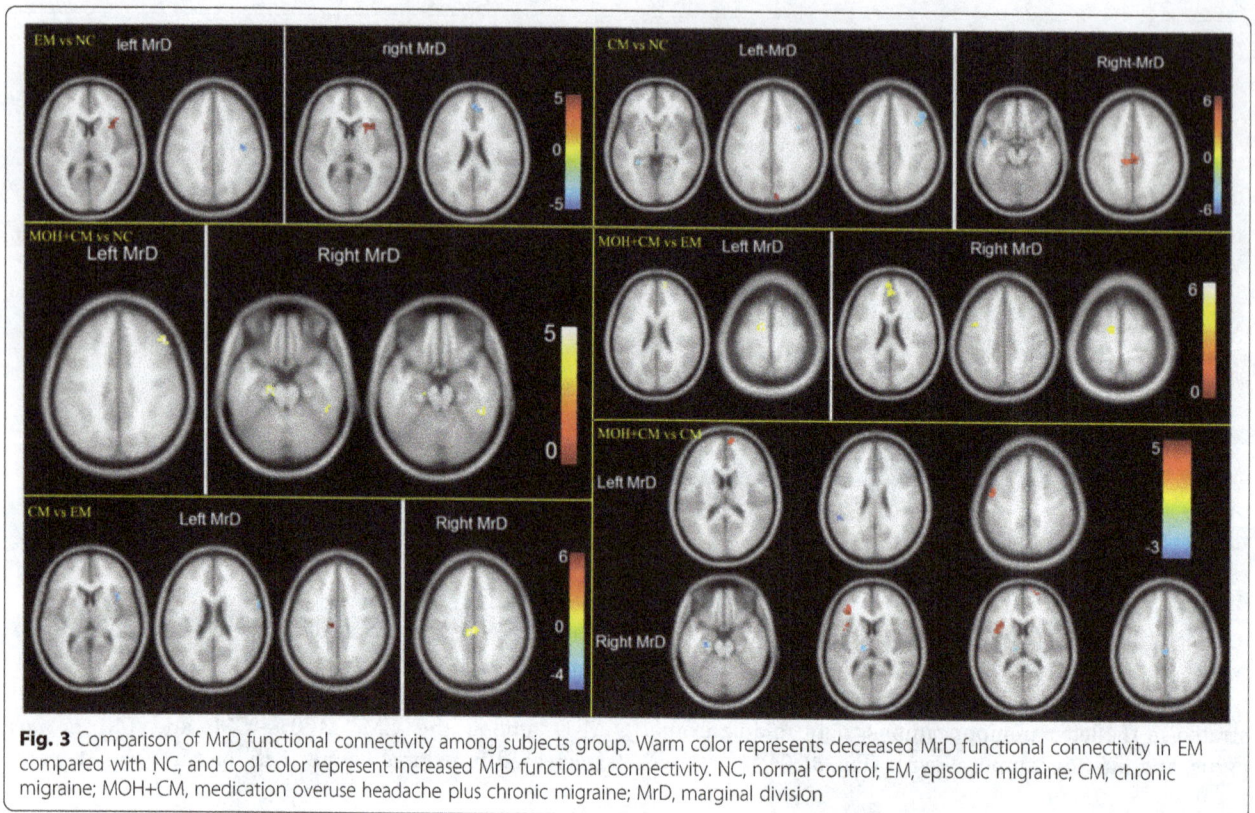

Fig. 3 Comparison of MrD functional connectivity among subjects group. Warm color represents decreased MrD functional connectivity in EM compared with NC, and cool color represent increased MrD functional connectivity. NC, normal control; EM, episodic migraine; CM, chronic migraine; MOH+CM, medication overuse headache plus chronic migraine; MrD, marginal division

in the left middle cingulum, and increased functional connectivity was observed in the right insula and precentral gyrus in the CM group compared with the EM group (Fig. 3).

In the MOH + CM group, decreased functional connectivity of MrD was demonstrated in the bilateral medial superior frontal gyrus, left precentral gyrus, and supplementary motor area compared with the EM group (Fig. 3). No increased functional connectivity of MrD was observed.

The decreased functional connectivity of MrD was detected in the left precentral gyrus, the triangular part of the inferior frontal gyrus, the insula, the right medial superior frontal gyrus, and the superior frontal gyrus, and increased functional connectivity was observed in the left superior temporal gyrus, hippocampus, thalamus, and right middle cingulum in the MOH + CM group compared with the CM group (Fig. 3, 4).

Discussion

Migraines are a common type of primary headaches with a reported prevalence of approximately 5.7 % in men and 17.0 % in women [23]. In China, the prevalence of migraine is 9.3 % of the general population [24]. Migraines are also a major cause of chronic headaches, with approximately 2.5 % of EM transformed to new-onset CM [25]. The prevalence rate of CM is 2 to 4 % of the general population [25], and that of MOH is 1 to 4 %

of the general population [26]. Therefore, chronicization of migraine is a worthy topic of further investigation.

The brain regions related with pain processing and modulation mainly included the prefrontal cortex, basal ganglia, thalamus, cingulate cortex, insula, cerebellum [27], and periaqueductal gray matter [28]. In this study, MrD was investigated to reveal its key roles in migraine chronicization using rs-fMRI.

Functional connectivity is actually the correlation analysis between the brain regions with MrD over the whole brain. The normal brain structure includes positive and negative functional connectivity to maintain the brain's functional balance. Altered functional connectivity may indicate the intrinsic pathophysiological changes for different brain disorders.

In this study, it was demonstrated that there was functional connectivity between other brain regions and MrD in the NCs and the patients with migraine. The normal connectivity pattern, such the positive associations with the bilateral basal ganglion nuclei, thalamus, insula, hippocampus, and medial frontal orbital cortex, and the negative associations with bilateral temporal lobes and middle frontal lobes, indicated that MrD was an important subcortical center. Previous report referred to it as a subcortical memory center. Interestingly, we found that MrD was also a subcortical pain center due to positive and negative associations with multiple brain

Table 3 Comparison of functional connectivity of MrD among CM group, MOH + CM group and EM group

Groups	Brain region	k value	P value	T value	x	y	z
CM vs. EM							
CM<EM							
Left	Cingulum_Mid_L	10	0.000	3.9	−9	−24	39
Right	Cingulum_Mid_L	42	0.000	5.0	−6	−27	39
CM>EM							
Left	Insula_R	17	0.000	5.0	39	15	6
	Precentral_R	12	0.000	4.7	66	3	21
MOH + CM vs.EM							
MOH + CM<EM							
Left	Frontal_Sup_Media_R	15	0.000	4.4	12	60	24
	Supp_Motor_Area_L	13	0.000	4.3	−12	−9	69
Right	Frontal_Sup_Media_L	53	0.000	5.1	−3	60	18
	Supp_Motor_Area_L	24	0.000	4.1	−9	−12	66
	Precentral_L	12	0.000	3.8	−39	0	45
MOH + CMvs.CM							
MOH + CM<CM							
Left	Precentral_L	19	0.000	4.9	−45	0	51
	Frontal_Sup_Media_R	11	0.000	4.4	9	60	18
Right	Frontal_Inf_Tri_L	16	0.000	4.8	−36	33	9
	Insula_L	42	0.000	4.6	−33	18	12
	Frontal_Sup_R	10	0.000	3.8	21	63	12
MOH + CM>CM							
Left	Temporal_Sup_L	10	0.000	3.9	−48	−42	24
Right	Hippocampus_L	13	0.000	4.8	−27	−18	−18
	Cingulum_Mid_R	14	0.000	4.1	3	−27	33
	Thalamus_L	10	0.000	3.7	−15	−18	9

R right hemisphere, L left hemisphere, Ant anterior, Mid middle, Media medial, Sup superior, Inf inferior, Tri triangular part

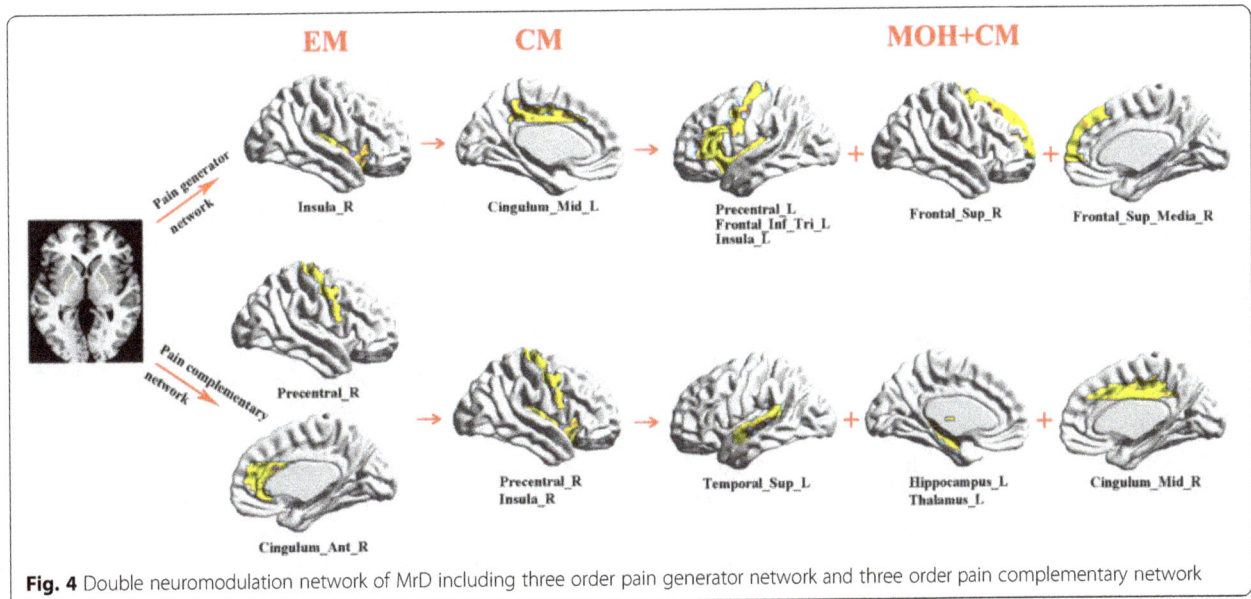

Fig. 4 Double neuromodulation network of MrD including three order pain generator network and three order pain complementary network

regions in different subtypes of headache. In this study, only the positive connectivity was demonstrated in the EM group, and both the positive and negative connectivities were confirmed in the CM and MOH + CM groups, which suggested that MrD demonstrated different pain modulation patterns in different subtypes of headache.

Between-groups analysis showed altered intrinsic functional connectivity in different subtypes of headache compared with NCs. The decreased functional connectivity of MrD was located in the right insula in the EM group, which was a component of the pain matrix. The insula seemed to play a leading role in the triggering of pain matrix network, and resulted in the subjective pain experience [29]. fMRI also demonstrated that the insula could process emotion and sensory-discriminative aspects of pain perception [30]. The impaired functional connectivity between MrD and the insula might disturb the balance of pain modulation of the insula in EM patients. Simultaneously, the functional connectivity was strengthened between the right precentral gyrus and the anterior cingulum cortex (ACC) and MrD. The increased connectivity could be understood as a positive feedback to maintain the concordance of the pain matrix network.

Compared with NCs, decreased functional connectivity was observed in the right cuneus and left middle cingulum in the CM group, which suggested that the cuneus and middle cingulum may be signature brain structures in chronic migraine, and may contribute to migraine chronicization. The cuneus is related to visual information processing [31], is responsible for the integration of the somatosensory information with other sensory stimuli and cognitive process [32], and could be activated with other pain-related brain regions [33]. The decreased functional connectivity between MrD and the cuneus may impair this integration, and facilitate migraine chronicization. The decreased functional connectivity between MrD and MCC was a new finding in CM patients compared previous studies [34–37] in which only the ACC was related to pain modulation, and the posterior cingulum cortex (PCC) was related to pain processing and cognitive impairment in migraineurs. The increased functional connectivity of MrD in the bilateral middle frontal gyrus, left hippocampus, and middle temporal gyrus indicated a dynamic compensation for the dysfunction of the pain-related brain regions in CM patients.

Only increased functional connectivity was confirmed in the left parahippocampus and right middle frontal and inferior temporal gyrus in the MOH + CM group, which indicated that the dysfunction of MrD could not be detected. The reasons for this may be explained as follows: (1) The negative functional connectivity of MrD was activated, and the impaired MrD network was compensated and strengthened; (2) Medication overuse may inhibit the modulation function of MrD and provide some protection for MrD. Therefore, the impairment of MrD connectivity was avoided. (3) The brain regions with increased functional connectivity may contribute to pain integration and protect the pain matrix.

Comparison of functional connectivity among different subtypes of headache demonstrated that MrD played a key role in migraine chronicization. The decreased functional connectivity of MrD could be detected from EM to CM, from EM to MOH + CM, and from CM to MOH + CM. Additionally, the increased FM could also be detected from EM to CM and from CM to MOH + CM. However, the increased functional connectivity was not revealed from EM to MOH + CM. The decreased connectivity pattern revealed the dysfunction of MrD, which could explain the role of MrD in migraine chronicization. Therefore, MrD can be regarded as a subcortical pain center. The increased connectivity indicated that MrD could maintain the concordance of the pain matrix network.

On the basis of rs-fMRI findings, it can be speculated that MrD plays a double role in the neuromodulation of migraine (Fig. 4). One type of neuromodulation is the negative pain network, which includes three-order pain generating networks, and the functional connectivity is decreased among these networks. The first-order pain generating network is the right insula, which is the EM generator (EMG) and demonstrates decreased functional connectivity with MrD. The second-order pain generating network is the left middle cingulate cortex (MCC), which is the CM generator (CMG) and also demonstrates decreased functional connectivity with MrD. These findings also suggested that the left MCC played a key role in migraine chronicization. The last-order pain-generating network is the MOH + CM generator (MOHG). This order pain network mainly included two brain regions: (1) the right superior frontal gyrus and medial superior frontal gyrus; (2) the left precentral gyrus, left pars triangularis of inferior frontal gyrus, and left insula.

The other neuromodulation is the positive pain network, which includes three-order pain complementary networks and the functional connectivity was strengthened among these networks. The first-order pain complementary network is located in the right precentral gyrus and right ACC, which may repair the dysfunction of MrD neuromodulation in EM patients. The second-order pain complementary network is mainly revealed in the right precentral gyrus and right insula, which could compensate for the dysfunction of MrD neuromodulation and prevent migraine chronicization. The last-order pain complementary network is involved in the left superior temporal gyrus, left hippocampus, left thalamus, and right MCC. These brain regions may improve the state of the pain network in MOH + CM patients.

The double neuromodulation network of MrD indicated that the three-order pain generating network and the three-order pain complementary network were the important neuromodulation patterns of MrD in migraines. The involved specific brain regions could be considered as target pain network biomarkers, and early-warning signals of neuromodulation in different subtypes of migraine.

There were some limitations in the present study. First, this study was a cross-sectional study, and the sample sizes of the EM and CM groups were relatively small. Future studies are needed to carry out longitudinal analysis to dynamically observe migraine chronicization and the real roles of MrD in this process. Second, task-based fMRIs should be performed to identify the key roles of MrD in pain modulation and transformation.

Conclusions

This study is the first to characterize the roles of MrD in the different subtypes of headache using rs-fMRI. The major findings are that the FC of MrD was demonstrated in the different subtypes of headache, and altered FC was revealed among different groups. These data indicated that MrD may play an important role in pain modulation and migraine chronicization, and the mechanism requires further investigation.

Abbreviations
CM: Chronic migraine; EM: Episodic migraine; MOH: Medication overuse headache; MrD: Marginal division; NC: Normal control

Acknowledgments
This work was supported by the National Natural Sciences Foundation of China (81371514), Special Financial Grant from the China Postdoctoral Science Foundation (2014 T70960) and the Foundation for Medical and health Sci & Tech innovation Project of Sanya (2016YW37).

Authors' contributions
Category 1: (a) Conception and Design: LM; SYS; SYY. (b) Acquisition of Data: ZYC; MQL; SFL; XYC. (c) Analysis and Interpretation of Data: ZYC. Category 2: (a) Drafting the Article: ZYC. (b) Revising It for Intellectual Content: LM; SYY. All authors read and approved the final manuscript.

Competing interests
The authors declare that they have no competing interests.

Author details
[1]Department of Radiology, Chinese PLA General Hospital, Beijing 100853, China. [2]Department of Neurology, Chinese PLA General Hospital, Beijing 100853, China. [3]Institute of Cognitive Neuroscience, South China Normal University, Guangzhou 510631, China.

References
1. Shu SY, Penny GR, Peterson GM (1988) The 'marginal division': a new subdivision in the neostriatum of the rat. J Chem Neuroanat 1:147–163
2. Shu SY, Bao X, Li S, Niu D, Xu Z, Li Y (1999) A new subdivision of mammalian neostriatum with functional implications to learning and memory. J Neurosci Res 58:242–253
3. Shu SY, McGinty JF, Peterson GM (1990) High density of zinc-containing and dynorphin B- and substance P-immunoreactive terminals in the marginal division of the rat striatum. Brain Res Bull 24:201–205
4. Shu SY, Bao XM, Zhang X (1991) Ultrastructural characteristics of substance P-immunoreactive terminals in marginal division of rat striatum. Chin Med J (Engl) 104:887–896
5. Talley EM, Rosin DL, Lee A, Guyenet PG, Lynch KR (1996) Distribution of alpha 2A-adrenergic receptor-like immunoreactivity in the rat central nervous system. J Comp Neurol 372:111–134
6. Shu SY, Wu YM, Bao XM, Wen ZB, Huang FH, Li SX, Fu QZ, Ning Q (2002) A new area in the human brain associated with learning and memory: immunohistochemical and functional MRI analysis. Mol Psychiatry 7:1018–1022
7. Wu YM, Shu SY, Bao XM, Wen ZB, Huang FH, Yang WK, Liu YH (2002) Role of the marginal division of human neostriatum in working memory capacity for numbers received through hearing: a functional magnetic resonance imaging study. Di Yi Jun Yi Da Xue Xue Bao 22:1096–1098
8. Zhang ZQ, Shu SY, Liu SH, Guo ZY, Wu YM, Bao XM, Zheng JL, Ma HZ (2008) Activated brain areas during simple and complex mental calculationjA functional MRI study. Sheng Li Xue Bao 60:504–510
9. Chudler EH, Dong WK (1995) The role of the basal ganglia in nociception and pain. Pain 60:3–38
10. Chudler EH, Sugiyama K, Dong WK (1993) Nociceptive responses in the neostriatum and globus pallidus of the anesthetized rat. J Neurophysiol 69: 1890–1903
11. Liu XM, Shu SY, Zeng CC, Cai YF, Zhang KH, Wang CX, Fang J (2011) The role of substance P in the marginal division of the neostriatum in learning and memory is mediated through the neurokinin 1 receptor in rats. Neurochem Res 36:1896–1902
12. Clark JW, Solomon GD, Senanayake PD, Gallagher C (1996) Substance P concentration and history of headache in relation to postlumbar puncture headache: towards prevention. J Neurol Neurosurg Psychiatry 60:681–683
13. Ma Y, Zhou C, Li G, Tian Y, Liu J, Yan L, Jiang Y, Tian S (2015) Effects on Spatial Cognition and Nociceptive Behavior Following Peripheral Nerve Injury in Rats with Lesion of the Striatal Marginal Division Induced by Kainic Acid. Neurochem Res 40:2357–2364
14. Wang C, Shu SY, Guo Z, Cai YF, Bao X, Zeng C, Wu B, Hu Z, Liu X (2011) Immunohistochemical localization of mu opioid receptor in the marginal division with comparison to patches in the neostriatum of the rat brain. J Biomed Sci 18:34
15. Zhang Z, Liu Y, Zhou B, Zheng J, Yao H, An N, Wang P, Guo Y, Dai H, Wang L, Shu S, Zhang X, Jiang T (2014) Altered functional connectivity of the marginal division in Alzheimer's disease. Curr Alzheimer Res 11:145–155
16. Chen Z, Li J, Liu M, Ma L (2013) Age-related changes in resting functional connectivity of the marginal division of the neostriatum in healthy adults. Nan Fang Yi Ke Da Xue Xue Bao 33:74–79
17. Chen Z, Li J, Liu M, Ma L (2013) Impact of gender on the marginal division of the neostriatum in health adults. Zhongguo Yi Xue Ke Xue Yuan Xue Bao 35:294–298
18. Chen Z, Ma L (2014) Right extremities pain caused by a malacia lesion in the left putamen:a resting functional magnetic resonance imaging of the marginal division of the human brain. Zhongguo Yi Xue Ke Xue Yuan Xue Bao 36:126–130
19. Headache Classification Committee of the International Headache Society (IHS) (2013) The International Classification of Headache Disorders, 3rd edition (beta version). Cephalalgia 33:629–808
20. Maier W, Buller R, Philipp M, Heuser I (1988) The Hamilton Anxiety Scale: reliability, validity and sensitivity to change in anxiety and depressive disorders. J Affect Disord 14:61–68
21. Hamilton M (1967) Development of a rating scale for primary depressive illness. Br J Soc Clin Psychol 6:278–296
22. Song XW, Dong ZY, Long XY, Li SF, Zuo XN, Zhu CZ, He Y, Yan CG, Zang YF (2011) REST: a toolkit for resting-state functional magnetic resonance imaging data processing. PLoS One 6:e25031
23. Scher AI, Gudmundsson LS, Sigurdsson S, Ghambaryan A, Aspelund T, Eiriksdottir G, van Buchem MA, Gudnason V, Launer LJ (2009) Migraine headache in middle age and late-life brain infarcts. JAMA 301:2563–2570
24. Yu S, Liu R, Zhao G, Yang X, Qiao X, Feng J, Fang Y, Cao X, He M, Steiner T (2012) The prevalence and burden of primary headaches in China: a population-based door-to-door survey. Headache 52:582–591
25. Lipton RB (2009) Tracing transformation: chronic migraine classification, progression, and epidemiology. Neurology 72:S3–S7

26. Wiendels NJ, Knuistingh Neven A, Rosendaal FR, Spinhoven P, Zitman FG, Assendelft WJ, Ferrari MD (2006) Chronic frequent headache in the general population: prevalence and associated factors. Cephalalgia 26:1434–1442

27. Bingel U, Quante M, Knab R, Bromm B, Weiller C, Buchel C (2002) Subcortical structures involved in pain processing: evidence from single-trial fMRI. Pain 99:313–321

28. Mainero C, Boshyan J, Hadjikhani N (2011) Altered functional magnetic resonance imaging resting-state connectivity in periaqueductal gray networks in migraine. Ann Neurol 70:838–845

29. Isnard J, Magnin M, Jung J, Mauguiere F, Garcia-Larrea L (2011) Does the insula tell our brain that we are in pain? Pain 152:946–951

30. Duerden EG, Albanese MC (2013) Localization of pain-related brain activation: a meta-analysis of neuroimaging data. Hum Brain Mapp 34:109–149

31. Calvert GA (2001) Crossmodal processing in the human brain: insights from functional neuroimaging studies. Cereb Cortex 11:1110–1123

32. Price DD (2000) Psychological and neural mechanisms of the affective dimension of pain. Science 288:1769–1772

33. de Leeuw R, Davis CE, Albuquerque R, Carlson CR, Andersen AH (2006) Brain activity during stimulation of the trigeminal nerve with noxious heat. Oral Surg Oral Med Oral Pathol Oral Radiol Endod 102:750–757

34. Kim JH, Kim S, Suh SI, Koh SB, Park KW, Oh K (2010) Interictal metabolic changes in episodic migraine: a voxel-based FDG-PET study. Cephalalgia 30:53–61

35. Valfre W, Rainero I, Bergui M, Pinessi L (2008) Voxel-based morphometry reveals gray matter abnormalities in migraine. Headache 48:109–117

36. Loggia ML, Edwards RR, Kim J, Vangel MG, Wasan AD, Gollub RL, Harris RE, Park K, Napadow V (2012) Disentangling linear and nonlinear brain responses to evoked deep tissue pain. Pain 153:2140–2151

37. Koppen H, Palm-Meinders I, Kruit M, Lim V, Nugroho A, Westhof I, Terwindt G, van Buchem M, Ferrari M, Hommel B (2011) The impact of a migraine attack and its after-effects on perceptual organization, attention, and working memory. Cephalalgia 31:1419–1427

13

Thalamo-cortical network activity between migraine attacks: Insights from MRI-based microstructural and functional resting-state network correlation analysis

Gianluca Coppola[1*], Antonio Di Renzo[1], Emanuele Tinelli[2], Chiara Lepre[3], Cherubino Di Lorenzo[4], Giorgio Di Lorenzo[5], Marco Scapeccia[2], Vincenzo Parisi[1], Mariano Serrao[6], Claudio Colonnese[2,7], Jean Schoenen[8] and Francesco Pierelli[6,7]

Abstract

Background: Resting state magnetic resonance imaging allows studying functionally interconnected brain networks. Here we were aimed to verify functional connectivity between brain networks at rest and its relationship with thalamic microstructure in migraine without aura (MO) patients between attacks.

Methods: Eighteen patients with untreated MO underwent 3 T MRI scans and were compared to a group of 19 healthy volunteers (HV). We used MRI to collect resting state data among two selected resting state networks, identified using group independent component (IC) analysis. Fractional anisotropy (FA) and mean diffusivity (MD) values of bilateral thalami were retrieved from a previous diffusion tensor imaging study on the same subjects and correlated with resting state ICs Z-scores.

Results: In comparison to HV, in MO we found significant reduced functional connectivity between the default mode network and the visuo-spatial system. Both HV and migraine patients selected ICs Z-scores correlated negatively with FA values of the thalamus bilaterally.

Conclusions: The present results are the first evidence supporting the hypothesis that an abnormal resting within networks connectivity associated with significant differences in baseline thalamic microstructure could contribute to interictal migraine pathophysiology.

Keywords: Migraine, Thalamus, Resting state, Fractional anisotropy, Magnetic resonance imaging

Background

During recent years, various experimental data suggested that the functional state of the migraineur's brain is altered between attacks. This was initially observed with clinical neurophysiology methods that disclosed for instance interictal deficient habituation of sensory responses attributable to abnormal thalamo-cortical interactions [1, 2], and abnormal brain responses to various neuromodulatory techniques [3]. Interictal functional abnormalities were confirmed also with functional imaging methods in response to both noxious [4, 5] and

innocuous stressors [6, 7]. Recently, several independent research groups showed that changes can also be demonstrated at rest, i.e. without any sensory input, in the microstructure of several brain areas [8], including the thalamus [9, 10]. The conjunction of neuroimaging and neurophysiological data can be considered as robust evidence favouring morphological and functional brain alterations as prominent features of migraine pathophysiology. Since the brain areas are part of interconnected cortical and subcortical networks, it seems of major interest to analyse during the interictal phase the functional connectivity between brain networks at rest and its relationship with the thalamic microstructure.

Among the various neuroimaging procedures, resting state functional MRI (RS-fMRI) analyses the spontaneous

* Correspondence: gianluca.coppola@gmail.com
[1]Research Unit of Neurophysiology of Vision and Neurophthalmology, G.B. Bietti Foundation-IRCCS, Via Livenza 3, 00198 Rome, Italy

BOLD signal modulations not attributable to explicit inputs or outputs [11] and allows studying among which distributed brain areas activity at rest is related [12]. A common method to identify spatial patterns of coherent spontaneous BOLD activity, so-called functional connectivity, is independent component analysis (ICA). ICA is a high-order statistical method to examine functional connectivity by deconvolving the cerebral signals into components that are maximally independent and that reflect specific interconnected neuroanatomical networks. Compared to other methods, ICA is devoid of any *a-priori* definition of seed regions of interest [11]. RS-fMRI ICA allows the study of group differences in the temporal relationship among independent spatially distributed networks/components [12]. With this method, spontaneous brain activity was shown to be organized in specific and distinct spatial patterns, or sets of resting-state networks [13, 14].

In recent years, several fMRI studies have assessed resting state functional connectivity in various networks in migraine patients. Most of them have used an *a-priori* selected seed-based analysis [15–21]. Between selected brain areas of the default mode network (DMN) both increased [20, 22] or decreased [23] connectivity was reported. Two studies by the same group of researchers used the single independent component approach without *a-priori* hypothesis [24, 25]. They found evidence for reduced DMN [25] and executive control network [24] connectivity in migraine without aura patients between attacks. To the best of our knowledge, there are no RS-fMRI studies using ICA to determine the functional connectivity between networks (not within) between migraine attacks. Moreover, RS-fMRI studies of subcortical and cortical nodes were not combined up to now with DTI studies to analyse in migraine patients the connectivity patterns between the thalamus and various functional cerebral networks at rest. We decided, therefore, to use ICA of the whole brain to search for changes in functional connectivity maps at rest in interictal episodic migraine without aura patients. In addition, the thalamo-cortical network was statistically inferred by correlating selected resting state independent component activity strength and thalamic anisotropy.

Methods
Subjects
We initially enrolled 32 episodic migraine patients without aura (MO, ICHD-3beta code 1.1) who attended our headache clinic in a time period of 2 years and agreed to undergo MRI. We discarded recordings of 14 patients who had an attack within 3 days before or after the recording session.

The final analysis dataset comprises thus 18 right-handed MO patients [26] who subsequently participated in a comprehensive battery of neuroimaging tests, including RS-fMRI. We have published elsewhere the results of the diffusion tensor imaging and voxel based morphometry studies performed on the initial 14 patients and used these data combined with those of 6 additional patients to search for correlations with RS-fMRI data [9, 27]. Patients underwent MRI scans during the interictal period (MO), defined as an absence of migraine attacks for at least three days before and after MRI. Inclusion criteria were as follows: no history of other neurological diseases, systemic hypertension, diabetes or other metabolic disorders, connective or autoimmune diseases, and any other type of primary (including chronic migraine) or secondary headache. Patients had uni/bilateral migraine headaches, but not fixed pain on the same side. In order to avoid confounding effects on neuroplasticity due to pharmacologic treatment, no preventive anti-migraine drugs were allowed during the preceding 3 months. The control group comprised 19 right-handed healthy volunteers (HV) made up of medical school students and healthcare professionals of comparable age and gender distribution to the experimental group. Control subjects did not have any overt medical conditions, personal or family history of migraine or epilepsy, or take regular medication. Female subjects were always scanned at mid-cycle. All scanning sessions were performed in the afternoon (4.00–7.00 p.m.).

None of the enrolled subjects had sleep deprivation or alcohol consumption the day preceding the scans. Caffeinated beverages were not allowed on the day of scanning. Further exclusion criteria for both HV and MO were evidence of brain lesions on structural magnetic resonance imaging. All participants received a complete description of the study and granted written informed consent. The ethical review board of the Faculty of Medicine, University of Rome, Italy, approved the project.

Imaging protocols
All images were acquired using a Siemens 3 T Verio MRI scanner with a 12-channel head coil and structural anatomic scans were performed using T1-weighted sagittal magnetization-prepared rapid gradient echo (MP-RAGE) series (TR: 1900 ms, TE: 2.93 ms, 176 sagittal slices, 0.508 x 0.508 x 1 mm^3 voxels).

We acquired an interleaved double-echo Turbo Spin Echo sequence proton density and T2-weighted images (repetition time: 3320 ms, echo time: 10/103 ms, matrix: 384×384, field of view: 220 mm, slice thickness: 4 mm, gap: 1.2 mm, 50 axial slices).

Functional MRI data were obtained using a T2*-weighted, echo-planar imaging (TR: 3000 ms, TE: 30 ms, 40 axial slices, 3.906 x 3.906 x 3 mm, 150 volumes).

Functional BOLD data were collected in a 7 min 30 s run, during which subjects were instructed to relax, avoid motion and keep their eyes closed.

Data processing and analyses

Image data processing was performed on a personal computer using statistical parametric mapping (SPM8) software package (Wellcome Trust Centre for Neuroimaging, London, UK; http://www.fil.ion.ucl.ac.uk/spm), GIFT v3.0 and FNC toolbox (http://mialab.mrn.org/) in Mat-Lab (http://www.mathworks.com/). The overall image data processing is based on the method already described elsewhere [12].

All images from a single subject were realigned using a 6-parameter rigid body process, replaced by a cubic spline interpolation. We did not perform slice time correction. Slice-timing correction is not mandatory because the haemodynamic response is longer than TR (about 30 s). Moreover, the actual EPI uses multiband sequences with simultaneous echo refocusing and parallel imaging (called GRAPPA by Siemens), that makes slice time correction obsolete. The structural (T1 – MPRAGE) and functional data were coregistered for each participant dataset, normalized into the standard Montreal Neurological Institute space, and then transformed into a common stereotactic space based on Talairach and Tournoux [28]. Finally, functional images were spatially smoothed with an 8 mm full width half-maximum Gaussian kernel on each direction.

Component identification and selection

Grouped spatial ICA was performed for all 37 participants (HV + MO) using the infomax algorithm [29]. Two separate group spatial ICAs were also carried out in HV and MO patients to ensure that the fluctuations of components at rest in each group of subjects were similar to those obtained in the total group of 37 subjects. GIFT software automatically decomposed data into 39 components. A modified version of the minimum description length (MDL) criterion was adopted to determine the number of components from the aggregate data set [30]. Single subject spatially or temporally independent maps were then back-reconstructed from the aggregate mixing matrix [31].

All 39 components were inspected after plotting to templates in GIFT, using a priori probabilistic maps, and those of interest whose patterns mainly consisted of gray matter rather than non-gray matter were selected. Components located in CSF or white matter, or with low correlation to gray matter, can be artifacts, such as eye movements, head motion, ballistic artifacts, and were discarded. With FNC toolbox in MatLab, after removing all the artifactual components and applying a p-value threshold of 0.01 (false discovery rate corrected), only two components survived for further analysis. Before performing correlation analyses, a band-pass Butterworth filter between 0.033 Hz and 0.13 Hz was applied on the two selected component time courses. Each IC consists of a temporal waveform and an associated spatial map; the latter is expressed in terms of Z-scores that reflect the degree to which a given voxel time-course correlates with the specific IC temporal waveform, i.e. a way to quantify the strength of the IC [32]. As a further step and in order to search for a correlation between regional RS-fMRI network changes and clinical features, the Z-max scores (voxel-wise analysis) of each IC network were extracted for each participant.

Diffusion weighted imaging of the thalami

Diffusion tensor imaging (DTI) was acquired using single shot echo-planar imaging, with a 12–channel head coil (TR 12200 ms, TE 94 ms, 72 axial slices, 2 mm thickness, isotropic voxels). Images from the same participants and during the same session were obtained with diffusion gradients applied along 30 non-collinear directions, effective b values of 0 and 1000 s/mm2 were used. Image data processing was performed with the FSL 4.0 software package (FMRIB Image Analysis Group, Oxford, England). Diffusion data were corrected for motion and distortions caused by eddy current artifacts; FMRIB's Diffusion Toolbox (FDT) was used for local fitting of diffusion tensors, and fractional anisotropy (FA) and mean diffusivity (MD) maps were created. Two regions of interest (ROI, from the "Harvard-Oxford Subcortical Structural Atlas" as distributed with FSL) were defined for each subject, covering totally right and left thalami on each slice (Fig. 1). The medial boundaries were determined on each slice using cerebro spinal fluid as a landmark; lateral limits were verified using FA maps to exclude the internal capsule. Mean FA and MD in each region for every subject were obtained by averaging the values of those voxels contained in the ROI.

We have previously published in extenso the results of the DTI analyses performed on the first 29 subjects, 15 HV and 14 MO [9].

Statistical analyses

Group differences for demographic data were estimated using ANOVA test.

We used a 2-sample t-test to detect significant differences in correlation values between the two independent components for HV vs MO. A conservative p value of $p < 0.05$ (correction for multiple comparisons with false discovery rate selected) was used as significance cut-off. Connectivity combinations with statistically significant ($p < 0.01$) lag values were assessed using a two sample t-test of the difference between averaged HV and MO patient lags. As a further step and in

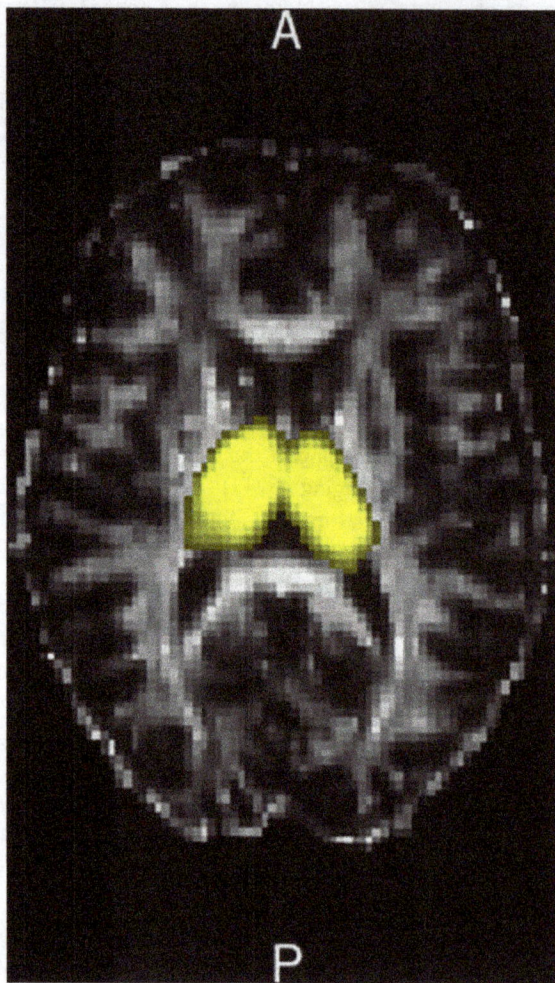

Fig. 1 Exemplary single subject axial representation of the diffusion tensor imaging FA map with the analyzed thalamic ROIs highlighted in yellow

Table 1 Clinical and demographic characteristics of healthy volunteers (HV) and migraine patients without aura scanned between (MO) attacks. Data are expressed as means ± SD

	HV (n = 19)	MO (n = 18)
Women (n)	12	12
Age (years)	29.7 ± 4.0	32.4 ± 7.2
Duration of migraine history (years)		14.1 ± 6.8
Attack frequency/month (n)		3.1 ± 2.1
Attack duration (hours)		27.3 ± 30.0
Visual analogue scale (n)		7.3 ± 0.9
Days from the last migraine attack (n)		20.8 ± 18.5

order to search for a correlation between regional RS-fMRI network changes and clinical features, the Z-max scores of each IC network were extracted for each participant.

Finally, we used Pearson's test to search for correlations between the MR DTI parameters FA and MD, individual IC Z-max scores and clinical variables such as severity of headache attacks [0–10], duration of migraine history [years], monthly attack frequency [n], attack duration [hours], days elapsed since the last migraine attack [n]. P values ≤ 0.05 were considered to indicate statistical significance.

Results

All subjects completed the study. Demographic and clinical data for the two groups are summarized in Table 1. Structural brain MRIs were normal in all participants. Specifically in migraine patients there were neither white matter lesions nor features suggestive of cortical atrophy.

Resting state fMRI

Significantly correlated components are represented in Fig. 2.

We found a significant difference in functional connectivity between independent components IC20 and IC15 in migraine patients between attacks respective to healthy volunteers. In fact, the correlation of independent component pair (IC20-IC15) is significantly lower in MO compared to HV (rho = 0.17 in MO vs rho = 0.41 in HV; FDR corrected, $p < 0.05$).

These components encompass respectively interconnected areas of the so-called default mode network (IC20) and a network composed of the visuo-spatial system and medial visual cortical areas (IC15), as seen on GIFT templates.

Although component directions slightly differed between HV and MO patient group, lag difference did not reach the level of significance.

There was no significant correlation between ICs Zmax-scores and clinical data.

Diffusion Tensor Imaging (DTI) data

The DTI results confirmed those published elsewhere on the first 29 subjects [9]. In MO patients the bilateral thalami have shown a significantly increased fractional anisotropy ($F_{(1,35)} = 4.99$, $p = 0.03$ and $F_{(1,35)} = 4.86$, $p = 0.03$ for the left and right thalamus respectively), but only a tendency to mean diffusivity change ($F_{(1,35)} = 2.50$, $p = 0.12$ and $F_{(1,35)} = 3.44$, $p = 0.07$ for the left and right thalamus respectively), than in HV.

Thalamo-cortical network correlation analysis

Pearson's correlation test disclosed that the IC15 Z-score correlated negatively with bilateral thalamic FA values in both HV (right $r = -0.547$, $p = 0.015$; left r = − 0.630,

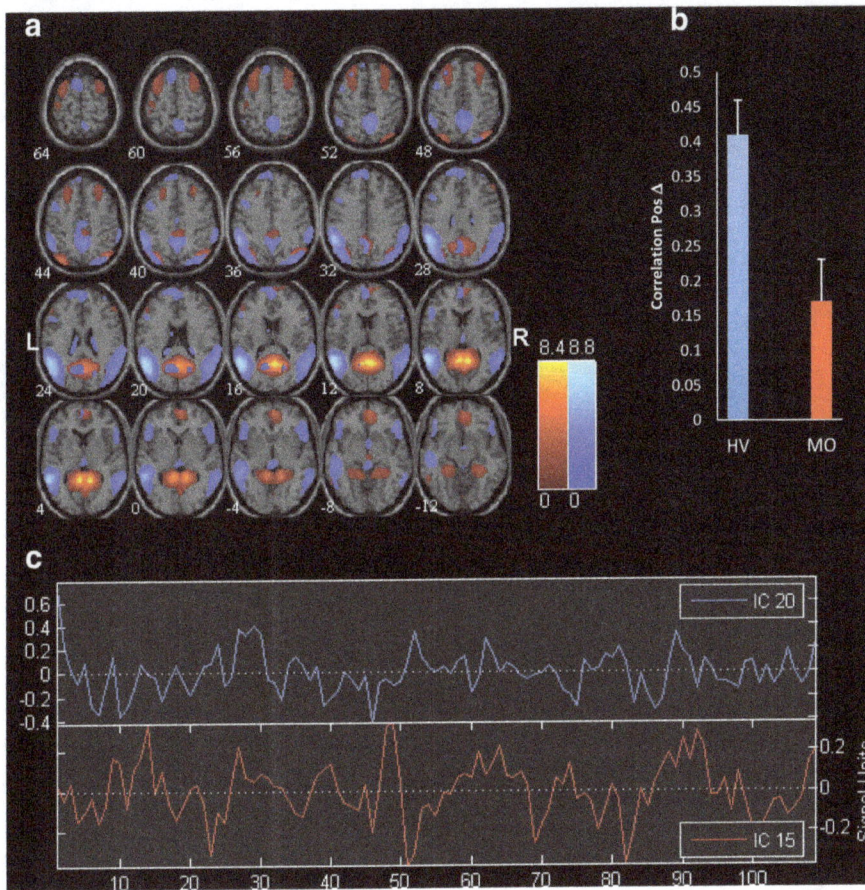

Fig. 2 a Representation of the two significant Independent Components (IC) functional connectivity networks differing in migraine patients scanned between attacks (MO) compared with healthy volunteers (HV) separated by independent component analysis (ICA). All images have been coregistered into the space of the MNI template. Brain areas are respectively coloured in hot metal scale (IC15) or in azure-blue (IC20). The numbers beneath each image refer to the z coordinate in Talairach space. **b** The bar graph reflects FDR corrected correlation between the 2 ICs, $p < 0.05$, in HV and MO. **c** Time course of spontaneous blood oxygen level dependent (BOLD) activity recorded during resting state and extracted from each of the two significant ICs

$p = 0.004$) and MO (right $r = -0.494$, $p = 0.037$; left $r = -0.636$, $p = 0.005$) (Fig. 3).

Discussion

Our study was specifically designed to search for differences in resting state networks and to test whether the resulting networks are correlated with thalamic microstructure in interictal migraine state. We found that functional connectivity of networks involved in in information processing, in cognitive, emotional, and, especially visual, attention processes differ between patients and healthy volunteers. We will discuss the possible neurobiological underpinnings of our findings and their potential relevance for migraine pathophysiology.

Resting state functional connectivity between attacks

Functional connectivity between the default mode network (IC 20) and a network composed of the visuo-spatial system and medial visual cortical areas (IC 15) is significantly reduced in migraine patients between attacks compared to HV.

The so-called default-mode network (DMN) encompasses a set of regions with relatively greater activity during "rest" than during active conditions [33]. The DMN includes the posterior cingulate gyrus, precuneus, medial prefrontal cortex, angular gyrus, and medial temporal lobe regions including the hippocampus and the lateral temporo-parietal area [34]. Although the exact functional role of the DMN is not completely understood, it is thought to be involved in retrieval of information from long-term memory and its manipulation for optimizing the sensorium and for problem solving and planning. The DMN is thus important in conscious experience as well as in maintaining a general low-level focus of attention for an event [35, 36]. Although the DMN is anatomically and functionally distinct from networks involved in sensory functions, comparative studies in animal and human studies have

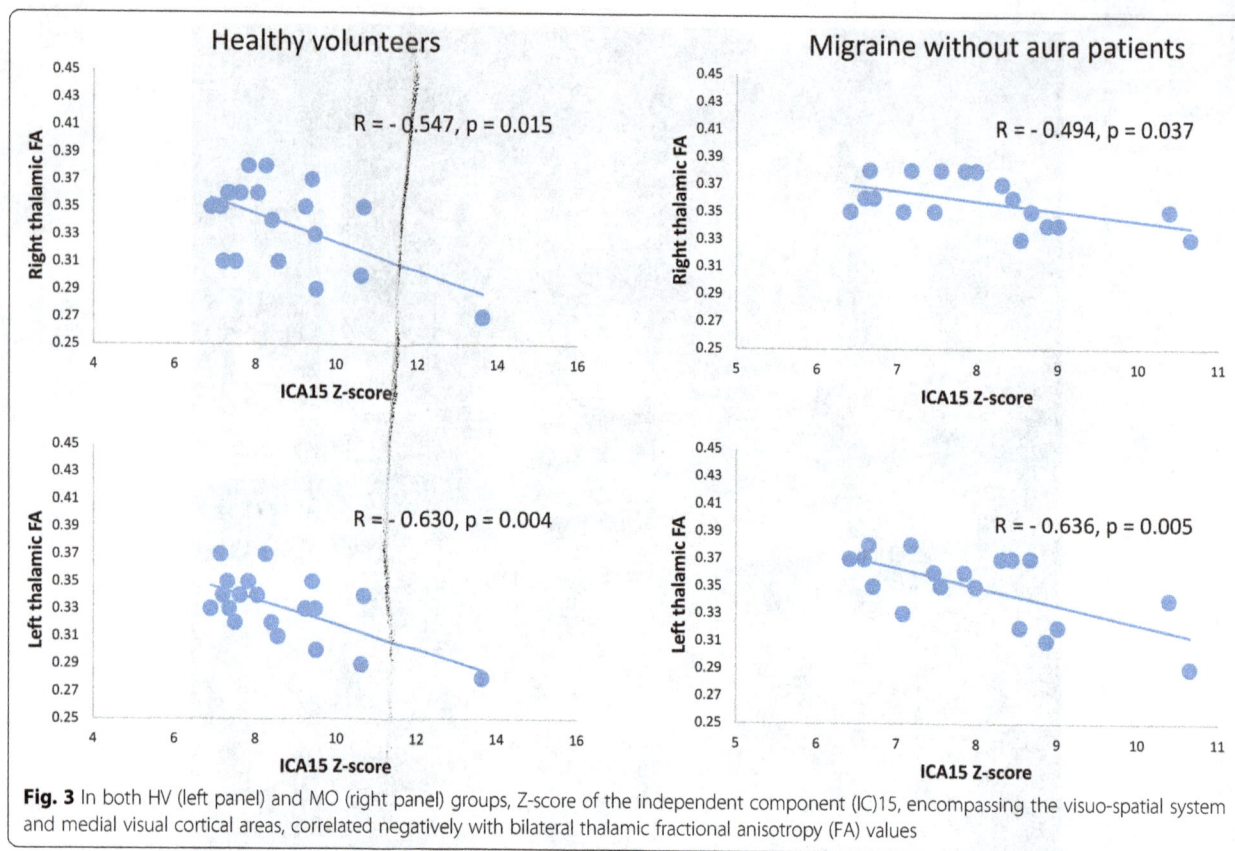

Fig. 3 In both HV (left panel) and MO (right panel) groups, Z-score of the independent component (IC)15, encompassing the visuo-spatial system and medial visual cortical areas, correlated negatively with bilateral thalamic fractional anisotropy (FA) values

shown that it is functionally correlated with all other resting state networks [14]. The visuo-spatial system comprises the posterior parietal cortex at the occipito-parietal junction, the precuneus, the posterior cingulate cortex and the frontal pole [13, 37]. Activity within this network in the resting state is associated with gathering information about our outer, and possibly inner, world [38], in episodic memory recall and orienting attention to salient novel or familiar stimuli and in emotional processing associated with episodic memory [39]. The medial visual cortical areas include the primary visual cortex as well as medial extrastriate regions such as lingual gyrus, inferior division of precuneus and lateral geniculate nucleus [13, 14]. This network is supposed to play a role in episodic memory, visual and visuo-spatial processing, reflections upon self and aspects of consciousness.

Given the brain networks involved and their known functions, the abnormalities we found in interictal migraine suggest a dysfunction of information gathering, evaluation and integration, and impaired short- as well as long- term memory processes. Moreover, because of the predominant involvement of visual areas/systems visuo-perceptual and visuo-spatial integration could be impaired in migraine between attacks. Whether these resting state fMRI abnormalities are the connectivity correlates of the subtle impairments in neuropsychological

performances, such as processing speed, verbal memory, and physiognomy recognition, previously reported in migraine between attacks remains to be determined [40–42]. It was shown that resting state spontaneous brain activity can be used to predict the task-response properties of brain regions [43]. It is thus of interest to verify if the reduced spontaneous network activity found here is correlated with the abnormal cognitive evoked potentials reported in migraine patients [44–49].

Thalamo-cortical interactions

We previously argued [9] that, in MO patients scanned between attacks, the pattern of increased anisotropy associated with normal MD may reflect shrinking of neuronal and glial cells and/or gain of directional organization in combination with a preserved cell density [50, 51]. Interestingly, data from animal models showed that cell shrinking may coincide with a reduced neuronal electric response [52, 53]. Therefore, since grey matter in the single thalamic sub-nuclei does not have a unique oriented fibre structure, the increased FA found in between attacks might also result from a decrease in neuron connections and thus dendritic arborization, which in turn may result in a reduced number of local circuits [54].

Here, the most striking finding is the correlation between MRI diffusion-weighted features of the thalamus and the functional connectivity between brain networks. In both HV and migraineurs between attacks, individual Z-scores of IC15, containing the visuo-spatial system and medial visual areas, correlated negatively with FA values of bilateral thalami, suggesting that the lower is the between networks connectivity the higher is the FA in the thalami bilaterally. However, this association between thalamic diffusion parameters and RS-fMRI is evident in examining each individual group, suggesting that the correlation between thalamic microstructure and RS-fMRI is a more general phenomenon related to the connectivity mechanisms. Nevertheless, we found significant differences in baseline thalamic microstructure – increased FA in MO – and in within networks connectivity – decreased connection in MO – between patients and healthy controls.

Overall, the results from the correlation analysis fit strikingly with evidence coming from neuroimaging studies showing a distinct functional connectivity between the thalamus and several areas within the visuo-spatial system and medial visual areas (e.g. posterior cingulate cortex, visual cortex, precuneus) [55–57]. Taken together the latter evidence with our present finding of no significant difference in the lag in intrinsic activity, an indirect estimation of the direction of the connection, between the pair of less interconnected networks (i.e. IC20-IC15), it is possible that the thalamic relay contributes the most to the cortical networks activity via the thalamocortical loops. Therefore, we hypothesize that a deficient thalamic activity in migraine between attacks, as highlighted by an increased FA [9], activates less the visuo-spatial system and medial visual cortical areas, which in turn leads to less activation of the DMN network (Fig. 4).

Clinical and experimental data indicate that the thalamus is a key structure in migraine pathophysiology. The thalamus was found to be implicated in many clinical [58–61] and neurophysiological features of migraine [62–64]. From animal experiments, it is known that the vast system of extrastriate and suprasylvian areas comprising the brain's most important networks receive extensive projections from the lateral posterior-pulvinar thalamic complex, including the intralaminar nuclei [65, 66], that were recently reported to be reduced in volume in migraine patients scanned when attack-free [10]. It is important to take into account that these nuclei receive the most significant overlap of different sensory modalities [67]. This is of particular interest for migraine since the majority of evoked potential studies between attacks have shown abnormalities, such as deficit of habituation, for most sensory modalities: non-painful and painful somatosensory, auditory and visual [1]. The only notable exception is olfaction, the only sensory modality not relayed in the thalamus, for which brain and behavioural responses habituate normally in migraineurs [5].

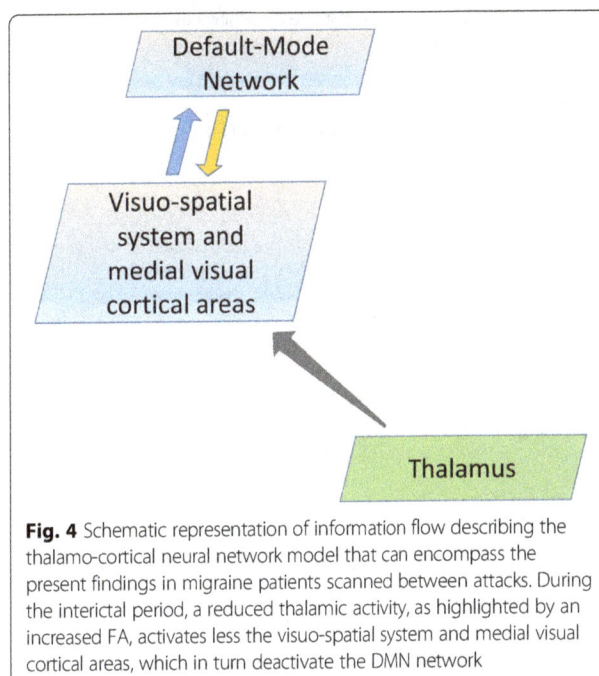

Fig. 4 Schematic representation of information flow describing the thalamo-cortical neural network model that can encompass the present findings in migraine patients scanned between attacks. During the interictal period, a reduced thalamic activity, as highlighted by an increased FA, activates less the visuo-spatial system and medial visual cortical areas, which in turn deactivate the DMN network

As with all studies, our findings need to be considered with our study limitations and strengths. The small number of patients could make our study underpowered to reveal more subtle findings, such as correlation between clinical features and functional connectivity, although our cohort was sufficient to disclose strong statistical significance. A strength of the present study is our approach to study the dependencies between pairs of functional networks, since it allowed us to examine weak, but significant, connectivity among strongly connected networks.

Conclusions

Overall, these results of RS-fMRI are in line with the concept of a global dysfunction in multisensory information processing and integration in migraine. The multimodal MRI data provide specifically structural and functional evidences for the involvement of the thalamus in the abnormal functional connectivity between different brain networks between attacks. Future work should attempt to clarify the role of the different networks with regard to migraine-associated multisensory phenomena, such as photophobia or allodynia, especially during the attack and in chronic migraine. It would also be of particular interest to verify whether the thalamocortical network dysfunctions are primary phenomena or secondary to a functional disconnection of the thalamus from the brainstem.

Abbreviations

3 T: 3 Tesla; DMN: Default mode network; DTI: Diffusion tensor imaging; EEG: Electroencephalography; FA: Fractional anisotropy; HV: Healthy volunteer; IC: Independent component; ICA: Independent component analysis; MD: Mean diffusivity; MO: Migraine without aura; MRI: Magnetic

resonance imaging; ROI: Region Of Interest; RS-fMRI: Resting state functional magnetic resonance imaging

Acknowledgment

Italian Ministry of Health and Fondazione Roma financially supported the research for this paper.

Authors' contributions

GC made substantial contributions to interpretation of data as well as in drafting the manuscript. GDL, VP, JS and FP were implied in the interpretation of data as well as in drafting the manuscript; CDL and MSe gave critical revision of the manuscript for important intellectual content. CC, CL, and MSc were implied in recording data. ADR and ET were implicated in analyzing data. All authors read and approved the final manuscript.

Competing interests

The authors declare that they have no competing interests.

Author details

[1]Research Unit of Neurophysiology of Vision and Neurophthalmology, G.B. Bietti Foundation-IRCCS, Via Livenza 3, 00198 Rome, Italy. [2]Department of Neurology and Psychiatry, Neuroradiology Section, "Sapienza" University of Rome, Rome, Italy. [3]Department of Medico-Surgical Sciences and Biotechnologies, Neurology Section, "Sapienza" University of Rome, Rome, Italy. [4]Don Carlo Gnocchi Onlus Foundation, Milan, Italy. [5]Laboratory of Psychophysiology, Psychiatric Clinic, Department of Systems Medicine, University of Rome "Tor Vergata", Rome, Italy. [6]Department of Medico-Surgical Sciences and Biotechnologies, "Sapienza" University of Rome Polo Pontino, Latina, Italy. [7]IRCCS Neuromed, Pozzilli, (IS), Italy. [8]Headache Research Unit, Department of Neurology-CHR Citadelle, University of Liège, Liège, Belgium.

References

1. Coppola G, Di Lorenzo C, Schoenen J, Pierelli F (2013) Habituation and sensitization in primary headaches. J Headache Pain 14:65
2. Magis D, Vigano A, Sava S et al (2013) Pearls and pitfalls: electrophysiology for primary headaches. Cephalalgia 33:526–539
3. Brighina F, Cosentino G, Fierro B (2013) Brain stimulation in migraine. Handb Clin Neurol 116:585–98. doi:10.1016/B978-0-444-53497-2.00047-4
4. Moulton EA, Becerra L, Maleki N et al (2011) Painful heat reveals hyperexcitability of the temporal pole in interictal and ictal migraine States. Cereb Cortex 21:435–448
5. Stankewitz A, Schulz E, May A (2013) Neuronal correlates of impaired habituation in response to repeated trigemino-nociceptive but not to olfactory input in migraineurs: An fMRI study. Cephalalgia 33:256–265
6. Demarquay G, Royet JP, Mick G, Ryvlin P (2008) Olfactory hypersensitivity in migraineurs: a H(2)(15)O-PET study. Cephalalgia 28:1069–80. doi:10.1111/j.1468-2982.2008.01672.x
7. Martín H, Sánchez del Rio M, de Silanes C et al (2011) Photoreactivity of the occipital cortex measured by functional magnetic resonance imaging-blood oxygenation level dependent in migraine patients and healthy volunteers: pathophysiological implications. Headache 51:1520–1528
8. Sprenger T, Borsook D (2012) Migraine changes the brain: neuroimaging makes its mark. Curr Opin Neurol 25:252–262
9. Coppola G, Tinelli E, Lepre C et al (2014) Dynamic changes in thalamic microstructure of migraine without aura patients: a diffusion tensor magnetic resonance imaging study. Eur J Neurol 21:287–e13. doi:10.1111/ene.12296
10. Magon S, May A, Stankewitz A et al (2015) Morphological abnormalities of thalamic subnuclei in migraine: A multicenter MRI study at 3 Tesla. J Neurosci 35:13800–13806
11. Fox M, Raichle ME (2007) Spontaneous fluctuations in brain activity observed with functional magnetic resonance imaging. Nat Rev 8:700–711
12. Jafri M, Pearlson GD, Stevens M, Calhoun VD (2008) A method for functional network connectivity among spatially independent resting-state components in schizophrenia. Neuroimage 39:1666–1681
13. Beckmann C, DeLuca M, Devlin JT, Smith SM (2005) Investigations into resting-state connectivity using independent component analysis. Philos Trans R Soc LondonSeries B Biol Sci 360:1001–1013

14. Mantini D, Perrucci MG, Del Gratta C et al (2007) Electrophysiological signatures of resting state networks in the human brain. Proc Natl Acad Sci U S A 104:13170–13175
15. Hadjikhani N, Ward N, Boshyan J et al (2013) The missing link: enhanced functional connectivity between amygdala and visceroceptive cortex in migraine. Cephalalgia 33:1264–1268
16. Jin C, Yuan K, Zhao L et al (2013) Structural and functional abnormalities in migraine patients without aura. NMR Biomed 26:58–64
17. Mainero C, Boshyan J, Hadjikhani N (2011) Altered functional magnetic resonance imaging resting-state connectivity in periaqueductal gray networks in migraine. Ann Neurol 70:838–845
18. Moulton E, Becerra L, Johnson A et al (2014) Altered hypothalamic functional connectivity with autonomic circuits and the locus coeruleus in migraine. PLoS One 9:10
19. Schwedt T, Larson-Prior L, Coalson RS et al (2014) Allodynia and descending pain modulation in migraine: a resting state functional connectivity analysis. Pain Med 15:154–165
20. Xue T, Yuan K, Zhao L et al (2012) Intrinsic brain network abnormalities in migraines without aura revealed in resting-state fMRI. PLoS One 7:10
21. Yuan K, Zhao L, Cheng P et al (2013) Altered structure and resting-state functional connectivity of the basal ganglia in migraine patients without aura. J Pain 14:836–844
22. Xue T, Yuan K, Cheng P et al (2013) Alterations of regional spontaneous neuronal activity and corresponding brain circuit changes during resting state in migraine without aura. NMR Biomed 26:1051–1058
23. Yu D, Yuan K, Zhao L et al (2012) Regional homogeneity abnormalities in patients with interictal migraine without aura: a resting-state study. NMR Biomed 25:806–812
24. Russo A, Tessitore A, Giordano A et al (2012) Executive resting-state network connectivity in migraine without aura. Cephalalgia 32:1041–1048
25. Tessitore A, Russo A, Giordano A et al (2013) Disrupted default mode network connectivity in migraine without aura. J Headache Pain 14:89
26. (2013) The International Classification of Headache Disorders, 3rd edition (beta version). Cephalalgia 33:629–808. doi: 10.1177/0333102413485658
27. Coppola G, Di Renzo A, Tinelli E et al (2015) Evidence for brain morphometric changes during the migraine cycle: A magnetic resonance-based morphometry study. Cephalalgia 35:783–791. doi:10.1177/0333102414559732
28. Talairach J, Tournoux P (1988) Co-planar Stereotaxic Atlas of the Human Brain. Georg Thieme Verlag, New York, Thieme
29. Bell A, Sejnowski TJ (1995) An information-maximization approach to blind separation and blind deconvolution. Neural Comput 7:1129–1159
30. Li YO, Adali T, Calhoun VD (2007) Estimating the number of independent components for functional magnetic resonance imaging data. Hum Brain Mapp 28:1251–1266
31. Calhoun VD, Adali T, Pearlson GD, Pekar JJ (2001) A method for making group inferences from functional MRI data using independent component analysis. Hum Brain Mapp 14:140–151
32. McKeown M, Makeig S, Brown GG et al (1998) Analysis of fMRI data by blind separation into independent spatial components. Hum Brain Mapp 6:160–188
33. Raichle M, MacLeod AM, Snyder AZ et al (2001) A default mode of brain function. Proc Natl Acad Sci U S A 98:676–682
34. Buckner R, Andrews-Hanna JR, Schacter DL (2008) The brain's default network: anatomy, function, and relevance to disease. Ann N Y Acad Sci 1124:1–38
35. Binder J, Frost JA, Hammeke TA et al (1999) Conceptual processing during the conscious resting state. A functional MRI study. J Cogn Neurosci 11:80–95
36. Carhart-Harris R, Friston KJ (2010) The default-mode, ego-functions and free-energy: a neurobiological account of Freudian ideas. Brain 133:1265–1283
37. Gusnard D, Raichle ME (2001) Searching for a baseline: functional imaging and the resting human brain. Nat Rev 2:685–694
38. Vogt B, Finch DM, Olson CR (1992) Functional heterogeneity in cingulate cortex: the anterior executive and posterior evaluative regions. Cereb Cortex 2:435–443
39. Maddock R (1999) The retrosplenial cortex and emotion: new insights from functional neuroimaging of the human brain. Trends Neurosci 22:310–316
40. Le Pira F, Lanaia F, Zappalà G et al (2004) Relationship between clinical variables and cognitive performances in migraineurs with and without aura. Funct Neurol 19:101–5

41. Suhr JA, Seng EK (2012) Neuropsychological functioning in migraine: clinical and research implications. Cephalalgia 32:39–54

42. Yetkin-Ozden S, Ekizoglu E, Baykan B (2015) Face Recognition in Patients with Migraine. Pain Pract 15:319–22

43. Fox M, Snyder AZ, Zacks JM, Raichle ME (2006) Coherent spontaneous activity accounts for trial-to-trial variability in human evoked brain responses. Nat Neurosci 9:23–25

44. Demarquay G, Caclin A, Brudon F et al (2011) Exacerbated attention orienting to auditory stimulation in migraine patients. Clin Neurophysiol 122:1755–1763

45. Iacovelli E, Tarantino S, De Ranieri C et al (2012) Psychophysiological mechanisms underlying spatial attention in children with primary headache. Brain Dev 34:640–647

46. Mickleborough M, Chapman CM, Toma AS et al (2013) Interictal neurocognitive processing of visual stimuli in migraine: evidence from event-related potentials. PLoS One 8:10

47. Mickleborough M, Chapman C, Toma A, Handy T (2014) Cognitive processing of visual images in migraine populations in between headache attacks. Brain Res 1582:167–175

48. Schoenen J, Timsit-berthier M (1993) Contingent negative variation: Methods and potential interest in headache. Cephalalgia 13:28–32

49. Wang W, Schoenen J, T-B M (1995) Cognitive functions in migraine without aura between attacks: a psychophysiological approach using the "oddball" paradigm. Neurophysiol Clin 25:3–11

50. Wieshmann UC, Clark CA, Symms MR et al (1999) Reduced anisotropy of water diffusion in structural cerebral abnormalities demonstrated with diffusion tensor imaging. Magn Reson Imaging 17:1269–1274

51. Mandl RC, Schnack HG, Zwiers MP et al (2008) Functional diffusion tensor imaging: measuring task-related fractional anisotropy changes in the human brain along white matter tracts. PLoS One 3:10

52. Tasaki I, Byrne PM (1992) Rapid structural changes in nerve fibers evoked by electric current pulses. Biochem Biophys Res Commun 188:559–564

53. Tasaki I (1999) Rapid structural changes in nerve fibers and cells associated with their excitation processes. Jpn J Physiol 49:125–138

54. Beaulieu C (2002) The basis of anisotropic water diffusion in the nervous system - a technical review. NMR Biomed 15:435–455. doi:10.1002/nbm.782

55. Zou Q, Long X, Zuo X et al (2009) Functional connectivity between the thalamus and visual cortex under eyes closed and eyes open conditions: a resting-state fMRI study. Hum Brain Mapp 30:3066–3078

56. Wang X, Xu M, Song Y et al (2014) The network property of the thalamus in the default mode network is correlated with trait mindfulness. Neuroscience 278:291–301

57. Ku J, Cho YW, Lee YS et al (2014) Functional connectivity alternation of the thalamus in restless legs syndrome patients during the asymptomatic period: a resting-state connectivity study using functional magnetic resonance imaging. Sleep Med 15:289–294

58. Burstein R, Jakubowski M, Garcia-Nicas E et al (2010) Thalamic sensitization transforms localized pain into widespread allodynia. Ann Neurol 68:81–91. doi:10.1002/ana.21994

59. Maleki N, Becerra L, Upadhyay J et al (2012) Direct optic nerve pulvinar connections defined by diffusion MR tractography in humans: implications for photophobia. Hum Brain Mapp 33:75–88

60. Noseda R, Kainz V, Jakubowski M et al (2010) A neural mechanism for exacerbation of headache by light. Nat Neurosci 13:239–245

61. Russo A, Marcelli V, Esposito F et al (2014) Abnormal thalamic function in patients with vestibular migraine. Neurology 82:2120–2126

62. Coppola G, De Pasqua V, Pierelli F, Schoenen J (2012) Effects of repetitive transcranial magnetic stimulation on somatosensory evoked potentials and high frequency oscillations in migraine. Cephalalgia 32:700–709

63. Coppola G, Iacovelli E, Bracaglia M et al (2013) Electrophysiological correlates of episodic migraine chronification: evidence for thalamic involvement. J Headache Pain 14:76

64. Coppola G, Bracaglia M, Di Lenola D et al (2016) Lateral inhibition in the somatosensory cortex during and between migraine without aura attacks: correlations with thalamocortical activity and clinical features. Cephalalgia 36:568–578. doi:10.1177/0333102415610873

65. Raczkowski D, Rosenquist AC (1983) Connections of the multiple visual cortical areas with the lateral posterior-pulvinar complex and adjacent thalamic nuclei in the cat. J Neurosci 3:1912–1942

66. Tong L, Kalil RE, Spear PD (1982) Thalamic projections to visual areas of the middle suprasylvian sulcus in the cat. J Comp Neurol 212:103–117

67. Cappe C, Morel A, Barone P, Rouiller EM (2009) The thalamocortical projection systems in primate: an anatomical support for multisensory and sensorimotor interplay. Cereb Cortex 19:2025–2037

14

Anodal transcranial direct current stimulation over the left temporal pole restores normal visual evoked potential habituation in interictal migraineurs

Francesca Cortese[1*], Francesco Pierelli[1,2], Ilaria Bove[1], Cherubino Di Lorenzo[3], Maurizio Evangelista[4], Armando Perrotta[2], Mariano Serrao[1], Vincenzo Parisi[5] and Gianluca Coppola[5]

Abstract

Background: Neuroimaging data has implicated the temporal pole (TP) in migraine pathophysiology; the density and functional activity of the TP were reported to fluctuate in accordance with the migraine cycle. Yet, the exact link between TP morpho-functional abnormalities and migraine is unknown. Here, we examined whether non-invasive anodal transcranial direct current stimulation (tDCS) ameliorates abnormal interictal multimodal sensory processing in patients with migraine.

Methods: We examined the habituation of visual evoked potentials and median nerve somatosensory evoked potentials (SSEP) before and immediately after 20-min anodal tDCS (2 mA) or sham stimulation delivered over the left TP in interictal migraineurs.

Results: Prior to tDCS, interictal migraineurs did not exhibit habituation in response to repetitive visual or somatosensory stimulation. After anodal tDCS but not sham stimulation, migraineurs exhibited normal habituation responses to visual stimulation; however, tDCS had no effect on SSEP habituation in migraineurs.

Conclusion: Our study shows for the first time that enhancing excitability of the TP with anodal tDCS normalizes abnormal interictal visual information processing in migraineurs. This finding has implications for the role of the TP in migraine, and specifically highlights the ventral stream of the visual pathway as a pathophysiological neural substrate for abnormal visual processing in migraine.

Keywords: Ventral stream, Visual system, Somatosensory system, Synaptic plasticity, Neurostimulation

Background

Migraine is a neurological disorder that is characterized by recurrent clinical attacks separated by variable-length headache-free intervals. Although the pathogenesis of migraine is far from completely understood, clinical neurophysiology and neuroimaging studies in recent decades have disclosed subtle functional and morphological abnormalities that manifest during the interictal phase and distinguish migraineurs from normal healthy

subjects [1–3]. Among the various subcortical and cortical areas implicated in migraine pathophysiology, emerging evidence highlights the temporal pole (TP) as a key neural substrate. In humans, the TP serves as a multimodal neural hub that receives and integrates various sensory modalities including olfactory, auditory, taste, and visual inputs. Moreover, the TP participates in the ventral visual stream (VVS) for visual information processing [4–6]. During an olfactory task, interictal migraineurs exhibited significantly higher brain glucose metabolism in the left TP compared to control subjects [7]. Moreover, BOLD signal in the TP in response to noxious stimulation was reduced in interictal patients compared to patients who were actively experiencing a

* Correspondence: francesca.cortese05@libero.it
[1]Department of Medico-Surgical Sciences and Biotechnologies, Sapienza University of Rome Polo Pontino, Corso della Repubblica, 79 – 04100, Latina, Italy
Full list of author information is available at the end of the article

migraine [8, 9]. In resting-state MRI studies comparing interictal migraineurs to healthy control subjects, decreased grey matter density was observed in the left TP [10] and the left TP exhibited decreased connectivity with components of the default-mode network [11]. Finally, the TP was implicated as an important area for differentiating patients with migraine from healthy control subjects in a cross-sectional brain MRI investigation [12]. Taken together, these findings suggest that the TP is both intricately related to the pathophysiology of migraine and sensitive to the cyclical recurrence of migraine attacks.

Transcranial direct current stimulation (tDCS) is a non-invasive technique for neuromodulation in humans that affects cortical excitability in a polarity-specific manner [13, 14]. Anodal polarization increases the excitability of cortical areas below electrodes, whereas cathodal polarization typically decreases cortical excitability [15]. A number of tDCS studies in different pain disorders [16, 17] have demonstrated that tDCS is well-tolerated by patients [18]. Anodal tDCS proved effective over either the motor cortex or the dorsolateral prefrontal cortex when used as prophylactic strategy both in episodic [19] and chronic [20, 21] migraine. Moreover, some studies reported that, in addition to the therapeutic effects, tDCS over the visual cortex also normalized interictal cortical hyperresponsivity in episodic migraine [22].

Nonetheless, to our knowledge, no study to date has targeted the TP for anodal tDCS in migraine, to enhance interictal temporal lobe activity and thereby interfere with an aspect of migraine pathophysiology. Thus, we examined whether anodal stimulation of the TP could restore normal function of the TP and thus physiological information processing in migraine. Moreover, given that the TP processes all kinds of sensorial information except for somatosensory information, we examined the habituation responses of evoked potentials to somatosensory stimuli (as a negative control) as well as visual stimuli.

Methods

Participants

Forty patients with migraine without aura (diagnosed in accordance with the International Classification of Headache Disorders III beta edition) were recruited from our headache clinic (Table 1). Of these, 4 patients were excluded because they did not meet the primary inclusion criteria (see below). Subjects were included if they were between 18 and 65 years of age and had at least a 1-year clinical history of migraine with 2–8 attacks per month. The use of preventive anti-migraine medication was not permitted during the 3 months preceding the study. The primary inclusion criterion was being attack-free for at least 3 days before and after each recording sessions, and was verified by headache diary and telephone or e-mail interview. Subjects were excluded from the study if they were regularly taking medication (e.g., antibiotics, corticosteroids, antidepressants, benzodiazepines, or prophylactic migraine medication) except for contraceptive pills; if they did not have a best-corrected visual acuity of >8/10; and if they had a history of other neurological disease, systemic hypertension, diabetes or other metabolic disease, autoimmune disease, or any other type of primary or secondary headache. Female participants were always recorded mid-menstrual cycle. All participants received a complete description of the study and provided written informed consent. The study was approved by a local ethical review board and was conducted in accordance with the Helsinki Declaration.

Experimental procedure

The 36 enrolled patients were equally randomized to receive anodal tDCS ($N = 18$) or sham tDCS ($N = 18$). Randomization was conducted using a secure web-based database. For all patients, visual evoked potential (VEP) and somatosensory evoked potential (SSEP) recordings were performed in a random order during a single session before and immediately after real or sham tDCS. All recordings were performed in the afternoon (between 14:00

Table 1 Descriptive statistics of clinical and demographic characteristics of migraine patients between attacks in the sham and real group

	Real (n = 18)	Sham (n = 18)	p value
Women (n)	13	11	0.495
Age (years)	28.6 ± 7.6	26.9 ± 4.9	0.430
Duration of migraine history (years)	15.6 ± 8.3	12.4 ± 7.0	0.220
Attack frequency/month (n)	5.0 ± 3.2	3.9 ± 2.1	0.231
Attack duration (hours)	17.1 ± 17.4	18.1 ± 14.8	0.854
Visual analogue scale (n)	7.0 ± 0.7	6.6 ± 1.2	0.230
Days from the last migraine attack (n)	8.5 ± 8.5	11.7 ± 13.0	0.388
Family history of migraine (%)	51.4	48.6	0.210
Acute medication intake/month (n)	2.0 ± 1.9	2.0 ± 1.8	0.996

Data are expressed as means ± SD

and 18:00) by the same investigators (F.C. and I.B.); these investigators were not involved in recruitment, inclusion, or randomization of subjects, and had no interactions with participants prior to the examination. All recordings were numbered anonymously and analysed offline in a blinded fashion by a single investigator (G.C.), who was not blinded to the order of the blocks.

tDCS

tDCS (2 mA, 20 min) was delivered using a constant current electrical stimulator (Brainstim®, EMSmedical) through a pair of surface electrodes: the anode was placed over the left temporal pole and the cathode was placed above the right shoulder. The electrodes were square in shape (25 cm^2), 6-mm thick, and covered in a saline-soaked sponge. Current was delivered at a density of 0.08 mA/cm^2, resulting in a total charge of 96 mC/cm^2. These parameters are below the threshold for possible tissue damage [14]. During stimulation, tDCS is not usually perceived except for occasional short-lasting itching sensations below the electrodes.

The stimulation site over the left temporal pole was determined by moving laterally 40% of the intra-auricular distance from the vertex and anteriorly 5% of the distance from inion to nasion [23, 24]. The target site was located approximately halfway between the T7 and FT7 EEG positions of the international 10–20 system. This positioning method, although less accurate than neuronavigation-based techniques, adequately correlates with MRI-guided stereotactic approaches [25, 26].

For sham tDCS, the electrode positions and stimulation intensity were the same as that used for anodal stimulation, but current was only applied for the first and last 30 s of the 20-min period. This was done so that patients would not easily be able to distinguish between real tDCS and sham tDCS sessions. Participants in the sham and real arms guessed the type of stimulation in 5 and 6 cases out of 18 respectively (chi^2 = 0.717, p = 1.0). The experimenters who applied tDCS (F.C. and I.B.) were also blind to the nature of the procedure (real versus sham tDCS); rather, a third experimenter (C.D.L.) pre-programmed the stimulator and ensured the randomization order.

VEP study

Subjects were seated in a semi-dark, acoustically isolated room in front of a TV monitor surrounded by a uniform luminance field of 5 cd/m^2. VEPs were elicited by monocular stimulation of the right eye. Visual stimuli were full-field checkerboard patterns (contrast, 80%; mean luminance, 50 cd/m^2) generated on the TV monitor and reversed in contrast at a reversal rate of 3.1 reversals per second. The viewing distance was 114 cm and single check edges subtended a visual angle of 15 min. Subjects were instructed to fixate with their right eye on a red dot in the middle of the screen while the contralateral eye was covered with a patch. VEPs were recorded from the scalp through silver cup electrodes positioned at Oz (active electrode) and at Fz (reference electrode as per the international 10–20 system). A ground electrode was placed on the right forearm. Signals were amplified by Digitimer™ D360 pre-amplifiers (band-pass, 0.05–2000 Hz; gain, 1000) and recorded on a CED™ power 1401 device (Cambridge Electronic Design Ltd., Cambridge, UK). A total of 600 consecutive sweeps (sweep duration, 200 ms) were collected and sampled at 4000 Hz. After offline application of a 100-Hz low-pass digital filter, cortical responses were partitioned into 6 sequential blocks of 100 (including at least 95 artefact-free sweeps). Responses in each block were averaged offline (block averages) using the Signal™ software package version 3.10 (CED Ltd). VEP latencies (N1, P1, and N2) and amplitudes (N1-P1 and P1-N2) were identified. Habituation was defined as the slope of the linear regression line for the 6 blocks.

SSEP study

SSEPs were elicited by electrical stimulation of the right median nerve at the wrist using a constant current square wave pulse (width, 0.1 ms; cathode proximal) with a stimulus intensity of 1.5-times the motor threshold and a repetition rate of 4.4 Hz. The active electrodes were placed over the contralateral parietal area (C3', 2 cm posterior to C3 as per the international 10–20 system; referenced to Fz), over the fifth cervical spinous process (Cv5; referenced to Fz), and over Erb's point ipsilateral to the stimulus (referenced to the contralateral side). The ground electrode was placed on the right arm. SSEP signals were amplified and recorded with the same hardware/software equipment described above for VEP recording.

Subjects were seated in a comfortable chair in a well-lit room with their eyes open. Subjects were asked to fix their attention on the stimulus-induced thumb movement. During continuous median-nerve stimulation at the wrist, 500 sweeps (sweep duration, 50 ms) were collected and sampled at 5000 Hz. A total of 500 artefact-free evoked responses were recorded and averaged for each subject (grand average). After digital filtering of the signal between 0 and 450 Hz, various SSEP components (N9, N13, N20, P25, and N33) and their respective peak-to-peak amplitudes (N9-p, N13-p, N20-P25, and P25-N33) were identified. Thereafter, based on the observation of a habituation effect from the 2nd block of 100 averaged responses onwards in previous studies [27, 28], the first 200 evoked responses were partitioned into 2 sequential blocks of 100 (including at least 95 artefact-free sweeps). Each block was averaged offline (block averages) and analysed for N20–P25 amplitudes. Habituation was expressed as the slope of the linear regression line for the 2 blocks [28].

For both VEPs and SSEPs, artefacts were automatically rejected using the Signal™ artefact rejection tool if the signal amplitude exceeded 90% of the analogue-to-digital converter (ADC) range. Signal was corrected offline for DC drift.

Statistical analysis

Data were collected and analysed in a blinded fashion by a single investigator (V.P.) using Statistica for Windows (StatSoft Inc., Tulsa, USA) version 8.0 software. Sample size calculations were based on a ketogenic diet clinical trial that examined the same evoked potentials [29] with a desired power of 0.80 and an α error of 0.05. Since our primary endpoint was to discover differences between the effects of real and sham tDCS on habituation, we used the amplitude habituations of the N1–P1 VEP and N20–P25 SSEP cortical components in the 2 conditions (before versus after ketogenic diet) to compute the sample size. The minimal required sample size was calculated to be 16 subjects for VEP habituation and 9 subjects for SSEP habituation.

A Kolmogorov-Smirnov test showed that VEP and SSEP component latencies and amplitudes had a normal distribution. General linear models approach was used to analyse the 'between-factor' × 'within-factors' interaction effect. The between-subject factor was 'group' (real tDCS versus sham tDCS) or 'time' (before stimulation versus after stimulation) and the within-subject factor was 'block'. Three models of repeated measures analysis of variance (ANOVA), two for VEPs (N1-P1 and P1-N2) and another for SSEPs, followed by univariate ANOVA, were used to investigate the interaction effect. Moreover, in order to analyse the slope of the linear regression (as a measure of habituation), we used a rm.-ANOVA with the between-subject factor 'group' (real tDCS versus sham tDCS) and the within-subject factor 'time' (before stimulation versus after stimulation). Univariate results were analysed only if Wilk's Lambda multivariate significance criterion was achieved. The sphericity of the covariance matrix was verified with the Mauchly Sphericity Test; in the case of

violation of the sphericity assumption, the Greenhouse-Geisser epsilon adjustment was used.

In the rm.-ANOVA and ANOVA models, partial eta2 (η_p^2) and observed power (op) were used as measures of effect size and power, respectively. To identify the comparison(s) contributing to major effects, we performed post hoc Tukey Honest Significant Difference (HSD) tests.

One-way ANOVA tests were used to compare the baseline grand averaged VEP and SSEP latencies and amplitudes between sham and real tDCS. Paired-sample t tests were used to compare the grand averaged VEP and SSEP latencies and amplitudes before vs. after both sham and real tDCS. P values less than 0.05 were considered statistically significant.

Results

Basic neurophysiological parameters

VEP and SSEP recordings were obtained from all participants. The grand averaged VEP latencies (N1, P1, and N2; Table 2) and SEP latencies (N9, N13, N20, P25, and N33; Table 3) as well as their corresponding amplitudes (VEP: N1–P1 and P1–N2; SSEP: N9, N13, N20–P25, and P25–N33) were not significantly different between real and sham tDCS groups ($P > 0.05$). Before stimulation, both groups showed positive slope values indicating a lack of habituation in response to visual (N1–P1: real tDCS = +0.112, sham tDCS = +0.059; P1–N2: real tDCS = +0.055, sham tDCS = +0.039) and somatosensory (real tDCS = +0.448, sham tDCS = +0.234) repetitive stimulations.

Effects of tDCS on neurophysiological parameters

The grand averaged VEP latencies (N1, P1, and N2; Table 2) and SSEP latencies (N9, N13, N20, P25, and N33; Table 3) as well as their corresponding amplitudes (VEP: N1–P1 and P1–N2; SSEP: N9, N13, N20–P25, and P25–N33) were not significantly different before and after stimulation in both the real and sham tDCS groups ($P > 0.05$).

Table 2 Latencies (in milliseconds) and amplitudes (µV) of VEPs in migraine patients' groups undergoing real or sham transcranial direct current stimulation (tDCS) before and after intervention

Electrophysiological parameters	Real (n = 18)		Sham (n = 18)	
	Before	After	Before	After
N1	80.3 ± 5.7	78.9 ± 6.4	78.4 ± 2.0	78.5 ± 3.1
P1	105.5 ± 6.1	105.2 ± 5.8	105.1 ± 4.3	106.7 ± 4.7
N2	146.1 ± 8.9	146.9 ± 9.7	150.7 ± 6.7	151.1 ± 6.8
N1-P1 1st amplitude block (µV)	8.3 ± 3.1	8.9 ± 3.6	7.2 ± 2.7	6.7 ± 2.4
N1-P1 amplitude slope	0.112 ± 0.315	- 0.236 ± 0.339 **	0.059 ± 0.241	0.038 ± 0.182
P1-N2 1st amplitude block (µV)	8.3 ± 3.1	8.9 ± 4.2	6.4 ± 3.4	6.3 ± 2.9
P1-N2 amplitude slope	0.055 ± 0.507	- 0.345 ± 0.569	0.039 ± 0.272	- 0.001 ± 0.269

Data are expressed as means ± SD. ** = $p < 0.01$ before vs. after the intervention

Table 3 Grand-average somatosensory evoked potentials (SSEPs) latencies and amplitudes in migraine patients' groups undergoing real or sham transcranial direct current stimulation (tDCS) before and after intervention

Electrophysiological parameters	Real (n = 18)		Sham (n = 18)	
	Before	After	Before	After
N9 (ms)	9.5 ± 0.6	9.7 ± 0.8	9.5 ± 0.6	9.6 ± 0.6
N13 (ms)	13.2 ± 0.8	13.3 ± 0.8	13.1 ± 0.7	13.2 ± 0.7
N20 (ms)	18.8 ± 0.9	19.0 ± 0.8	18.6 ± 1.1	18.8 ± 1.1
P25 (ms)	23.6 ± 2.2	23.9 ± 2.1	22.9 ± 2.2	23.2 ± 2.2
N33 (ms)	31.5 ± 2.6	31.5 ± 1.6	31.9 ± 2.1	31.5 ± 1.3
N9-p (µV)	4.1 ± 1.6	3.8 ± 1.4	3.5 ± 1.4	3.5 ± 1.9
N13-p (µV)	2.0 ± 0.8	2.0 ± 0.6	2.0 ± 0.6	1.8 ± 0.7
N20-P25 (µV)	2.3 ± 1.3	2.4 ± 1.5	2.3 ± 0.7	2.1 ± 0.9
P25-N33 (µV)	1.3 ± 0.5	1.3 ± 0.9	1.2 ± 0.5	1.0 ± 0.5
N20-P25 1st amplitude (µV)	2.4 ± 1.1	2.2 ± 1.2	2.3 ± 0.7	2.2 ± 0.6
N20-P25 amplitude slope	0.448 ± 0.710	0.315 ± 0.543	0.234 ± 0.406	0.213 ± 0.481

Data are expressed as means ± SD

In the rm.-ANOVA model using the VEP N1–P1 peak-to-peak block amplitude as the dependent variable, the multivariate test was significant for the 'group' × 'time' × 'block' interaction effect ($F_{5,340}$ = 3.290, p = 0.006). The univariate rm.-ANOVA for N1–P1 peak-to-peak amplitudes confirmed a significant interaction factor effect (Greenhouse-Geisser epsilon adjustment applied, $F_{4.1282.1}$ = 3.29, ε = 0.83, p = 0.01, partial $\eta2$ = 0.05, op = 0.89) in the multivariate test. At the post-hoc analysis 1st N1-P1 VEP amplitude block did not differ between before and after both stimulations. The linear regression N1–P1 slope of VEP

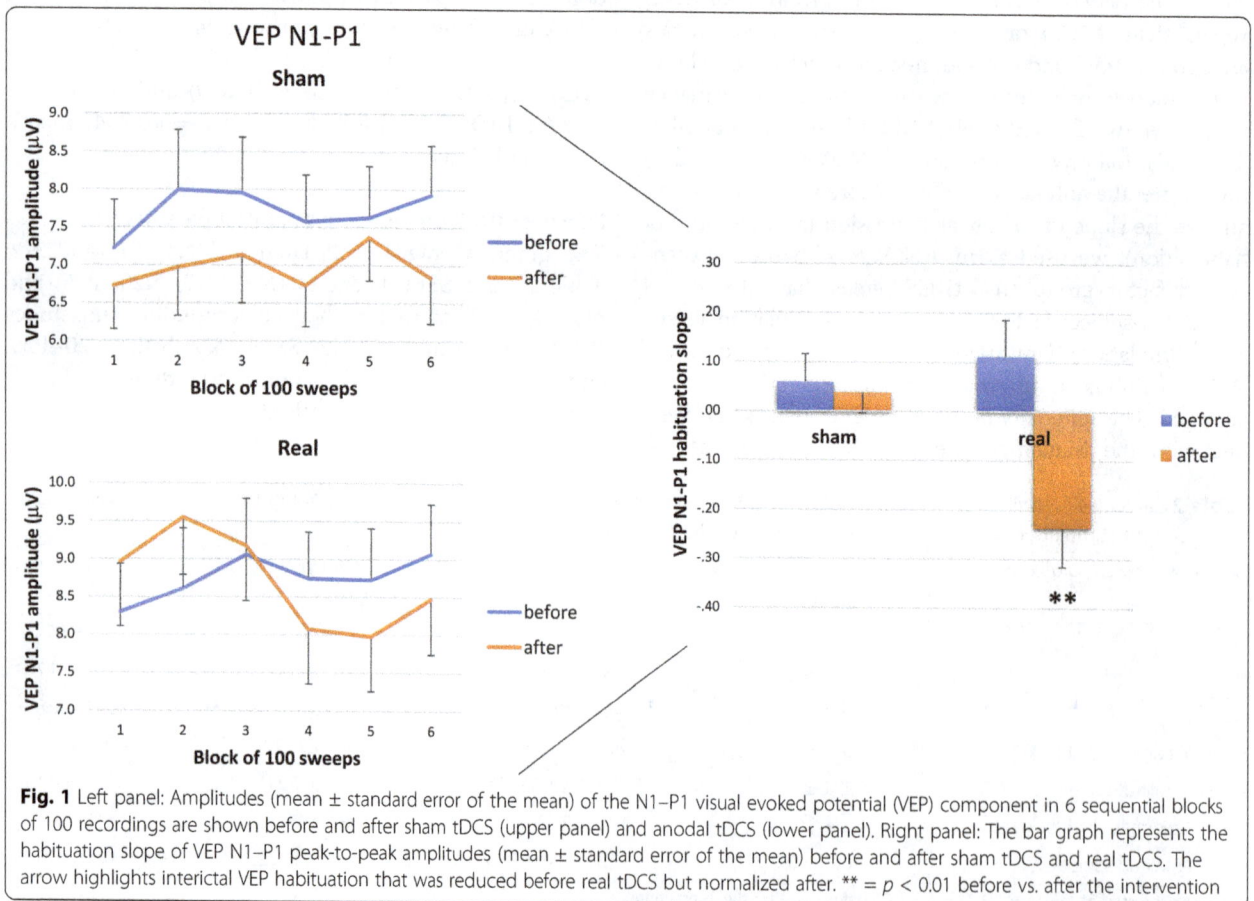

Fig. 1 Left panel: Amplitudes (mean ± standard error of the mean) of the N1–P1 visual evoked potential (VEP) component in 6 sequential blocks of 100 recordings are shown before and after sham tDCS (upper panel) and anodal tDCS (lower panel). Right panel: The bar graph represents the habituation slope of VEP N1–P1 peak-to-peak amplitudes (mean ± standard error of the mean) before and after sham tDCS and real tDCS. The arrow highlights interictal VEP habituation that was reduced before real tDCS but normalized after. ** = p < 0.01 before vs. after the intervention

Anodal transcranial direct current stimulation over the left temporal pole restores normal visual evoked...

115

amplitudes over all blocks was significantly different between before and after stimulation ($F_{1,34}$ = 5.21, p = 0.029, partial η2 = 0.133, op = 0.60; raw data are shown in Fig. 1). A post-hoc analysis showed that the slope of VEP amplitudes from block 1 to block 6 was positive before the intervention in both the real tDCS (+0.112) and sham tDCS (+0.059) groups, whereas after the intervention these values were negative in the real tDCS group (–0.236, p = 0.003 versus before stimulation) but positive in the sham tDCS group (+0.038, p > 0.05 versus before stimulation) (Fig. 1, right panel).

In the rm.-ANOVA model using the VEP P1–N2 peak-to-peak block amplitude as the dependent variable, the 'group' × 'time' × 'block' interaction effect was not significant ($F_{5,340}$ = 1.55, p = 0.171) in the multivariate test (Fig. 2).

In the rm.-ANOVA model using the SSEP N20–P25 peak-to-peak block amplitude as the dependent variable, the 'group' × 'time' × 'block' interaction effect was not significant ($F_{1,68}$ = 0.19, p = 0.659) in the multivariate test (Fig. 3).

Discussion

The present study mainly revealed that a single session of anodal tDCS over the left temporal pole restored normal visual but not somatosensory habituation in interictal migraineurs.

Neurophysiological studies have shown that interictal migraineurs exhibit dysfunctional sensory information processing in the form of habituation deficits in response to various sensory inputs, including visual and somatosensory inputs [2]. Recent neuroimaging studies have revealed subtle microstructural alterations in the brains of patients with migraine in areas associated with the ictal-interictal cycle. Among these studies, some evidence highlights a pathophysiological role for the TP in migraine [7–12].

The TP region encompasses the most anterior segment of the temporal lobe and receives extensive inputs from visual regions of the thalamus [30, 31]. Additionally, the TP is highly interconnected with the amygdala, hippocampus, superior temporal gyrus, hypothalamus, occipitobasal cortex, prefrontal regions, and insula, suggesting its participation in autonomic regulation, memory, and emotional processing [32, 33]. The TP is considered a multisensory associative cortex because it is also connected to the main sensory systems of the temporal lobe, including the visual, auditory, olfactory, and gustative systems, but not the somatosensory system [32, 34]. Indeed, neuroimaging studies have

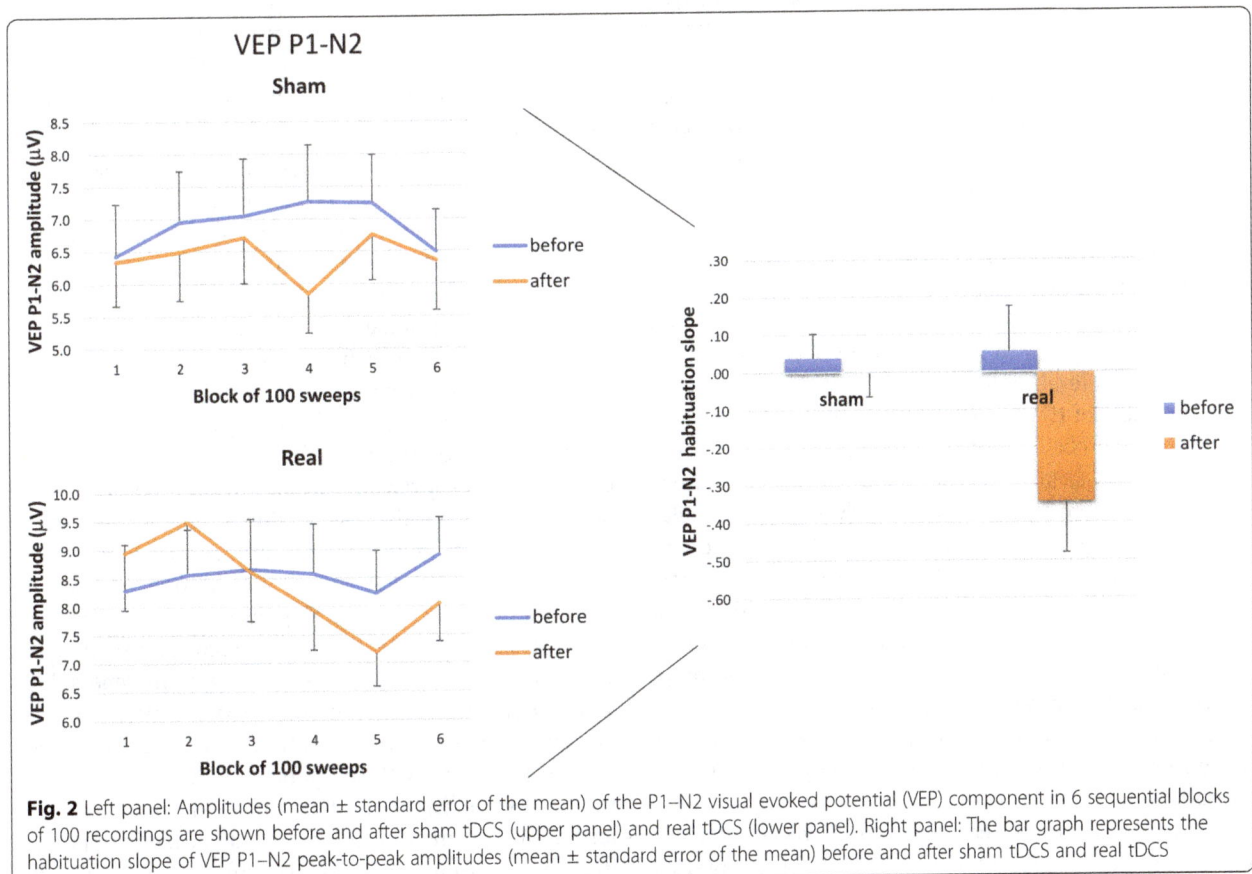

Fig. 2 Left panel: Amplitudes (mean ± standard error of the mean) of the P1–N2 visual evoked potential (VEP) component in 6 sequential blocks of 100 recordings are shown before and after sham tDCS (upper panel) and real tDCS (lower panel). Right panel: The bar graph represents the habituation slope of VEP P1–N2 peak-to-peak amplitudes (mean ± standard error of the mean) before and after sham tDCS and real tDCS

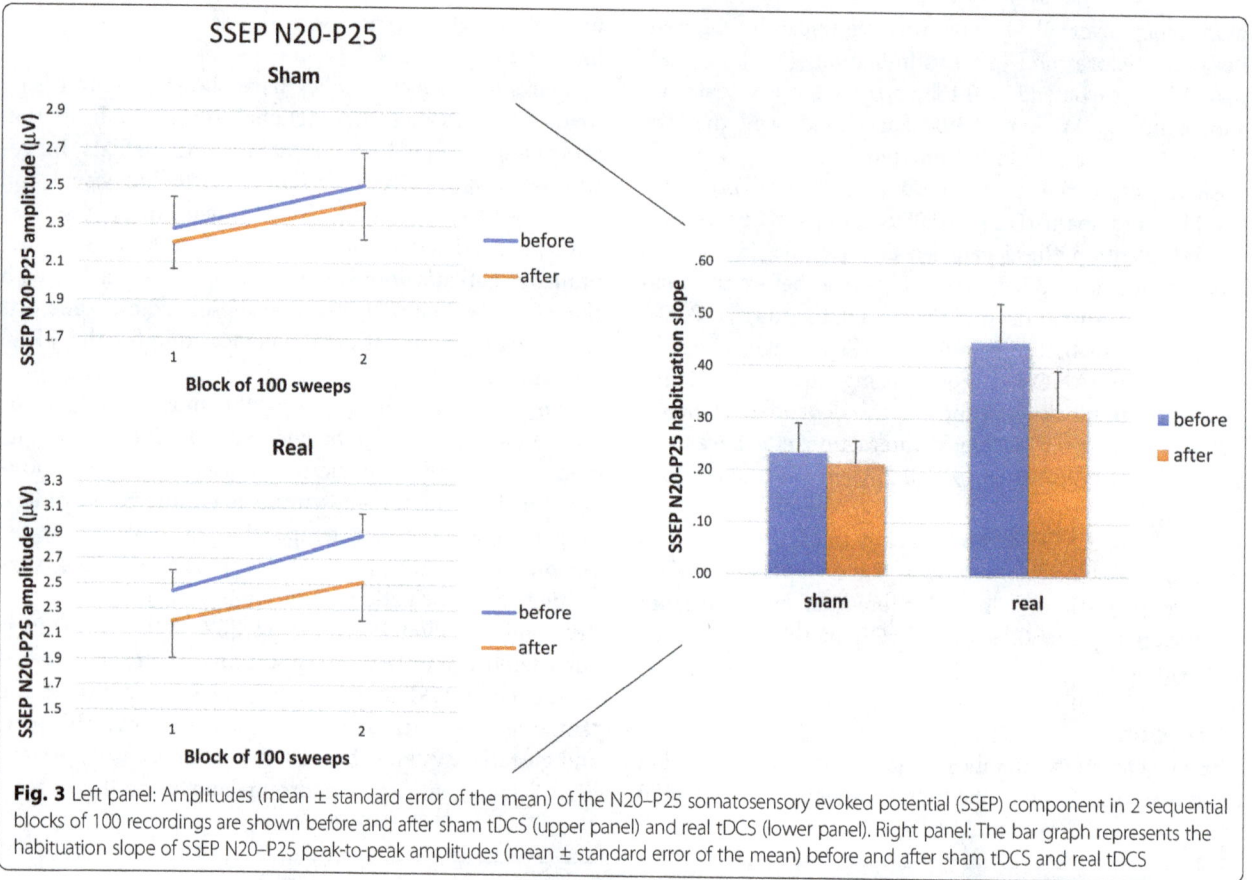

Fig. 3 Left panel: Amplitudes (mean ± standard error of the mean) of the N20–P25 somatosensory evoked potential (SSEP) component in 2 sequential blocks of 100 recordings are shown before and after sham tDCS (upper panel) and real tDCS (lower panel). Right panel: The bar graph represents the habituation slope of SSEP N20–P25 peak-to-peak amplitudes (mean ± standard error of the mean) before and after sham tDCS and real tDCS

demonstrated subregional activation of the TP in response to specific sensory stimuli, with the ventromedial aspect of the TP having a predominant role in higher order visual information processing [34] as part of the VVS.

Our finding that anodal (excitatory) stimulation of the left TP restored physiological visual information processing but not somatosensory processing in interictal migraineurs is largely consistent with the abovementioned roles of the left TP in high-level multimodal perceptual processing. A selective effect of tDCS over the TP on visual information processing is probably related to the role of the TP in the VVS and its lack of participation in somatosensory elaboration. Interestingly, another study observed similar normalization of abnormal interictal VEP habituation in response to the application of tDCS over the occipital cortex in migraineurs [22]. This can be explained either by a direct interconnection between the TP and occipital cortex along the VVS or an indirect effect of the tDCS on brain structures that positively modulate both cortices.

The VVS is involved in visual recognition and in the assignment or retrieval of a given meaning for visual information [35]. After early activation of the occipital area, the complexity of representation of visual information increases as information flows to the anterior regions of the VVS, with the TP located at the end of the stream and sending backward facilitatory projections to the occipital cortex to optimize sensory processing (e.g., improve perception and learning) [35, 36]. Consistent with this evidence, we observed that the enhancement of TP activity with anodal tDCS improved VEP amplitude habituation, a basic form of learning [37], without affecting initial baseline excitability (reflected by non-significant changes in 1st block VEP amplitudes). In habituation paradigms, early and late responses can behave differently as a result of regulation by different mechanisms; according to the dual-process theory, increasing responsiveness (sensitization) competes with decreasing responsiveness (habituation) to determine final behavioural outcomes. Facilitation occurs at the beginning of the stimulus session and accounts for an initial temporary increase in response amplitude, whereas habituation occurs throughout the recording session and accounts for delayed decreases in responsiveness [38]. Therefore, our results regarding the selective effect of anodal tDCS on delayed habituation in migraineurs appear to be in line with the putative mechanism of tDCS; that is, the ability of tDCS to affect the potentiation of long-term learning processes and synaptic plasticity underlying learning and memory [39]. Alternatively, it has been shown that anodal tDCS exerts modulatory effects on thalamo-cortical circuits by increasing functional coupling between the thalamus and cortex [17, 40]. These experimental observations are of particular interest in migraine because independent research groups have previously reported reduced functional [41, 42] and morphological [43, 44] thalamic integrity coupled with decreased intracortical inhibition during visual stimulation in migraineurs [45, 46]. We thus can hypothesize that an alternative mechanism of action for anodal tDCS in the present study is increased thalamo-cortical activity, which in turn increased delayed inhibitory mechanisms to restore normal VEP habituation.

Irrespective of the mechanism, the observation that tDCS over the left TP is able to restore normal VEP habituation in interictal migraineurs leads to hypothesize that together with the visual, motor, and dorsolateral prefrontal cortices [19, 20], the TP could represent a novel target for tDCS as a prophylactic strategy for treating migraine [47].

This study had some limitations. For example, we only stimulated the left TP, such that we cannot know whether anodal tDCS of the right TP would have yielded similar results. Several studies have shown divergent functional roles of the left and right TP, where the right TP is more involved in elaborating socio-emotional implications of multisensory perceptual stimuli [48] while the left TP is mostly implicated in perceptual decoding, semantic processing, and conceptualization [34]. Nonetheless, both the left and right TPs are joined via the interior white commissure to advance multimodal perceptual analysis [32], such that the relevance of the right TP cannot be discounted. Furthermore, the positioning method we used is accurate, although not as accurate as neuronavigation-based techniques, which are unfortunately only available for neurosurgical procedures in our clinic. Another shortcoming of the present study is the lack of inclusion of a healthy control group undergoing the same stimulations, although this would not add anything to the results of the study because the healthy subjects usually already habituate normally at the baseline, i.e. we cannot normalize the already normal information processing.

Conclusions

In conclusion, anodal but not sham tDCS selectively enhanced visual but not somatosensory habituation in interictal migraineurs probably by restoring normal inhibitory activity of the left TP. We propose that this effect can be explained by either a direct interference with short- and long-term synaptic plasticity mechanisms or an indirect potentiation of the thalamo-cortical circuit. Further studies are needed to determine whether TP stimulation also normalizes the habituation response to other sensory inputs, such as auditory and nociceptive inputs. Regardless of the underlying cellular and molecular mechanisms of our observed effect, we propose that the TP should be considered as a key site of involvement in the pathophysiology of migraine and as a potential therapeutic target. Clinical studies are needed to clarify whether repeated sessions of anodal tDCS improve TP function and connectivity in patients with migraine to ultimately reduce the number and severity of migraine attacks.

Abbreviations
EEG: Electroencephalogram; MO: Migraine without aura; SSEP: Somatosensory evoked potential; tDCS: transcranial direct current stimulation; TP: Temporal pole; VEP: Visual evoked potential; VVS: Ventral visual stream

Acknowledgments
The Italian Ministry of Health and Fondazione Roma provided financial support for this study.

Authors' contributions
FC and GC made substantial contributions to interpretation of data as well as in drafting the manuscript. FP, AP, MS, VP, and ME were implied in the interpretation of data as well as in drafting the manuscript. CDL was implicate in patients' recruitment and in setting stimulator's parameters. IB and FC were implied in recording the data; GC was implicated in analysing data. All authors read and approved the final manuscript.

Competing interests
The authors declare that they have no competing interests.

Author details
[1]Department of Medico-Surgical Sciences and Biotechnologies, Sapienza University of Rome Polo Pontino, Corso della Repubblica, 79 – 04100, Latina, Italy. [2]INM Neuromed IRCCS, Pozzilli (IS), Italy. [3]Don Carlo Gnocchi, Onlus Foundation, Milan, Italy. [4]Università Cattolica del Sacro Cuore/CIC, Istituto di Anestesiologia, Rianimazione e Terapia del Dolore, Rome, Italy. [5]G. B. Bietti Foundation IRCCS, Research Unit of Neurophysiology of Vision and Neuro-Ophthalmology, Rome, Italy.

References
1. Sprenger T, Borsook D (2012) Migraine changes the brain: neuroimaging makes its mark. Curr Opin Neurol 25:252–262
2. Coppola G, Di Lorenzo C, Schoenen J, Pierelli F (2013) Habituation and sensitization in primary headaches. J Headache Pain 14:65
3. Lai TH, Protsenko E, Cheng YC et al (2015) Neural plasticity in common forms of chronic headaches. Neural Plast 2015:205985
4. Shapiro K, Hillstrom AP, Husain M (2002) Control of visuotemporal attention by inferior parietal and superior temporal cortex. Curr Biol 12:1320–1325
5. Kravitz DJ, Saleem KS, Baker CI et al (2013) The ventral visual pathway: an expanded neural framework for the processing of object quality. Trends Cogn Sci 17:26–49
6. Patterson K, Nestor PJ, Rogers TT (2007) Where do you know what you know? The representation of semantic knowledge in the human brain. Nat Rev 8:976–987
7. Demarquay G, Royet JP, Mick G, Ryvlin P (2008) Olfactory hypersensitivity in migraineurs: a H(2)(15)O-PET study. Cephalalgia 28:1069–1080
8. Moulton EA, Becerra L, Maleki N et al (2011) Painful heat reveals hyperexcitability of the temporal pole in interictal and ictal migraine states. Cereb cortex (New York, NY 1991) 21:435–448
9. Stankewitz A, May A (2011) Increased limbic and brainstem activity during migraine attacks following olfactory stimulation. Neurology 77:476–482
10. Coppola G, Di Renzo A, Tinelli E et al (2015) Evidence for brain morphometric changes during the migraine cycle: a magnetic resonance-based morphometry study. Cephalalgia 35:783–791

11. Tessitore A, Russo A, Giordano A et al (2013) Disrupted default mode network connectivity in migraine without aura. J Headache Pain 14:89

12. Schwedt TJ, Berisha V, Chong CD (2015) Temporal lobe cortical thickness correlations differentiate the migraine brain from the healthy brain. PLoS One 10:e0116687

13. Priori A, Berardelli A, Rona S et al (1998) Polarization of the human motor cortex through the scalp. Neuroreport 9:2257–2260

14. Nitsche MA, Cohen LG, Wassermann EM et al (2008) Transcranial direct current stimulation: state of the art 2008. Brain Stimul 1:206–223

15. Brunoni AR, Nitsche MA, Bolognini N et al (2012) Clinical research with transcranial direct current stimulation (tDCS): challenges and future directions. Brain Stimul 5:175–195

16. Zaghi S, Heine N, Fregni F (2009) Brain stimulation for the treatment of pain: a review of costs, clinical effects, and mechanisms of treatment for three different central neuromodulatory approaches. J Pain Manag 2:339–352

17. DaSilva AF, Truong DQ, DosSantos MF et al (2015) State-of-art neuroanatomical target analysis of high-definition and conventional tDCS montages used for migraine and pain control. Front Neuroanat 9:89

18. Bikson M, Grossman P, Thomas C et al (2016) Safety of Transcranial direct current stimulation: evidence based update 2016. Brain Stimul 9:641–661

19. Auvichayapat P, Janyacharoen T, Rotenberg A et al (2012) Migraine prophylaxis by anodal transcranial direct current stimulation, a randomized, placebo-controlled trial. J Med Assoc Thail 95:1003–1012

20. Dasilva A, Mendonca ME, Zaghi S et al (2012) tDCS-induced analgesia and electrical fields in pain-related neural networks in chronic migraine. Headache 52:1283–1295

21. Andrade SM, de Brito Aranha REL, de Oliveira EA et al (2017) Transcranial direct current stimulation over the primary motor vs prefrontal cortex in refractory chronic migraine: a pilot randomized controlled trial. J Neurol Sci 378:225–232

22. Viganò A, D'Elia TS, Sava SL et al (2013) Transcranial direct current stimulation (tDCS) of the visual cortex: a proof-of-concept study based on interictal electrophysiological abnormalities in migraine. J Headache Pain 14:23

23. Gallate J, Chi R, Ellwood S, Snyder A (2009) Reducing false memories by magnetic pulse stimulation. Neurosci Lett 449:151–154

24. Chi RP, Fregni F, Snyder AW (2010) Visual memory improved by non-invasive brain stimulation. Brain Res 1353:168–175

25. Herwig U, Satrapi P, Schönfeldt-Lecuona C (2003) Using the international 10-20 EEG system for positioning of transcranial magnetic stimulation. Brain Topogr 16:95–99

26. Sparing R, Buelte D, Meister IG et al (2008) Transcranial magnetic stimulation and the challenge of coil placement: a comparison of conventional and stereotaxic neuronavigational strategies. Hum Brain Mapp 29:82–96

27. Ozkul Y, Uckardes A (2002) Median nerve somatosensory evoked potentials in migraine. Eur J Neurol 9:227–232

28. Coppola G, Iacovelli E, Bracaglia M et al (2013) Electrophysiological correlates of episodic migraine chronification: evidence for thalamic involvement. J Headache Pain 14:76

29. Di Lorenzo C, Coppola G, Bracaglia M et al (2016) Cortical functional correlates of responsiveness to short-lasting preventive intervention with ketogenic diet in migraine: a multimodal evoked potentials study. J Headache Pain 17:58

30. Markowitsch HJ, Emmans D, Irle E et al (1985) Cortical and subcortical afferent connections of the primate's temporal pole: a study of rhesus monkeys, squirrel monkeys, and marmosets. J Comp Neurol 242:425–458

31. Cusick CG, Scripter JL, Darensbourg JG, Weber JT (1993) Chemoarchitectonic subdivisions of the visual pulvinar in monkeys and their connectional relations with the middle temporal and rostral dorsolateral visual areas, MT and DLr. J Comp Neurol 336:1–30

32. Chabardès S, Kahane P, Minotti L et al (2002) Anatomy of the temporal pole region. Epileptic Disord 4(Suppl 1):S9–15

33. Olson IR, Plotzker A, Ezzyat Y (2007) The enigmatic temporal pole: a review of findings on social and emotional processing. Brain 130:1718–1731

34. Pascual B, Masdeu JC, Hollenbeck M et al (2015) Large-scale brain networks of the human left temporal pole: a functional connectivity MRI study. Cereb Cortex 25:680–702

35. Pehrs C, Zaki J, Schlochtermeier LH et al (2017) The temporal pole top-down modulates the ventral visual stream during social cognition. Cereb Cortex 27:777–792

36. Bar M (2003) A cortical mechanism for triggering top-down facilitation in visual object recognition. J Cogn Neurosci 15:600–609

37. Harris JD (1943) Habituatory response decrement in the intact organism. Psychol Bull 40:385–422

38. Rankin CH, Abrams T, Barry RJ et al (2009) Habituation revisited: an updated and revised description of the behavioral characteristics of habituation. Neurobiol Learn Mem 92:135–138

39. Rioult-Pedotti MS, Friedman D, Donoghue JP (2000) Learning-induced LTP in neocortex. Science 290:533–536

40. Polanía R, Paulus W, Nitsche MA (2012) Modulating cortico-striatal and thalamo-cortical functional connectivity with transcranial direct current stimulation. Hum Brain Mapp 33:2499–2508

41. Hodkinson DJ, Wilcox SL, Veggeberg R et al (2016) Increased amplitude of Thalamocortical low-frequency oscillations in patients with migraine. J Neurosci 36:8026–8036

42. Porcaro C, Di Lorenzo G, Seri S et al (2016) Impaired brainstem and thalamic high-frequency oscillatory EEG activity in migraine between attacks. Cephalalgia. doi:10.1177/0333102416657146

43. Coppola G, Tinelli E, Lepre C et al (2014) Dynamic changes in thalamic microstructure of migraine without aura patients: a diffusion tensor magnetic resonance imaging study. Eur J Neurol 21:287–e13

44. Magon S, May A, Stankewitz A et al (2015) Morphological abnormalities of thalamic subnuclei in migraine: a multicenter MRI study at 3 Tesla. J Neurosci 35:13800–13806

45. Höffken O, Stude P, Lenz M et al (2009) Visual paired-pulse stimulation reveals enhanced visual cortex excitability in migraineurs. Eur J Neurosci 30:714–720

46. Coppola G, Parisi V, Di Lorenzo C et al (2013) Lateral inhibition in visual cortex of migraine patients between attacks. J Headache Pain 14:20

47. Martelletti P, Jensen RH, Antal A et al (2013) Neuromodulation of chronic headaches: position statement from the European headache federation. J Headache Pain 14:86

48. Tippett LJ, Miller LA, Farah MJ (2000) Prosopamnesia: a selective impairment in face learning. Cogn Neuropsychol 17:241–255

15

Functional connectivity and cognitive impairment in migraine with and without aura

Viviana Lo Buono[1*], Lilla Bonanno[1], Francesco Corallo[1], Laura Rosa Pisani[1], Riccardo Lo Presti[1], Rosario Grugno[1], Giuseppe Di Lorenzo[1], Placido Bramanti[1] and Silvia Marino[1,2]

Abstract

Background: Several fMRI studies in migraine assessed resting state functional connectivity in different networks suggesting that this neurological condition was associated with brain functional alteration. The aim of present study was to explore the association between cognitive functions and cerebral functional connectivity, in default mode network, in migraine patients without and with aura, during interictal episodic attack.

Methods: Twenty-eight migraine patients (14 without and 14 with aura) and 14 matched normal controls, were consecutively recruited. A battery of standardized neuropsychological test was administered to evaluate cognitive functions and all subjects underwent a resting state with high field fMRI examination.

Results: Migraine patients did not show abnormalities in neuropsychological evaluation, while, we found a specific alteration in cortical network, if we compared migraine with and without aura. We observed, in migraine with aura, an increased connectivity in left angular gyrus, left supramarginal gyrus, right precentral gyrus, right postcentral gyrus, right insular cortex.

Conclusion: Our findings showed in migraine patients an alteration in functional connectivity architecture. We think that our results could be useful to better understand migraine pathogenesis.

Keywords: Migraine, Cognitive functions, Functional connectivity, default mode network

Background

Migraine is a common episodic neurological disorder with a complex physiopathology. It is characterized by typical unilateral, often severe, pain throbbing with associated features such as hypersensitivity to multiple stimuli, including visual (photophobia), auditory (phonophobia), and sensory (cutaneous allodynia) stimuli during migraine attacks [1]. Indeed, about one third of patients had experience of aura associated to visual, motor, or somatosensory symptoms during attacks [2, 3].

Migraine is a very common and debilitating disease that causes significant limitations in daily life with effects on emotional-behavioral and relational aspects [4].

Neuropsychological studies suggests that migraine affect also cognitive functions during attacks and interictal periods [5], even though it is unclear the association between cognitive dysfunctions and migraine. Migraineurs could present executive dysfunction which presumably reflects frontal lobe abnormalities [6], or alteration in memory areas. However, while several authors reported significant lower performances in migraine patients, others did not confirm these findings. In other cases authorsdescribed the presence of cognitive deficit only after a long disease duration [7, 8].

Several fMRI studies in migraine assessed resting state functional connectivity in various networks suggesting an association with cortical functional alteration [9]. In particular, some authors reported increased connectivity in specifics cerebral areas, such as right rostral anterior cingulate cortex, prefrontal cortex, orbitofrontal cortex and supplementary motor area [10]. This altered connectivity

* Correspondence: viv.lobuono@gmail.com
[1]IRCCS Centro Neurolesi "Bonino-Pulejo", S.S. 113 Via Palermo, C.da Casazza, 98124 Messina, Italy

could indicate intrinsic pathophysiological changes in migraine, even if only a very few studies explored the different functional connectivity in migraine with (MA) and without aura (MO) [11].

The aim of present study was to explore the association between cognitive functions and cerebral functional connectivity (FC) between MO and MA, during interictal episodic attack.

Methods

Twenty-eight migraine patients (14 without aura and 14 with aura) and 14 sex and age matched health controls (HC), were enrolled. Aura included temporary visual or sensory disturbances nausea, and sensitivity to light and sound. The patients were recruited from migraine ambulatory. The diagnosis of definite MA or MO was performed by two neurologist, specialist in headache disorders, blinded to MRI and neuropsychological findings, according to International Headache Society criteria [12] (Headache Classification Committee of the International Headache, 2013).

Control subjects were volunteers recruited from local communities, with no history of neurological diseases. They did not suffer from migraine or headache and were free from medication intake. The study protocol was approved by the Local Ethics Committee according to Declaration of Helsinki. All patients gave written consent to study. All information related to migraine was collected by interviews and examination of medical records. All patients had a clinic diagnosis for at least 10 years. We excluded patients with: 1) other types of headache; 2) vascular disease or trauma; 3) history of major psychiatric disorders; 4) presence of metabolic disorders; 5) other neurological conditions.

Demographic and clinical characteristics were also collected (Table 1). The type of medication, during attack, in patient included: simple analgesics (18/24), simple triptens (4/24), and combination analgesics (6/24).

Table 1 Socio-demographic characteristics of patients with aura (n = 14) without aura (n = 14) and controls (n = 14)

	Aura (Mean ± SD)	No Aura (Mean ± SD)	HC (Mean ± SD)
Age	41.28 ± 13.44	40.75 ± 11.82	41.75 ± 12.82
Years of education	15.8 ± 3.2	16.7 ± 4.2	16.2 ± 4.1
Disease duration	10.9 ± 3.7	12.3 ± 5.8	
Attack frequency/month (n)	5.05 ± 2.31	6.07 ± 2.81	
Single-Attack duration (hours)	3.58 ± 2.27	4.21 ± 2.99	
Days to next migraine attack after examination			

Legend: *SD* standard deviation

A battery of standardized neuropsychological test to evaluate cognitive functions, was administered by two psychologists, blinded to patients/controls status, diagnosis and MRI findings. Processing speed was assessed using the Trail Making Test, Part A (TMT-A), [13]. Attentional set-shifting was measured using the Trail Making Test, Part B (TMT-B). Memory was assessed using the Rey Auditory Verbal Learning Test (RAVLT) [14]. Language was assessed with semantic and phonemic verbal fluency test [15]. Wisconsin Card Sorting test (WCST) was used for executive function and cognitive flexibility. Finally, Hamilton Rating Scale for depression (HAM-D) and Hamilton Rating Scale for anxiety (HAM-A) were used to asses anxiety and depressive symptoms [16, 17].

All patient underwent to a MRI examination with a scanner operating at 3.0 T (Achieva, Philips Healthcare, Best, The Netherlands), by using a 32-channel SENSE head coil. MRI scans were performed in the interictal stage at least 3 days after migraine attack. For each subject, T1 [TR = 8 ms, TE = 4 ms, slice thickness/gap = 1/0 mm, number of slices = 173, field of view 240 mm], T2-weighted [TR = 3.0 s, TE = 80 ms, slice thickness/gap = 3.0/0.3 mm, number of slices = 30, field of view 230 mm] were acquired. The scan parameters of the resting-state functional magnetic resonance imaging (fMRI) scan were as follows: TR = 3.0 s; TE = 35 msec; flip angle = 90°; and voxel size 1.9 · 1.9 · 4.0 mm, scan duration 10 min. During the resting-state scan, participants were instructed to lie still with their eyes closed and not to fall asleep.

Neuropsychological testing and MRI scanning were performed on same day.

Resting state analysis

fMRI-analysis was performed with FSL (FMRIB's Software Library, www.fmrib.ox.ac.uk/fsl). The following pre-processing procedure was applied: employing different modules of the FSL-software package. The preprocessing of the resting-state data consisted of motion correction (MCFLIRT) [18], brain extraction [19], spatial smoothing using a Gaussian kernel with a full width at a half maximum of 8 mm. After preprocessing, the functional images were registered to the corresponding high-resolution echo planar images, (co-registered to T1-weighted images,) which were registered to the 2 mm isotropic MNI-152 standard space image [18]. These registration parameters were combined to obtain registration matrix from native (fMRI) space to MNI space and its inverse (from MNI space to native space). Independent component analysis (ICA) was carried out using MELODIC toolbox implementing probabilistic independent component analysis (PICA) [20]. Variance normalization was used and IC maps were thresholded using an alternative hypothesis test based on fitting a Gaussian/gamma mixture model to distribution of voxel intensities within spatial maps and controlling the local false-discovery rate at $p < 0.5$ [20]. The selection of clusters of interest obtained of MELODIC analysis implied the presence of anatomically relevant areas in each group component map that reproduced the layouts of the main physiological resting state network jointly and consistently across subjects. The artefact components were removed manually from analysis and for all groups we considered IC of the DMN, one of the main networks that are consistently identified when an individual is at wakeful rest and not performing an attention-demanding task. This network includes the precuneus, posterior cingulate cortex (PCC), medial prefrontal cortex, medial temporal lobe and angular gyrus. For inter group analysis was carried out using dual regression (FSL technique) that allows for voxel-wise comparisons of resting-state [21, 22]. This allow, a) to separate fMRI data sets using the group-ICA spatial maps in a linear model fit against, resulting in matrices (time-course matrices) describing the temporal dynamics for each component and subject, and b) estimate subject-specific spatial maps using these time-course matrices. The dual regression analysis was performed with variance normalization because reflects differences in both activity and spatial spread of the network. As a statistical analysis the different component maps are collected across subjects into single 4D files and tested voxel-wise for statistically significant differences between the groups using FSL randomize non parametric permutation testing, with 5000 permutations, using a threshold-free cluster enhanced (TFCE) technique to control for multiple comparisons [23] and corrected for multiple comparisons (across space) within the permutation framework. Age and gender also included in this analysis as nuisance variable. The Harvard-Oxford Cortical structural atlas were used to identify the anatomical characteristics of the resulting PICA maps. Fslstats and fslmaths tools were used to calculate the number of non-zero voxels in the selected difference maps, and their t-score values.

Results

Demographic characteristics

Inter group analysis by U Mann Whitney test no highlighted differences between characteristics and clinical scores of patients (Table 1). There were no differences between MA and MO patients in age, ($p = 0.84$), education ($p = 0.35$) and disease duration ($p = 0.27$). Both groups did not show abnormalities in neuropsychological evaluation (Table 2).

Table 2 Cognitive performances of the migraine patients

Test	Aura	No Aura	Controls groups	Cut-off
Attention				
Attentive Matrix	44.60 ± 4.80	45.51 ± 6.91	43.35 ± 7.87	30
Language				
Fluency Phonemic	32.08 ± 11.72	35.35 ± 10.9	30.85 ± 6.63	17
Fluency Semantic	36.25 ± 6.64	36.28 ± 5.86	37.42 ± 5.74	25
Memory				
RAVLT (Immediate recall)	40.86 ± 25.01	36.28 ± 5.86	38.17 ± 4.59	28.53
RAVLT (Delayed recall)	8.2 ± 2.45	9.23 ± 3.10	6.85 ± 1.65	4.69
Executive Functions				
Trial Making Test-A	42.62 ± 25.01	48.73 ± 55.20	55.28 ± 15.52	93
Trial Making Test-B	123.35 ± 56.28	155.14 ± 70.16	126.64 ± 30.49	282

Resting state

MA vs MO

MA group showed increased functional connectivity if compared to MO group (blue area, p values are color coded from 0.05 FWE corrected (dark blue) to <0.0001 FWE corrected (light blue). Increased in functional connectivity was found in left angular gyrus, left supramarginal gyrus, right precentral gyrus, right postcentral gyrus, right insular cortex (Fig. 1a, full list of structures are showed in Table 3). No significant voxels for MA < MO were found.

MA vs HC

Patients showed increased functional connectivity (blue area, p values are color coded from 0.05 FWE corrected (dark blue) to <0.0001 FWE corrected (light blue)) in bilateral frontal pole, right paracingulate gyrus, in right first and second Heschl's gyrus, planum temporale, left in first and second Heschl's gyrus, planum temporale and superior temporal gyrus (Fig. 1b, full list of structures in Table 4). No significant voxels for MA < HC were found.

MO vs HC

Cerebral regions showed increased functional connectivity in the DMN included right lingual gyrus, occipital fusiform gyrus, occipital pole and cingulate gyrus and, in the left side, increase connectivity in lingual gyrus, occipital fusiform gyrus, occipital pole and cingulate gyrus

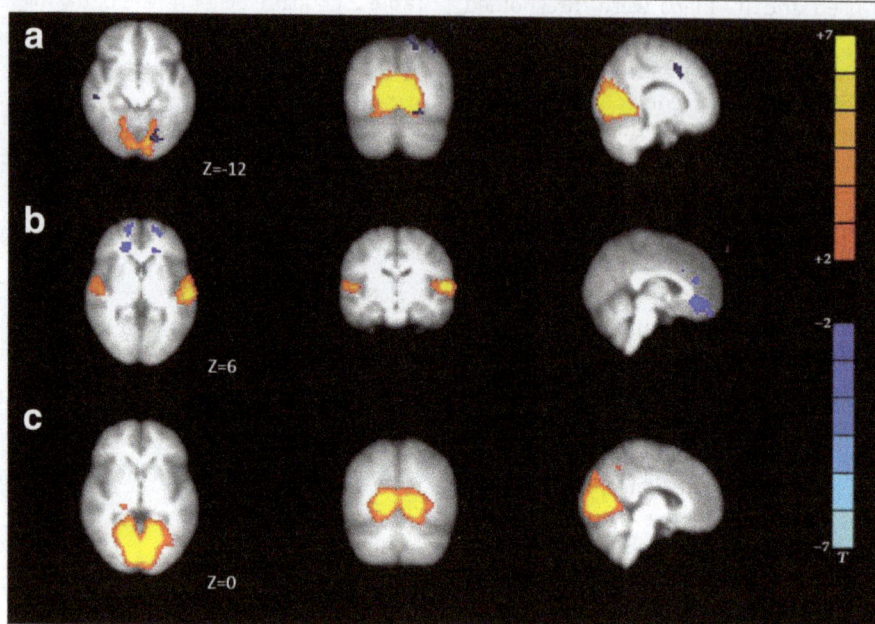

Fig. 1 *Functional connectivity average DMN of groups:* **a.** MA > MO group; **b.** MA > HC; **c.** MO > HC group. MA patients showed increased functional connectivity compared MO (*blue areas*, p values are color coded from 0.05 FWE corrected (*dark blue*) to <0.0001 FWE corrected (*light blue*), full list of structures in Table 2). Axial images are overlaid on transverse slices of MNI-152 standard anatomical image. The left side of the brain corresponds to the right hemisphere and vice versa. Z-coordinates of each slice in the MNI-152 standard space are given

(Fig. 1c, full list of structures in Table 5) in both groups. No significant voxels for MO < HC were found.

Discussion

Recently, several studies investigated the activity of resting state network in migraine and showed alterations in brain functional reorganization. Altered functional connectivity was found in cognitive cerebral networks, such as executive control network, default mode network,

visual network. It seem to be associated to disease duration, gender, and migraine chronicity [24–26]. The DMN is a cerebral network related to different regions with relatively greater activity during rest-state than during active conditions [27, 28]. It refers to an interconnected group of brain structures that are hypothesized to be part of a functional system. Although the exact functional role of DMN is not completely know, it is thought to be involved in several cognitive processes, such as memory, problem solving and planning [2, 29]. In DMN, there are heteromodal association areas, which have a high number of connections with brain regions involved in integration processes, including pain matrics. In chronic pain DMN is altered [30], and this is possibly due to the increase of baseline activity of other cognitive,

Table 3 Increased functional connectivity in MA compared with MO

Brain Structure	Peak voxel coordinates (MNI)			Peak T-score
	x	y	z	
Right Central Opercular Cortex	48	-6	6	3.89
Right Insular cortex	42	−9	6	4.97
Right first and second Heschl's Gyrus	45	−12	6	4.12
Left Central Opercular Cortex	−45	−9	6	3.17
Left first and second Heschl's Gyrus	−51	−15	6	3.75
Left Superior Temporal gyrus	−69	−27	6	3.41
Right Lingual gyrus	18	−66	−12	4.61
Right Occipital fusiform gyrus	18	−75	−12	5.48
Left occipital pole	−12	−93	−12	6.60
Left Lingual gyrus	−12	−84	−12	6.82

Harvard-Oxford Cortical structural atlas
For each peak voxel x-, y-, and z-coordinates in the MNI − 152 standard space image are given

Table 4 Increased functional connectivity in MA compared with HC group

Brain Structure	Peak voxel coordinates (MNI)			Peak T-score
	x	y	z	
Right Heschi's	54	-15	6	4.20
Right Planum temporale	54	−21	6	3.97
Left Heschi's gyrus	−54	−15	6	3.80
Left Planum temporale	−57	−21	6	3.51
Left Superior temporal gyrus	−57	−33	6	3.75

Harvard-Oxford Cortical structural atlas
For each peak voxel x-, y-, and z-coordinates in the MNI-152 standard space image are given

Table 5 Increased functional connectivity in MO compared with HC group

Brain Structure	Peak voxel coordinates (MNI)			Peak T-score
	x	y	z	
Right Lingual gyrus	18	−54	0	3.54
Right Occipital fusiform gyrus	21	−75	0	3.21
Right Occipital pole	9	−93	0	4.85
Right Cingulate gyrus	18	−45	0	2.8
Left Lingual gyrus	−18	−54	0	4.0
Left Occipital fusiform gyrus	−21	−75	0	3.1
Left Occipital pole	−9	−93	0	4.57
Left Cingulate gyrus	−12	−45	0	3.5

Harvard-Oxford Cortical structural atlas
For each peak voxel x-, y-, and z-coordinates in the MNI-152 standard space image are given

salience, or sensorimotor networks. Over time, chronic pain becomes an intrinsic brain activity occurring even in the absence of explicit brain input or output: thus, the alterations in patient's brain at "rest" could be considered as a different or altered DMN organization [31]. In our study we identified specific alterations, during resting state examination, in cortical DMN if we compared MA, MO and HC. Our findings showed an increase of functional connectivity, in MA, in frontal and parietal lobes, in particular in angular, supramarginal gyrus, somatosensory association cortex, postcentral gyrus and primary somatosensory cortex. Since pain is inherently salient it is rational to speculate that the intrinsic connectivity in this network may be changed in chronic pain patients, like migraine subjects. In addition, in MA patients, we found an altered connectivity in insular cortex. It is know that insula is involved in triggering of pain matrix network and in the subjective pain experience [32]. It is also implicated in cognitive, affective, and regulatory functions, including interoceptive awareness, emotional responses, empathic and attentional processes [33]. The insula seems to be a cortical hub, to process complex sensory and emotional aspects in the migraine condition [34], through connections in frontal, temporal and parietal cortex, basal ganglia, thalamus and limbic structures. It is important to understand if functional connectivity abnormalities in this network could be correlated to minimal impairments in neuropsychological performances, such as processing speed, verbal memory, as reported in migraine in interictal attack period. In fact, although MA showed a cognitive performance lower than MO in executive functions, we did not find a significant impairment in two groups. In other word, in our patients, connectivity altered in DMN dwas not associate to neuropsychological variables and cognitive performances.

Moreover, we found in MA a greater cortical hyperexcitability than MO: resting-state abnormal activity could

play a key role in the pathogenesis knowledge of migraine attacks with aura [35]. In particular, alterations of the DMN functional connectivity in migraine may lead to changes in pain modulating network, which could be considered as a neuroimaging biomarkers for disease pathophysiology.

Conclusions

The importance of various frequencies of BOLD fluctuations is not yet known, even if recently few studies started to explore this feature, especially in pain conditions. Brain dysfunction affecting intrinsic connectivity in migraine, possibly reflecting the impact of long lasting and constant pain on brain function.

Although our study was limited to a small sample size, our results confirmed that brain functional connectivity in migraine patients showed an alteration of DMN connectivity, suggesting that pain has a widespread impact on brain function, since modify the complex brain networks and beyond pain perception. Although migraine is one of the most investigated neurologic disorders, specific neuroimaging biomarker for its pathophysiology has not been found.Altered intrinsic functional connectivity architecture was identified in migraine patients and our finding could provide a new perspective to understand the pathogenesis of MA and MO migraine, in order to find a more appropriate therapeutic management.

Authors' contributions
VLB contributed to study conception and design, acquisition of data, analysis and interpretation of data, drafting of manuscript and critical revision; LB has made substantial contributions to the statistical analysis of data. FC and LRP have performed the clinical data collection. RL, RG, GDL have made substantial contributions to interpretation of data. PB and SM have been involved in analysis and interpretation data and in the drafting of manuscript and critical revision. All authors read and approved the final manuscript.

Competing interests
The authors have no competing interests to report.

Author details
[1]IRCCS Centro Neurolesi "Bonino-Pulejo", S.S. 113 Via Palermo, C.da Casazza, 98124 Messina, Italy. [2]Department of Biomedical and Dental Sciences and Morphological and Functional Imaging, University of Messina, Messina, Italy.

References
1. Schwedt TJ (2013) Multisensory integration in migraine. Curr Opin Neurol 26(3):248
2. Tessitore A, Russo A, Giordano A, Conte F, Corbo D, De Stefano M, Cirillo S, Cirillo M, Esposito F, Tedeschi G (2013) Disrupted default mode network connectivity in migraine without aura. J Headache Pain 14:89
3. Rasmussen BK, Olesen J (1992) Migraine with aura and migraine without aura: an epidemiological study. Cephalalgia 12(4):221–228
4. Corallo F, De Cola MC, Lo Buono V, Grugno R, Pintabona G, Presti L et al (2015) Assessment of anxiety, depressive disorders and pain intensity in migraine and tension headache patients. Acta Med Austriaca 31:615
5. Santangelo G, Russo A, Trojano L, Falco F, Marcuccio L, Siciliano M, Conte F, Garramone TA, Tedeschi G (2016) Cognitive dysfunctions and psychological

symptoms in migraine without aura: a cross-sectional study. J Headache Pain 17(1):76

6. Le Pira F, Reggio E, Quattrocchi G, Sanfilippo C, Maci T, Cavallaro T, Zappia M (2014) Executive dysfunctions in migraine with and without aura: what is the role of white matter lesions? Headache 54(1):125–130

7. Pearson AJ, Chronicle EP, Maylor EA, Bruce LA (2006) Cognitive function is not impaired in people with a long history of migraine: a blinded study. Cephalalgia 26:74–80

8. Kalaydjian A, Zandi PP, Swartz KL, Eaton WW, Lyketsos C (2007) How migraines impact cognitive function findings from the Baltimore ECA. Neurology 68(17):1417–1424

9. Zhang J, Su J, Wang M, Zhao Y, Yao Q, Zhang Q, Wu YL (2016) Increased default mode network connectivity and increased regional homogeneity in migraineurs without aura. J Headache Pain 17(1):98

10. Yu D, Yuan K, Zhao L, Zhao L, Dong M, Liu P, Wang G, Liu J, Sun J, Zhou G, von Deneen KM, Liang F, Qin W, Tian J (2012) Regional homogeneity abnormalities in patients with interictal migraine without aura: a resting-state study. JNMR Biomed 25(5):806–812

11. Faragó P, Tuka B, Tóth E, Szabó N, Király A, Csete G et al (2017) Interictal brain activity differs in migraine with and without aura: resting state fMRI study. J Headache Pain 18(1):8

12. Headache Classification Committee of the International Headache S (2013) The international classification of headache disorders, 3rd edition (beta version). Cephalalgia 33(9):629–808

13. Tombaugh TN (2004) Trail making test a and B: normative data stratified by age and education. Arch Clin Neuropsychol 19(2):203–214

14. Schmidt M (1996) Rey auditory verbal learning test: a handbook. Western Psychological Services, Los Angeles, p 1996

15. Troyer AK, Moscovitch M, Winocur G (1997) Clustering and switching as two components of verbal fluency: evidence from younger and older healthy adults. Neuropsychology 11(1):138

16. Hamilton M (1959) The assessment of anxiety states by rating. Br J Med Psychol 32(1):50–55

17. Hamilton M (1960) A rating scale for depression. J Neurol Neurosurg Psychiatry 23(1):56–62

18. Jenkinson M, Bannister P, Brady M, Smith S (2002) Improved optimization for the robust and accurate linear registration and motion correction of brain images. NeuroImage 17:825–841

19. Smith SM (2002) Fast robust automated brain extraction. Hum Brain Mapp 17:143–155

20. Beckmann CF, Smith SM (2004) Probabilistic independent component analysis for functional magnetic resonance imaging. IEEE TransMedImaging 23:137–152

21. Filippini N, MacIntosh BJ, Hough MG, Goodwin GM, Frisoni GB, Smith SM, Matthews PM, Beckmann CF, Mackay CE (2009 Apr 28) Distinct patterns of brain activity in young carriers of the APOE-epsilon4 allele. Proc Natl AcadSci USA 106(17):7209–7214

22. Abou-Elseoud A, Starck T, Remes J, Nikkinen J, Tervonen O, Kiviniemi V (2010) The effect of model order selection in group PICA. Hum BrainMapp 31:1207–1216

23. Nichols TE, Holmes AP (2002) Non parametric permutation tests for functional neuroimaging: a primer with examples. HumBrainMapp 15:1–25 Filippini N, MacIntosh BJ, Hough MG, Goodwin GM, Frisoni GB, Smith SM, ... Mackay CE (2009) Distinct patterns of brain activity in young carriers of the APOE-ε4 allele. Proc Natl Acad Sci 106(17):7209-7214

24. Guidetti V, Faedda N, Siniatchkin M (2016) Migraine in childhood: biobehavioural or psychosomatic disorder? J Headache Pain 17(1):82

25. Liu J, Zhao L, Li G, Xiong S, Nan J, Li J, Yuan K, von Deneen KM, Liang F, Qin W, Tian J (2012) Hierarchical alteration of brain structural and functional networks in female migraine sufferers. PLoS One 7(12):e51250

26. Mainero C, Boshyan J, Hadjikhani N (2011) Altered functional magnetic resonance imaging resting-state connectivity in periaqueductal gray networks in migraine. Ann Neurol 70:838–845

27. Buckner RL, Andrews-Hanna JR, Schacter DL (2008) The brain's default network. Ann N Y Acad Sci 1124(1):1–38

28. Raichle ME, MacLeod AM, Snyder AZ, Powers WJ, Gusnard DA, Shulman GL (2001) A default mode of brain function. Proc Natl Acad Sci 98(2):676–682

29. Coppola G, Di Renzo A, Tinelli E, Lepre C, Di Lorenzo C, Di Lorenzo G et al (2016) Thalamo-cortical network activity between migraine attacks: insights from MRI-based microstructural and functional resting-state network correlation analysis. J Headache Pain 17(1):100

30. Baliki MN, Geha PY, Apkarian AV, Chialvo DR (2008) Beyond feeling: chronic pain hurts the brain, disrupting the default-mode network dynamics. J Neurosci 28(6):1398–1403

31. Foss JM, Apkarian AV, Chialvo DR (2006) Dynamics of pain: fractal dimension of temporal variability of spontaneous pain differentiates between pain states. J Neurophysiol 95(2):730–736

32. Starr CJ, Sawaki L, Wittenberg GF, Burdette JH, Oshiro Y, Quevedo AS, Coghill RC (2009) Roles of the insular cortex in the modulation of pain: insights from brain lesions. J Neurosci 29(9):2684–2694

33. Menon V, Uddin LQ (2010) Saliency, switching, attention and control: a network model of insula function. Brain Struct Funct 214(5–6):655–667

34. Borsook D, Veggeberg R, Erpelding N, Borra R, Linnman C, Burstein R, Becerra L (2015) The Insula a "hub of activity" in migraine. Neuroscientist 22(6):632–652

35. Liu H, Ge H, Xiang J, Miao A, Tang L, Wu T et al (2015) Resting state brain activity in patients with migraine: a magnetoencephalography study. J Headache Pain 16(1):1–10

16

Volume expansion of periaqueductal gray in episodic migraine: a pilot MRI structural imaging study

Zhiye Chen[1,2,3], Xiaoyan Chen[2], Mengqi Liu[1,3], Shuangfeng Liu[1], Lin Ma[1*] and Shengyuan Yu[2*] 🔾

Abstract

Background: The periaqueductal gray (PAG) dysfunction was recognized in migraine, and the nonspecific PAG lesions were also observed in episodic migraine (EM) recently. However, the PAG volume change was not totally detected in EM up to now. Herein, the aim of this study was to investigate altered PAG volume in EM patients based on high resolution brain structural image.

Methods: The brain structural images were obtained from 18 normal controls (NC), 18 EM patients and 16 chronic migraine (CM) on 3.0 T MR system. PAG template was created based on the ICBM152 gray matter template using MRIcron, and the individual PAG was created by applying the deformation field to the PAG template after structural image segment. One-way analysis of covariance, partial correlation analysis and Receiver operating characteristics (ROC) curve were applied.

Results: EM had a larger PAG volume (0.35 ± 0.02 ml) than that (0.32 ± 0.02 ml) of NC ($P = 0.017$). The PAG volume of CM (0.33 ± 0.02 ml) was negatively related to the VAS score ($P = 0.03$). ROC analysis demonstrated that PAG volume has higher diagnostic efficacy (AUC, 0.731; Sensitivity, 0.556; Specificity, 0.889) for NC vs. EM compared with that NC vs. CM (AUC, 0.634; Sensitivity, 0.438; Specificity, 0.833) and EM vs. CM (AUC, 0.618; Sensitivity, 0.813; Specificity, 0.556).

Conclusion: PAG volume expansion may be the direct impairment evidence on the brain in EM, and could be considered as a diagnostic and evaluated imaging biomarker in migraine.

Keywords: Chronic migraine, Episodic migraine, Periaqueductal gray, Magnetic resonance imaging, Volume measurement

Background

The Migraine is a common type of primary headaches with a reported prevalence of approximately 5.7% in men and 17.0% in women [1], and affect 12% of the population worldwide [2]. The neuromechanism of migraine has been the key focus of research [3]. Of all the target "generator" of migraine attacks, the PAG region has been the key observed brain structure.

Periaqueductal gray (PAG) was a center with powerful descending antinociceptive neuronal network in midbrain [4, 5], and PAG activation was modulated by expectation

of pain [6] and placebo analgesia [7]. PAG could exert a dual control, including inhibition and facilitation, on nociceptive transmission in the dorsal horn and trigeminal nucleus [8] by descending PAG-RVM (rostral ventromedial medulla) pathway contributing to central sensitization and development of secondary hyperalgesia [8, 9]. A previous study [10] confirmed PAG dysfunction in migraine, and functional MRI studies demonstrated that the PAG dysfunction was associated with increased iron deposition, which may play a role in the genesis or pathophysiology of MOH [4, 11, 12] The PAG dysfunction changes might explain the neuromechanism of migraine, however, the PAG structure change was not elucidated completely.

PAG abnormalities can be detected in migraine patients with brain T2-visible lesion using voxel-based morphometry (VBM), which mainly identified increased

* Correspondence: cjr.malin@vip.163.com; yusy1963@126.com
[1]Department of Radiology, Chinese PLA General Hospital, Fuxing Road 28, Beijing 100853, China
[2]Department of Neurology, Chinese PLA General Hospital, Fuxing Road 28, Beijing 100853, China

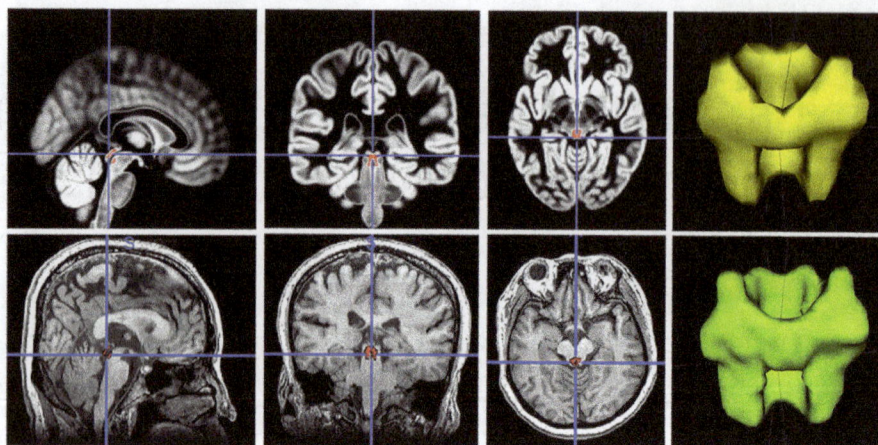

Fig. 1 The creation of PAG template and individual PAG. Top line represents the PAG template created by MRIcron based on mni_icbm152_gm_tal_nlin_asym_09a template. Bottom line represents the individual PAG created by deformation field. The last column represent three-dimensional reconstructed image of PAG template and individual PAG, which were created by ITK-SNAP (version 3.6.0 beta) (http://www.itksnap.org)

PAG density in migraine brain [13]. The altered PAG density indicated the volume change without modulation in VBM, which did not represent the true volume change [14]. Therefore, the true PAG volume abnormalities were not investigated in episodic migraine.

Although PAG was a very small region in the midbrain, and the PAG volume changes had indirectly been assessed by VBM [13, 15, 16], which represent the volume changes in statistical level while not the true volume changes. Therefore, the PAG volume measurement was important for the accurate structural assessment of PAG. In our previous study, the PAG volume measurement using automated PAG segment had been applied to the medication-overuse patients [17].

In the current study, we hypothesize that migraine patients without T2-visible lesions may present PAG volume changes. To address this hypothesis, we prospectively obtained conventional T2WI and high resolution structural images from 18 episodic migraine (EM) patients, 16 chronic migraine (CM) patients and 18 age- and sex-matched normal controls without T2-visible lesions on the brain to calculate and analyze PAG volume change using an automated three dimensional volume mapping measurement.

Methods

Subjects

Written informed consent was obtained from all participants according to the approval of the ethics committee of the local institutional review board. Eighteen EM patients without aura and 16 chronic migraine (CM) patients without aura were recruited from the International Headache Center, Department of Neurology, Chinese PLA General Hospital. The diagnostic criteria of EM and CM should meet the following conditions: (1) EM is

defined as migraine attack days being less than 15 days per month [18]. The definition of migraine refers to 1.1 Migraine without aura and 1.2 Migraine with aura in ICHD-III beta [19]; (2) diagnosis of 1.3 CM, and 1.1 and 1.2 migraine based on the International Classification of Headache Disorders, third Edition (beta version) (ICHD-III beta) [19]; (3) no migraine preventive medication used in the past 3 months; The patients should be excluded if they meet the following conditions: (1) with any chronic disorders such as hypertension, diabetes mellitus and cerebrovascular disease; (2) with alcohol, nicotine, or other substance abuse; (3) with any cerebral disorder.

Eighteen NCs were recruited from the hospital's staff and their relatives. NCs should never have any primary headache disorders or other types of headache in the past year,

Table 1 The clinical characteristics of normal controls, EM patients and CM patients

	NC	EM	CM
Num(M/F)	18 (4/14)	18 (4/14)	16 (4/12)
Age(year)	39.11 ± 9.99	33.39 ± 10.99	42.44 ± 8.65
DD(year)	NA	12.44 ± 8.07	11.25 ± 9.30
VAS	NA	8.33 ± 1.50	7.88 ± 1.45
MIDSA	NA	16.00 ± 17.94	101.81 ± 53.95
Frequence(month)	NA	3.75 ± 2.67	24.81 ± 6.32
HAMA	9.67 ± 3.16	15.67 ± 9.85	21.62 ± 10.98
HAMD	15.89 ± 2.89	10.89 ± 7.26	16.31 ± 10.52
MoCA	26.89 ± 2.47	29.16 ± 1.47	22.94 ± 5.37
Volume	0.32 ± 0.02	0.35 ± 0.02	0.33 ± 0.02

NC normal control, *EM* episodic migraine, *CM* chronic migraine, *DD* disease duration, *VAS* visual analogue scale, *MIDSA* migraine disability assessment scale, *HAMA* Hamilton Anxiety Scale, *HAMD* Hamilton Depression Scale, *MoCA* Montreal Cognitive Assessment, *NA* not available

Table 2 The comparison of PAG volume among groups using one-way analysis of covariance

	Mean difference (95% CI)*	Std. Error.	Sig.[a]
NC vs. EM	−0.023(−0.041 ~ −0.004)	0.009	0.017
NC vs. CM	−0.013(−0.032 ~ 0.006)	0.009	0.170
EM vs. cm	0.01(−0.01 ~ 0.03)	0.010	0.327

*The mean difference is significant at the.05 level
[a]Adjustment for multiple comparisons: Least Significant Difference (equivalent to no adjustments), and covariates appearing in the model are evaluated at the following values: Age = 38.15

and fulfil the same exclusion criteria. Additionally, the anxiety, depression, and cognitive function of all the participants were assessed by using the Hamilton Anxiety Scale (HAMA) [20], the Hamilton Depression Scale (HAMD) [21], and the Montreal Cognitive Assessment (MoCA) Beijing Version (www.mocatest.org). MRI scans were taken in the interictal stage at least three days after a migraine attack for EM patients. All the patients were given with the Visual Analogue Scale (VAS) and the Migraine Disability Assessment Scale (MIDAS). All the subjects underwent conventional MRI examination to exclude the subjects with cerebral infarction, malacia, or occupying lesions. Alcohol, nicotine, caffeine, and other substances were avoided for at least 12 h before MRI examination.

MRI acquisition

Images were acquired on a GE 3.0 T MR system and a conventional eight-channel quadrature head coil was used. All subjects were instructed to lie in a supine position, and formed padding was used to limit head movement. The structural images were generated by a three-dimensional T1-weighted fast spoiled gradient recalled echo (3D T1-FSPGR) sequence, and the scanning parameters were set as follows: TR (repetition time) = 6.3 ms, TE (echo time) = 2.8 ms, flip angle = 15o, FOV (field of view) = 25.6 cm × 25.6 cm, Matrix = 256 × 256, NEX (number of acquisition) = 1. All imaging protocols were identical for all subjects.

MR image processing

All MR structural image data were processed using Statistical Parametric Mapping 12 (SPM 12) (http://www.fil.ion.ucl.ac.uk/spm/) running under MATLAB 7.6 (The Mathworks, Natick, MA, USA). The image processing included following steps: (1) Create PAG template based on mni_icbm152_gm_tal_nlin_asym_09a template using MRIcron; (2) Create individual PAG mask by apply the deformation field (generated by new segment) to the PAG template using run-back strategy; (3)

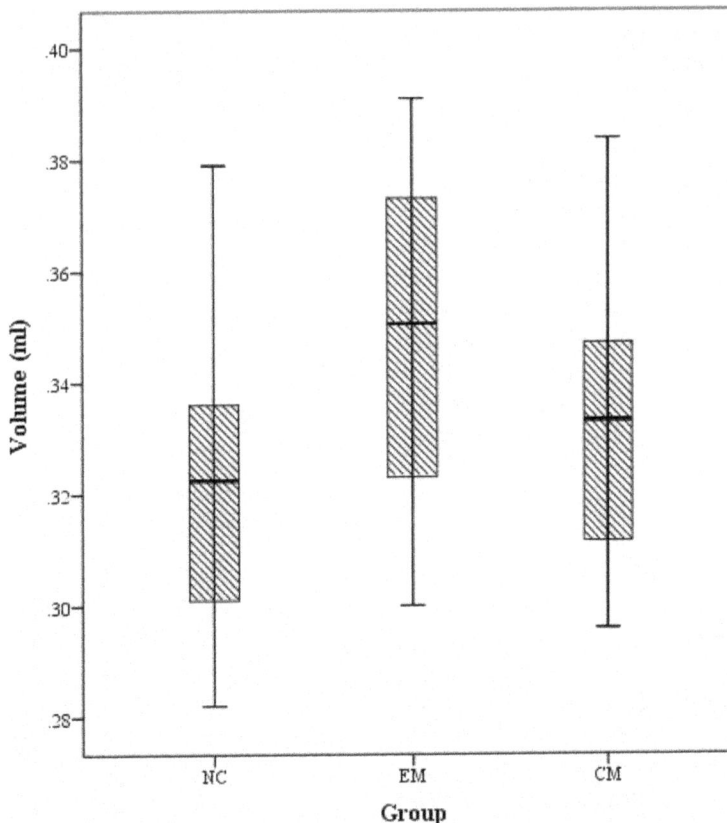

Fig. 2 PAG volume of NC, EM and CM patients, whose mean PAG volume is 0.32 ml, 0.35 ml and 0.33 ml, respectively

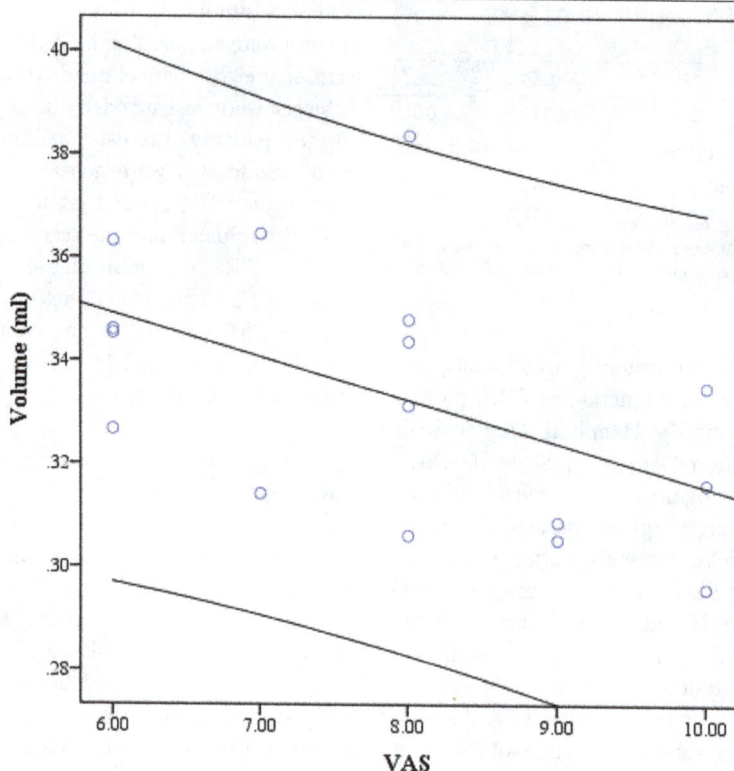

Fig. 3 The scatter plot between PAG volume and VAS score in CM, and a negative correlation was revealed ($P = 0.03$)

compute the PAG volume by ITK-SNAP (version 3.6.0 beta) (http://www.itksnap.org) (Fig. 1).

Statistical analysis
The statistical analysis was performed by using PASW Statistics 18.0. One-way analysis of covariance was performed among each group with age as covariate. Partial correlation were performed between the PAG volume and the clinical variables with age as covariate. Significant difference was set at a P value of <0.05. Receiver operating characteristics (ROC) curve was applied to evaluate the diagnostic efficacy of PAG volume, and area under the curve (AUC) was recognized reasonable diagnostic valuable with AUC set at >0.7.

Results
Demography and neuropsychological test
Demographic and clinical data are summarized in Table 1. Eighteen EM patients (F/M = 14/4), 16 CM patients (F/M = 14/2) and 18 NCs (F/M = 14/4) were enrolled. There was a significant difference for age between EM (33.39 ± 10.69 years old) and CM (42.44 ± 8.65 years old). There was a significant difference for HAMA between NC (9.67 ± 3.16) and EM (15.67 ± 9.85), HAMD between EM (15.67 ± 9.85) and CM (16.31 ± 10.52), MoCA among NC (26.89 ± 2.47),

EM (29.16 ± 1.47), and CM (22.94 ± 5.37). Significant difference was revealed for MIDSA ($P = 0.000$) and onset frequence ($P = 0.000$) between EM and CM (Table 1).

Comparison of PAG volume among NC, EM and CM groups
Table 2 demonstrated that there was a significant difference for PAG volume between NC (0.32 ± 0.02 ml) and EM (0.35 ± 0.02 ml) ($P = 0.017$). Figure 2 indicated that PAG volume of CM (0.33 ± 0.02 ml) fell in between NC and EM, and showed no significance ($P > 0.05$).

Table 3 The partial correlation analysis between PAG volume and clinical variables

	EM		CM	
	r	P value	r	P value
DD(year)	0.10	0.36	0.002	0.49
VAS	0.043	0.44	−0.493	0.03
MIDSA	0.094	0.36	−0.291	0.14
Frequence(month)	−0.24	0.17	0.293	0.14
HAMA	0.028	0.46	0.115	0.34
HAMD	0.222	0.20	−0.286	0.15
MoCA	0.058	0.41	−0.025	0.47

Table 4 ROC curve analysis among groups

	Cut-off Value	AUC	Sensitivity	Specificity
NC vs. EM	0.349	0.731	0.556	0.889
NC vs. CM	0.341	0.634	0.438	0.833
EM vs. CM	0.349	0.618	0.813	0.556

Partial correlation analysis between clinical variables and PAG volume

Partial correlation analysis (with age as covariable) showed significant negative correlation of VAS score with PAG volume in CM ($P = 0.03$) (Fig.e 3), and the other clinical variables showed no significant correlation with PAG volume in EM and CM (Table 3).

ROC curve analysis among NC, EM and CM groups

Table 4 indicated that PAG volume had a larger AUC in NC vs. EM (0.731) compared with NC vs. CM (0.634) and EM vs. CM (0.618) (Fig. 4). The cut-off value of PAG volume was set as 0.349 ml with sensitivity 0.556 and specificity 0.889 in distinguish EM from NC.

Discussion

In this study, the individual PAG was created by applying the deformation field [22] to the PAG template, and it could be used to compute the true PAG volume. Figure 1 provided a good profile for the PAG template and individual PAG segment, which was completely consistent with the actual PAG location and size.

This study demonstrated that EM had the largest PAG volume, and it was significantly larger than that of NC,

which indicated that the PAG volume expansion may take part in the migraine attack. Previous studies demonstrated that PAG lesions may lead to migraine attack [23–25], and functional MRI studies also demonstrated that the PAG network was disrupted in migraine [26, 27]. Therefore, it could be considered that PAG structural change might be the cause of migraine, and PAG volume expansion might be the result of disrupted PAG network in migraine.

Although there was no significant difference on PAG volume within NC-CM and EM-CM groups, the PAG volume of CM showed a slightly reduced tendency compared with EM and slightly increased tendency compared with NC. Therefore, it may speculate that PAG volume reducement may exist in the transformation of EM to CM, and the neuromechanism should be further investigated.

Partial correlation demonstrated that only PAG volume in CM was negatively related to the VAS score, which indicated the PAG volume changes may be associated with VAS score. In EM patients, PAG volume showed no any correlation with the clinical variable, and this point indicated PAG volume expansion may be the direct impairment in EM and may be associated with pathological substrates [13]. The previous study presented that T2-visible load, age, and disease duration may be associated with gray matter volume by VBM methods. Therefore, this study provided a new viewpoint that PAG volume expansion in the migraine patients without T2-visible may be the specific imaging appearance in the midbrain, and it may be an independent

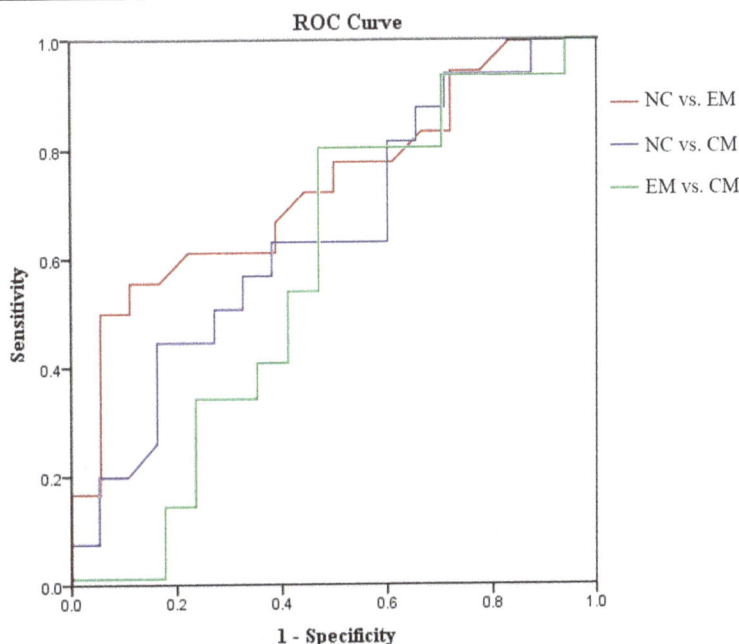

Fig. 4 ROC curve among each group, and NC vs. EM had a largest area under the curve (0.731)

brain changes in migraine, which was not infected by T2-load and other clinical factors. Herein, we could speculate that the gray matter changes in migraine may be classified as two patterns: PAG volume expansion and extra-PAG volume reducement based on the current study and previous studies [13, 15, 16].

ROC curve demonstrated that PAG volume expansion may provide a fair level for the diagnosis of EM from NC (AUC = 0.731), and it was not enough to distinguish CM from NC and CM from EM because of lower AUC. Although PAG volume had a fair diagnostic efficacy for EM from NC, and it presented a slightly higher specificity (0.889) and a slightly lower sensitivity (0.556). Based on the Fig. 2, the overlap was observed in between NC and EM, which may decreased the sensitivity for PAG volume as a biomarker. However, it was reasonable to believe that the PAG volume expansion may be inclined to the diagnosis of EM.

Although PAG is a very small structural in the midbrain, this study provided an automated PAG volume measurement methods, and which could be routinely used for the PAG volume measurement in clinical practice. PAG volume expansion could not only be considered as a potential diagnostic imaging biomarker for EM, but also might be considered as a treatment response prognosis for EM just as PAG volume reducement associated with treatment response in medication-overuse headache [16]. The main limit of this study was that the sample of this study was relative small, and it would be necessary to increase the sample size in the future study.

Conclusion

In conclusion, PAG volume expansion may directly underlie the impairment evidence on the brain in EM, and could be considered as the imaging biomarker for diagnose and evaluation for the migraine.

Abbreviations
CM: Chronic migraine; EM: Episodic migraine; NC: Normal controls; PAG: Periaqueductal gray

Acknowledgments
This work was supported by the Special Financial Grant from the China Postdoctoral Science Foundation (2014 T70960) and the Foundation for Medical and health Sci & Tech innovation Project of Sanya (2016YW37).

Authors' contributions
Category 1: (a) conception and design: LM, SYY. (b) Acquisition of Data: ZYC, MQL, SFL, XYC. (c) analysis and interpretation of data: ZYC. Category 2: (a) drafting the article: ZYC. (b) revising it for intellectual content: LM, SYY. All authors read and approved the final manuscript.

Competing interests
The authors declare that they have no competing interests.

Author details
[1]Department of Radiology, Chinese PLA General Hospital, Fuxing Road 28, Beijing 100853, China. [2]Department of Neurology, Chinese PLA General Hospital, Fuxing Road 28, Beijing 100853, China. [3]Department of Radiology, Hainan Branch of Chinese PLA General Hospital, Sanya 572013, China.

References
1. Scher AI, Gudmundsson LS, Sigurdsson S, Ghambaryan A, Aspelund T, Eiriksdottir G et al (2009) Migraine headache in middle age and late-life brain infarcts. JAMA 301:2563–2570
2. Gomez-Beldarrain M, Oroz I, Zapirain BG, Ruanova BF, Fernandez YG, Cabrera A et al (2015) Right fronto-insular white matter tracts link cognitive reserve and pain in migraine patients. J Headache Pain. 17:4
3. Chen Z, Chen X, Liu M, Liu S, Shu S, Ma L, Yu S (2016) Altered functional connectivity of the marginal division in migraine: a resting-state fMRI study. J Headache Pain. 17:89
4. Welch KM, Nagesh V, Aurora SK, Gelman N (2001) Periaqueductal gray matter dysfunction in migraine: cause or the burden of illness? Headache 41:629–637
5. Smith GST, Savery D, Marden C, Costa JJL, Averill S, Priestley JV, Rattray M (1994) Distribution of messenger RNAs encoding enkephalin, substance P, somatostatin, galanin, vasoactive intestinal polypeptide, neuropeptide Y, and calcitonin gene-related peptide in the midbrain periaqueductal grey in the rat. J Comp Neurol 350:23–40
6. Fairhurst M, Wiech K, Dunckley P, Tracey I. (2006) Anticipatory brainstem activity predicts neural processing of pain in humans. European Journal of Pain. 10:S83b–S
7. Wager TD, Scott DJ, Zubieta JK (2007) Placebo effects on human mu-opioid activity during pain. Proc Natl Acad Sci U S A 104:11056–11061
8. Heinricher MM, Tavares I, Leith JL, Lumb BM (2009) Descending control of nociception: specificity, recruitment and plasticity. Brain Res Rev 60:214–225
9. Fields H (2004) State-dependent opioid control of pain. Nat Rev Neurosci 5:565–575
10. Raskin NH, Yoshio H, Sharon L (1987) Headache may arise from perturbation of brain. Headache 27:416–420
11. Kruit MC, Launer LJ, Overbosch J, van Buchem MA, Ferrari MD (2009) Iron accumulation in deep brain nuclei in migraine: a population-based magnetic resonance imaging study. Cephalalgia 29:351–359
12. Tepper SJ, Lowe MJ, Beall E, Phillips MD, Liu K, Stillman MJ et al (2012) Iron deposition in pain-regulatory nuclei in episodic migraine and chronic daily headache by MRI. Headache 52:236–243
13. Rocca MA, Ceccarelli A, Falini A, Colombo B, Tortorella P, Bernasconi L et al (2006) Brain gray matter changes in migraine patients with T2-visible lesions: a 3-T MRI study. Stroke 37:1765–1770
14. Radua J, Canales-Rodriguez EJ, Pomarol-Clotet E, Salvador R (2014) Validity of modulation and optimal settings for advanced voxel-based morphometry. NeuroImage 86:81–90
15. Riederer F, Marti M, Luechinger R, Lanzenberger R, von Meyenburg J, Gantenbein AR et al (2012) Grey matter changes associated with medication-overuse headache: correlations with disease related disability and anxiety. World J Biol Psychiatry 13:517–525
16. Riederer F, Gantenbein AR, Marti M, Luechinger R, Kollias S, Sandor PS (2013) Decrease of gray matter volume in the midbrain is associated with treatment response in medication-overuse headache: possible influence of orbitofrontal cortex. J Neurosci 33:15343–15349
17. Chen Z, Chen X, Liu M, Liu S, Ma L, Yu S (2017) Volume gain of periaqueductal gray in medication-overuse headache. J Headache Pain. 18:12
18. Burshtein R, Burshtein A, Burshtein J, Rosen N (2015) Are episodic and chronic migraine one disease or two? Curr Pain Headache Rep 19:53
19. Headache Classification Committee of the International Headache S (2013) The international classification of headache disorders, 3rd edition (beta version). Cephalalgia 33:629–808
20. Maier W, Buller R, Philipp M, Heuser I (1988) The Hamilton anxiety scale: reliability, validity and sensitivity to change in anxiety and depressive disorders. J Affect Disord 14:61–68
21. Hamilton M (1967) Development of a rating scale for primary depressive illness. Br J Soc Clin Psychol 6:278–296
22. Ashburner J (2007) A fast diffeomorphic image registration algorithm. NeuroImage 38:95–113

23. Haas DC, Kent PF, Friedman DI (1993) Headache caused by a single lesion of multiple sclerosis in the periaqueductal gray area. Headache 33:452–455
24. Wang Y, Wang XS (2013) Migraine-like headache from an infarction in the periaqueductal gray area of the midbrain. Pain Med 14:948–949
25. Chen Z, Chen X, Liu M, Liu S, Ma L, Yu S (2016) Nonspecific periaqueductal gray lesions on T2WI in episodic migraine. J Headache Pain 17:101
26. Mainero C, Boshyan J, Hadjikhani N (2011) Altered functional magnetic resonance imaging resting-state connectivity in periaqueductal gray networks in migraine. Ann Neurol 70:838–845
27. Li Z, Liu M, Lan L, Zeng F, Makris N, Liang Y et al (2016) Altered periaqueductal gray resting state functional connectivity in migraine and the modulation effect of treatment. Sci Rep 6:20298

17

Measurement and implications of the distance between the sphenopalatine ganglion and nasal mucosa: a neuroimaging study

Joan Crespi[1,2,3]* ◎, Daniel Bratbak[2,4], David Dodick[2,5], Manjit Matharu[6], Kent Are Jamtøy[2,7], Irina Aschehoug[2] and Erling Tronvik[1,2,3]

Abstract

Background: Historical reports describe the sphenopalatine ganglion (SPG) as positioned directly under the nasal mucosa. This is the basis for the topical intranasal administration of local anaesthetic (LA) towards the sphenopalatine foramen (SPF) which is hypothesized to diffuse a distance as short as 1 mm. Nonetheless, the SPG is located in the sphenopalatine fossa, encapsulated in connective tissue, surrounded by fat tissue and separated from the nasal cavity by a bony wall. The sphenopalatine fossa communicates with the nasal cavity through the SPF, which contains neurovascular structures packed with connective tissue and is covered by mucosa in the nasal cavity. Endoscopically the SPF does not appear open. It has hitherto not been demonstrated that LA reaches the SPG using this approach.

Methods: Our group has previously identified the SPG on 3 T–MRI images merged with CT. This enabled us to measure the distance from the SPG to the nasal mucosa covering the SPF in 20 Caucasian subjects on both sides ($n = 40$ ganglia). This distance was measured by two physicians. Interobserver variability was evaluated using the intraclass correlation coefficient (ICC).

Results: The mean distance from the SPG to the closest point of the nasal cavity directly over the mucosa covering the SPF was 6.77 mm (SD 1.75; range, 4.00–11.60). The interobserver variability was excellent (ICC 0.978; 95% CI: 0.939–0.990, $p < 0.001$).

Conclusions: The distance between the SPG and nasal mucosa over the SPF is longer than previously assumed. These results challenge the assumption that the intranasal topical application of LA close to the SPF can passively diffuse to the SPG.

Keywords: Sphenopalatine ganglion, Pterygopalatine ganglion, Local anaesthetics, Intranasal, Block

Background

The sphenopalatine ganglion (SPG) has been a target for treatment of headache disorders for more than a century [1]. Different approaches, including the direct application of pharmacological substances or neurolysis, have been used in an attempt to block the sphenopalatine ganglion to treat a broad range of headache and facial pain disorders such as cluster headache, migraine, trigeminal neuralgia, postherpetic trigeminal neuralgia, post-traumatic headache, post-dural puncture headache, and hemicrania continua [2, 3]. Attempts at pharmacological blockade include direct percutaneous injections towards the SPG or topical intranasal administration. While it appears reasonable to posit that a substance will reach the SPG with an image-guided injection, the ability of a substance to passively diffuse and reach the SPG after intranasal application is uncertain. This is especially true since there is not readily available clinical biomarker to verify that the target (SPG) has been engaged and blocked.

* Correspondence: Joan.crespi@ntnu.no
[1]Department of Neurology, St Olav's University Hospital, Edvards Grieg's gate 8, 7030 Trondheim, Norway
[2]Department of Neuromedicine and Movement Science, NTNU (University of Science and Technology), Trondheim, Norway

The first RCT evaluating the intranasal administration of local anaesthetics (INALA) was published in 1996 demonstrated a significant acute treatment effect in patients with migraine [4]. In 1999 these results were confirmed in a second RCT by the same group [5], resulting in a Level C recommendation for INALA for acute migraine treatment [6]. Both studies hypothesized that the mechanism of action for INALA is neural blockade of the SPG. In order to reach the SPG, the local anaesthetics (LA) must diffuse from the intranasal cavity. The authors argue that this is reasonable since the SPG is ≤ 1 mm below the nasal mucosa in the area of the sphenopalatine foramen (SPF), citing the work of Sluder from 1909 [7]. In line with this hypothesis and evidence base, the application of intranasal LA as close as possible to the SPF became a widely adopted procedure in clinical practice and drove the commercial development, marketing, and availability of intransal catheter devices designed to provide application of LA near the SPF.

Advanced imaging techniques allows the opportunity to determine the actual distance from the SPF to the SPG in living subjects. The aim of this study is to measure the distances between the nasal mucosa over the SPF and the SPG in 20 (40 sides) patients on fused MRI/CT images. We also review the literature on the efficacy of INALA for the treatment of headache and discuss the evidence that a drug applied intranasally over the SPF will freely diffuse to and engage the SPG.

Methods

Our investigation has formerly identified the SPG on MRI in living humans [8]. In this study, the relative location of the SPG to bony landmarks in radiological images (fusioned CT and MRI images) was compared and found to be equivalent to the distances obtained in an anatomical cadaveric study by Keller [9]. By using the same image sets we were able to measure the distance from the nasal mucosa covering the SPF to the SPG on 20 living humans ($n = 40$ ganglia). The distance was measured by two physicians (JC, DFB). The 20 patients included in this study had been formerly included in two other trials where they underwent a block of the SPG using a new neuronavigation technique at St. Olavs Hospital, Trondheim, Norway, between October 2013 and February 2016. Ten patients had intractable chronic cluster headache [10] and ten patients had intractable chronic migraine [11]. All patients were examined with CT and MRI scans covering the region of the sphenopalatine fossa and neighboring regions. None of the patients eligible for inclusion were excluded. None of the patients had received previous injections towards the SPG, which might have altered the anatomy of the sphenopalatine fossa.

MR scans were performed on a 3 T scanner (Magnetom Skyra, Siemens, Germany). Technical parameters were as follows: Sagittal T2 weighted: Repetition time (TR) range 3780, echo time (TE) 111, slice thickness 2 mm, matrix 0.4 × 0.4 × 2.0 mm, field of view (FOV) 210, number of acquisitions 3; sagittal T1 weighted: TR range 710, TE 10, slice thickness 2 mm, matrix 0.4 × 0.4 × 2.0 mm, FOV 210, number of acquisitions 2; axial T2 weighted: TR range 4160, TE 110, slice thickness 2 mm, matrix 0.4 × 0.4 × 2.0 mm, FOV 220, number of acquisitions 2; and axial T1 weighted: TR range 710, TE 7.9, slice thickness 2 mm, matrix 0.4 × 0.4 × 2.0 mm, FOV 210, number of acquisitions 2. All CT scans were performed using a helical CT scanner (Somatom sensation 64, Siemens, Germany) set at effective mAs 63, 120 kV, slice thickness1 mm, reconstruction increment 0.7 mm, collimation 12 × 0.6 mm, Kernel U 70, window width 450 HU and window centre 50 HU. Fusion of MR and CT images was performed using Brainlab iPlan 3.0 (Brainlab AG, Feldkirchen, Germany).

Both studies were approved by the regional ethics committee (ref. 2012/164 and 2014/962), the Norwegian Medicines Agency (EUDRACT nr: 2012–000248-91 and 2014–001852-43) and registered at ClinicalTrial.gov (NCT02019017 and NCT02259075). Written informed consent was obtained from all patients.

The SPG was localized in T2 weighted images. The closest point of the nasal mucosa covering the SPF was localized on CT-scan images and not in MRI in order to reduce the partial volume effect.

Statistical analysis

SPSS version 24.0 (SPSS Inc., Chicago, Illinois, USA) was used in the data analyses.

Data distributions were expressed as means and standard deviations (SD), results are given as mean ± standard deviation if not otherwise stated. Interobserver variability was evaluated using the intraclass correlation coefficient (ICC). A post hoc analysis for intra-individual variability was assessed using an independent samples t-test.

Results

Table 1 illustrates the demographic characteristics of the 20 patients examined in this study.

The mean distance from the SPG to the closest point of the nasal cavity directly over the mucosa covering the SPF was 6.77 mm (SD 1.75; range, 4.00–11.60). The interobserver variability was excellent (ICC 0.978; 95% CI: 0.939–0.990, $p < 0.001$). There was no significant difference between the average distances in the right and left sides, with a mean difference right-left of – 0.58 mm (95% CI: -1.76-0.60, $p = 0.327$).

The SPG was localized in MRI scans in all patients. Fig. 1 shows axial images (T1 weighted MRI and CT) through the SPG in one of the patients of the study.

Table 1 Demographics of the sample

	All patients ($n = 20$)
Number of females/males	15/5
Mean age, years ± SD (range)	44.8 ± 13.0 (24–68)
Number of Caucasians	20/20
Primary headache	20/20
• Chronic cluster headache	10/20
• Chronic migraine	10/20

Discussion

This is the first study to measure the distance between the mucosa overlying the SPF and the SPG in living humans. The mean distance of 6.77 mm is higher than the distance described in cadaveric studies, possibly as a result of dessication of post-mortem tissue.

It has been assumed that a LA applied intranasally in the proximity of the SPF can reach the SPG [1, 4, 5, 12, 13]. An important prerequisite for such a hypothesis is that the distance between the surface of the nasal mucosa and the SPG is sufficiently short. Sluder estimated the distance to be as little as 1 mm and this has been cited among many advocating for the therapeutic effect of INALA [7]. However, Sluder also acknowledged that the SPG may rest up to 9 mm from the SPF and that there is considerable variability between individuals [7]. Unfortunately, the methodology used to assess the localization of the SPG was not described nor was the size or demographics of the sample defined. Penteshina analysed 70 SPG and found significant individual differences in the structure and topography of the SPG [14]. SPG's size was stable (3 to 5 mm) but its position in relation to the anterior foramen of the Vidian canal, SPF, palatine bone and maxillary nerve were variable. In this study, the SPG was located 3–4 mm from the nasal mucosa membrane in 35 cadavers, but in 20 cases, it was at a depth

of 10 mm and surrounded by fatty tissue. In some cases, the SPG was located in the Vidian canal making the SPG inaccessible to INALA [14]. Only in 15 out of 70 ganglia was the SPG closely adjacent to the nasal mucosa membrane [14].

In addition to the distance between the nasal mucosa and the SPG, there are several barriers through which LA must diffuse through to reach the SPG, including nasal mucosa; neurovascular structures connective tissue filling the SPF and adipose tissue in the sphenopalatine fossa between the SPF and the SPG (Fig. 2).

The nasal cavity and the sphenopalatine fossa are divided by the vertical wing of the palatine bone with neurovascular structures entering and exiting the nasal cavity through the SPF. The SPF is covered by mucosa and it does not present as an open foramen that communicates with the sphenopalatine fossa (Fig. 3). Since LA cannot transverse through bone, it has to pass through the foramen alongside the vascular structures. LA entering the vascular structures may enter the systemic circulation and be transported away from the SPG. Some studies raise the question whether the observed effect of INALA might be due to systemic absorption of the anesthetic rather than a block of the SPG [15–17]. After passing through the SPF, LA would enter the sphenopalatine fossa, which is filled with adipose tissue requiring diffusion of the LA through adipose and connective tissue in order to reach the SPG.

Rusu et al. performed dissections of the sphenopalatine fossa in 20 human cadavers and observed that 30% of the SPGs did not appear as single macroscopic structures, but had two distinctive partitions (one superior and one inferior) [18]. In addition, all patients had neuronal clusters and neuronal cords within the proximity of the SPG (intrinsic intraneural dispersed sphenopalatine microganglia), which were not apparent macroscopically.

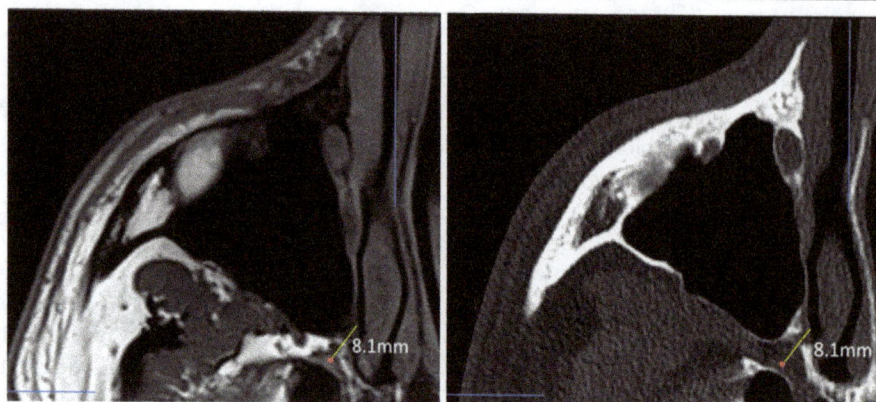

Fig. 1 Axial images through the SPG in one of the patients. Left: T1 weighted MRI. Right: CT scan. Both images show the same anatomical plane. The SPG (red dot) is first localized in the MRI scan and the closest point of the nasal mucosa through the SPF is localized in fusioned CT images. In this example, the distance was 8.1 mm (yellow line). Notice the typical crescent form of the SPG anterior to the opening of the Vidian canal

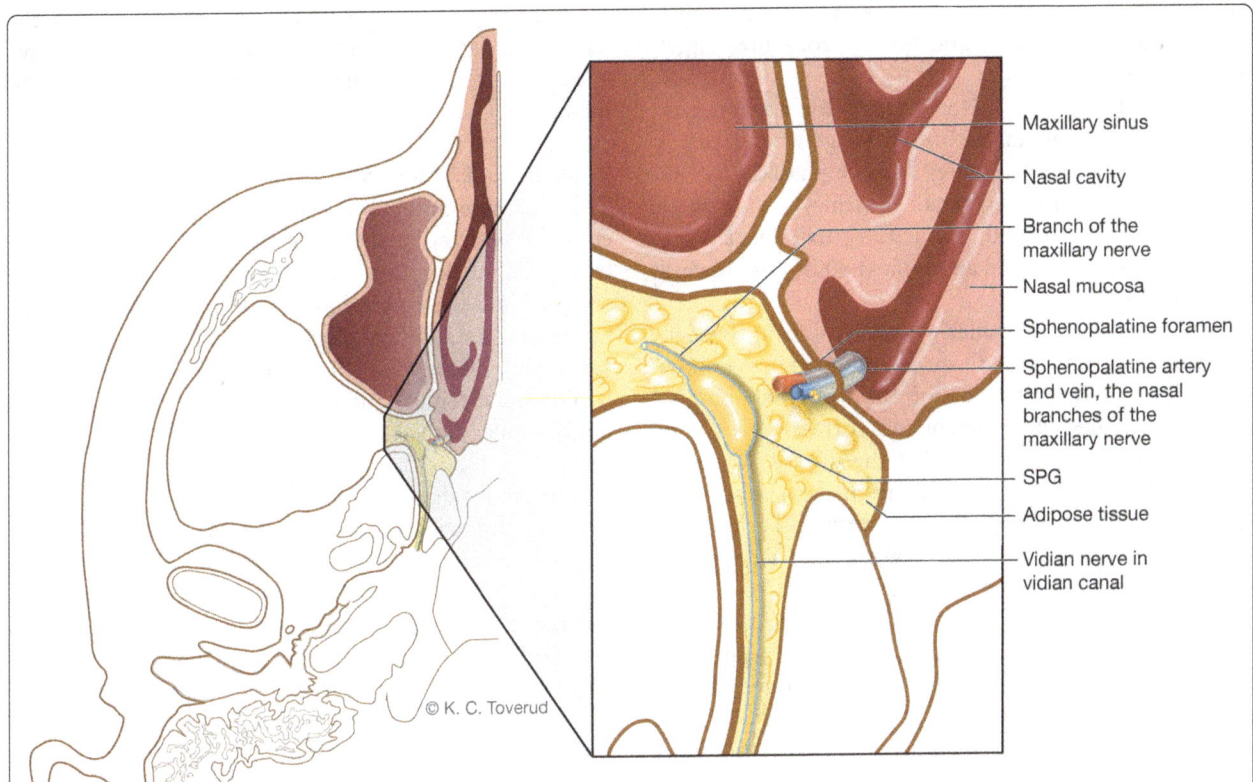

Fig. 2 Illustration of the relation between the nasal cavity and the sphenopalatine fossa (axial plane). In order to reach the SPG, a drug applied intranasally over the sphenopalatine foramen will have to diffuse through mucosa, the sphenopalatine foramen, which is packed with neuro-vascular structures and connective tissue, and the fat tissue filling the sphenopalatine fossa. SPF: sphenopalatine foramen; SPG: sphenopalatine ganglion

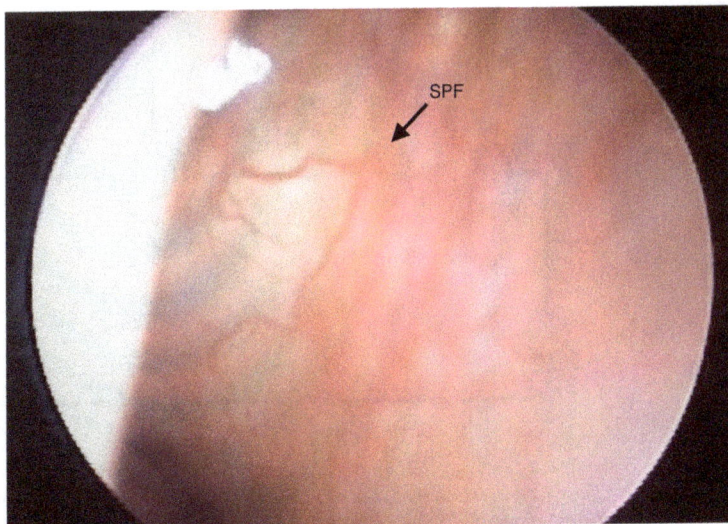

Fig. 3 Rhinoscopy showing the mucosa over the sphenopalatine foramen (SPF) and the sphenopalatine artery (arrow). The SPF does not appear as an open foramen communicating directly with the sphenopalatine fossa. The SPF is covered by mucosa and packed with neurovascular structures and connective tissue

These factors may account for the therapeutic failure observed in some patients undergoing procedures targeting the SPG [18, 19].

The SPF lies lateral in the wall of the nasopharynx, which constitutes an anatomical challenge when trying to gain access to it. Some authors have emphasized the importance of a proper technique to achieve a transnasal block of the SPG [5, 20], particularly that the patient's head is properly extended and rotated 30 degrees towards the desired side.

Most commercially available catheters do not visually localize the SPG, either through endoscopy or fluoroscopy. The blind application of LA may therefore not approximate the SPF. Alherabi et al. dissected 16 lateral nasal walls and documented that the distance from the nasal sill to the SPF varies widely from 55 to 76 mm and the range of the angle of elevation formed between the SPF to the nasal sill is 11–12 degrees [21]. The authors describe that the standard reference points to localize the SPF are widely different and of little practical help. Other groups have also described the anatomical variation of the SPF [22]. The size of the foramen is also variable. Prades et al. measured the SPF in 12 skulls and reported a mean height of 6.1 mm (5.2–6.8 mm) and a mean width of 2.5 mm (2.4–2.5 mm) [23]. In most

approaches, LA are applied to a larger area within the nasal cavity and therefore the concentration would have to be high to allow enough substance to diffuse close to the SPG.

Rationale for LA block of the SPG

The trigemino-autonomic reflex, where parasympathetic efferents with synapses in the SPG activate meningeal trigeminal nociceptors, is thought to be important in several headache conditions [24]. A postulated mechanism to understand why blocking the SPG may be effective is by reducing the efferent release of neuropeptides on dural nociceptors and thereby reducing afferent trigeminovascular activity (Fig. 4).

Alternative mechanisms of action

The positive effect of the transnasal topical block in headache shown in several studies could be due to a trigeminal block rather than a block of the SPG. This possible mechanism has already been suggested in cluster headache by Barre [20], Raskin [25] and Robbins [26]. Barre proposed several possible mechanisms of action of cocaine in cluster headache: local blockade of neural transmission of nerves in the vicinity of the Vidian Nerve, SPG or maxillary division of the trigeminal

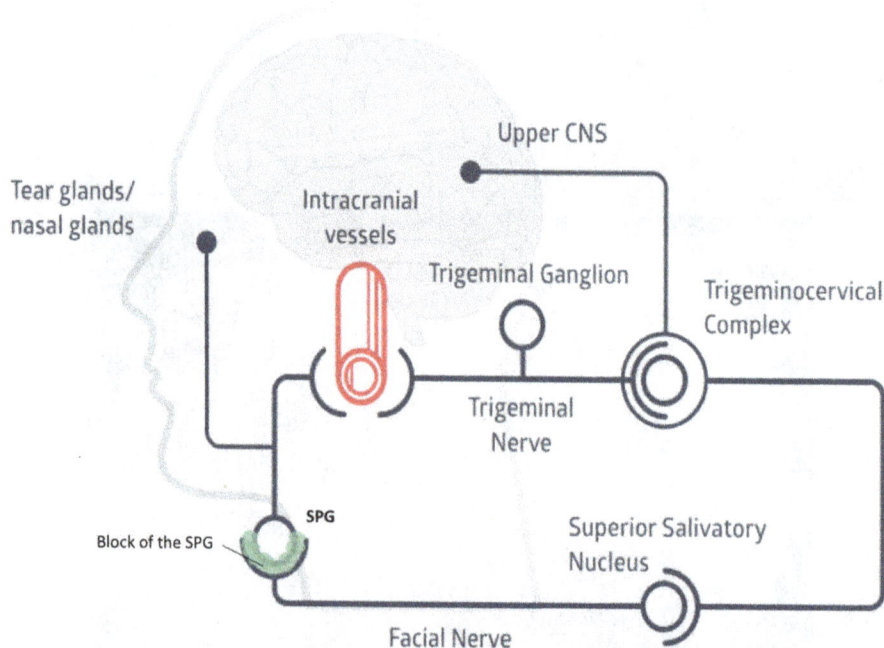

Fig. 4 Diagram showing the involvement of the sphenopalatine ganglion (SPG) in the physiopathology of trigeminoautonomic headaches. The afferent part of this loop is mediated by the trigeminal nerve, which sends nociceptive signals from the dural blood vessels to the trigeminocervical complex. This information projects to higher brain structures, resulting in cephalic pain. The efferent part of this loop conveys mostly through the superior salivatory nucleus, exiting the brain stem via the facial nerve and reaching the sphenopalatine ganglion through the greater petrosal nerve. Postganglionic fibres exit the sphenopalatine nerve towards the dural vessels, closing the loop. Blocking the SPG might reduce the afferent input of signals towards the trigeminal system and reduce the activation of the trigeminocervical complex. CNS: central nervous system

nerve; via its sympathomimetic effects in inducing local or regional vasoconstriction secondary to the development of sensitization to catecholamines; or a combination of both of the above [20]. Later observations that cocaine and lidocaine appear to be similarly effective in cluster headache led to some authors favoring the anesthetic effect over the vasoconstrictor hypothesis [27].

It is known that applying a local anesthetic intranasally blocks first and second trigeminal nerve endings in the nasal mucosa, which is a standard technique used in transnasal surgery. Hardebo et al. described in a series of 24 patients that when intranasal lidocaine was effective, pain was usually reduced in the orbital and nasal region [27]. Schueler et al. described that the maxillary and mandibular branches of the trigeminal nerve in rats have both intra and extracranial receptive fields and that its stimulation could release CGRP [28]. Thus, one cannot exclude a trigeminal block or systemic absorption as a possible explanation for the observed effect.

Review of evidence on intranasal administration of LA in headache

Most studies evaluating the administration of topical intranasal LA are of poor quality. A total of 9 RCTs have been conducted using INALAs (Table 2). Three were negative for the primary endpoint [29–31]. While these studies have claimed that the SPG was the target, it is unclear whether the study drug reached the SPG. Even though most of the procedures administrating intranasal LA are well tolerated and considered to be safe, adverse events have been reported [2]. The most frequently reported serious adverse event is epistaxis. Most of the adverse events are transient and include bitter taste, oropharyngeal numbness, ipsilateral nostril and eye burning sensation, nasal discomfort, diplopia and reduced buccal opening. Cady et al. using the Tx360° catheter, found that the most common side effects were lacrimation, unpleasant taste and mouth numbness [13, 32].

When one applies LA intranasally, most of the volume will descend to the pharynx and the patient will often swallow the fluid, commonly complaining of a bitter taste after the procedure [15]. As a consequence, the final volume of LA that will remain on the surface of the SPF to passively diffuse to the SPG is likely to be small. The bitter taste of most LA constitutes a problem for blinding. This issue has not been properly assessed and might constitute an important bias in several studies.

Different techniques for intranasal administration of LA
The technique which has been most commonly used is the one described by Barre [20] (Table 2). New intranasal catheters that claim to offer higher tolerability have been developed [2]. Other indirect and blind techniques

have been described for the use of INALA [15, 26, 33–35, 30, 36, 37] but the same limitations and anatomical restrictions discussed above still apply.

Limitations
Some limitations of the study are its relatively small sample (20 subjects) and that the gender ratio is skewed (m:f 1:3). All examined patients are Caucasians. The method used in this article to identify the SPG on MRI images [8] is not an established method. The presence of autonomic symptoms pre- and posttreatment was not recorded in these group of patients.

Future perspectives
Different studies have used different LA, or combinations of them. The concentration of the LA also varies across the studies (Table 2). Some have mixed LA with corticosteroids or with other analgesics. Different LA have different pharmacological properties that might influence their ability to reach the SPG by free diffusion. The volumes of local anesthetic have varied between 0.3 and 2 ml. Such important aspects as which drug (or combination), which concentration and volume would be most suitable, have not been properly assessed in the literature. The technique used to apply the LA in the proximity of the SPF varies in the different studies. Further studies that assess the pharmacological and anatomical basis to support that a drug applied over or in the proximity of the SPF, will actually reach the SPG by free diffusion, are warranted.

Conclusion
SPG blockade through the intranasal injection of LA has been employed widely as an acute and preventive treatment for a variety of primary and secondary headache disorders. However, the evidence is mixed and inconclusive. The rationale to justify this approach has been the assumption that the SPG lies directly under the nasal mucosa. In this study on living humans, we show that the distance between the SPG and the nasal mucosa over the SPF is significantly longer than previously assumed. Moreover, the bony and mucosal anatomy, combined with the connective and adipose tissue that fills the sphenopalatine fossa, challenge the assumption that intranasal topical application of LA may reach the SPG. Whether these anatomical considerations discussed above have clinical implications is not known. Further research using biomarker evidence to confirm whether the SPG has been blocked after the local intranasal application of LA, and high quality RCTs with adequate placebo to protect the blind, are necessary to assess the veracity and efficacy of this procedure.

Table 2 Summary of studies evaluating topical intranasal administration of LA in pain disorders of the head and face

Author	Drug	Concentration	Volume	Condition	RCT	Effect	Nr of patients	Technique	Ref.
Sluder	Cocaine	4–70%	A drop	Meckel's ganglion neuralgia	No	Positive effect in a series of patients	5	Applicator, surgery	[7]
	Alcohol	–	A drop						
	formaldehyde	0.4%	N/S						
	Silver nitrate	2%	N/S						
Barre	Cocaine	5–10%	N/S	CH	No	Positive effect in a series of patients	11	Barre's technique[a]	[20]
Kittrelle	Cocaine	5%	–	CH (NTG-induced)	No	>75% reduction in headache intensity within 3 min, in 4 of 5 patients with lidocaine	5	Barre's technique[a]	[12]
	lidocaine	4%	1 ml						
Hardebo	Cocaine	10%	0.3 ml	CH	No	Lidocaine and cocaine equally effective	24	Nasal droper	[27]
	Lidocaine	4%	0.5–0.8 ml						
Robbins	Lidocaine	4%	4–6 sprays	CH	No	54% mild to moderate relief after treatment	30	Spray	[26]
Kudrow	Lidocaine	4%	0.4 ml	Migraine	No	Migraine attacks aborted in 12 of 23 patients	23	Barre's technique[a]	[38]
Maizels	Lidocaine	4%	0.5 ml	Migraine	Yes	55% of patients that received lidocaine had at least 50% reduction of headache within 15 min (primary endpoint)	81	Barre's technique[a]	[4]
Maizels	Lidocaine	4%	0.5 ml	Migraine	Yes	Randomized trial with open-label follow-up. Controlled trial: 35.8% of patients had headache relieved to mild or none 15 min. After treatment.	131	Barre's technique[a]	[5]
Maizels	Lidocaine	4%	0.5 ml	Migraine	No	Prevention of the development of headache following aura.	1	Barre's technique[a]	[39]
Saberski	Lidocaine	20%	N/S	Postherpetic neuralgia	No	Decrease of the pain (therapy repeated 11 times)	1	Applicator dipped in anaesthetic	[40]
Costa	Lidocaine	10%	1 ml	CH (NTG-induced)	Yes	All patients responded to both anaesthetics with complete cessation of induced pain (31.3 ± 13.1 min for cocaine and 37.0 ± 7.8 for lidocaine. For saline, pain severity increased initially and resolved with a latency of 59.3 ± 12.3 min.	15	Cotton swab under rhinoscopy	[34]
	Cocaine	10%	1 ml						
Blanda	Lidocaine	4%	1 ml	Migraine	Yes	The study was negative for the main outcome measure (decrease of ≥50% of initial pain score or an absolute pain score ≤ 2.5 cm at 5 min.	49	Barre	[29]
Windsor	Lidocaine	2%	1–2 ml	Herpes keratitis	No	Relief of pain in one case report	1	Applicator developed by the authors	[15]
Chae	Lidocaine	2%	N/S	Post-traumatic headache	No		2	N/S	[41]

Table 2 Summary of studies evaluating topical intranasal administration of LA in pain disorders of the head and face (*Continued*)

Author	Drug	Concentration	Volume	Condition	RCT	Effect	Nr of patients	Technique	Ref.
Cohen	Lidocaine	4%	N/S	Postdural puncture headache	No	Reduction of VAS scale within 15 min in both patients (from 8/10 to 0/10 in the first and from 10/10 to 2/10 in the second)	13	Applicator saturated	[42]
Bakbak	Lidocaine	10%	2 ml	CH	No	Relieve of pain and autonomic symptoms	1	Cotton-tipped applicator	[43]
Pfaffenrath	Lidocaine Ketorolac	6%	0,1 ml 0,1 ml	Migraine	Yes	Primary endpoint not met: proportion of pain-free patients two hours after treatment. Improvement of several secondary endpoints.	140	Spray	[30]
Candido	Ropivacaine Dexamethasone	0,5% –	0,5 ml –	1 TN, 1 CM, 1 post-herpetic neuralgia	No	All 3 patients reported pain relief within the first 15 min. Post-treatment.	3	Tx360®	[44]
Cady	Bupivacaine	0,5%	0,3 ml	Chronic migraine	Yes	Reduction of pain compared to placebo at 15 min, 30 min and 24 h compared to placebo (primary endpoint). Decreased HIT-6 score compared to placebo at 1 and 6 months.	38	Tx360®	[30]
Mohammadkarimi	Lidocaine	10%	1 puff	Acute headache	Yes	Significant reduction of mean pain scores at 1 min (primary endpoint). The effect was sustained at 30 min	90	Spray	[37]
Cohen	Lidocaine	5%	N/S	Postdural puncture headache	No	Relief of pain in a series of patients	32	Applicator saturated	[45]
Cady	Bupivacaine	0,5%	0,3 ml	Chronic migraine	Yes	Primary endpoint: statistically significant reduction of NRS scores. A comparison of the number of headache days during the baseline period and 1 month post-treatment was not significant.	38	Tx360®	[32]
Schaffer	Bupivacaine	0,5%	0,3 ml	Acute headache	Yes	Primary endpoint (50% reduction in pain at 15 min) negative.	93	Tx360®	[31]
Androlaukis	Bupivacaine	0,5%	0,6 ml	Hemicrania continua	No	Reduction in average intensity and frequency of headaches and autonomic symptoms.	1	Tx360®	[3]
Dance	Lidocaine	4%	N/S	Migraine (pediatric patients age 7–18)	No	Reduction of pain scores (only abstract available).	85	Allevio®	[46]

LA local anesthetic, *SPF* sphenopalatine foramen, *RCT* randomized clinical trial, *CH* cluster headache, *N/S* not specified, *TN* trigeminal neuralgia, *CM* chronic migraine, *NTG* nitroglycerine
[a]Barre's technique: the patient lies supine with extended neck (45 degrees) and head rotated 30 degrees ipsilateral to the pain. After the desired volume of anesthetic is applied, the patient should stay in the described position for 30 s. [3–5, 7, 12, 13, 15, 20, 26, 27, 29–32, 34, 37–46]

Clinical implications

- The distance from the nasal mucosa to the sphenopalatine ganglion (SPG) appears to be longer than previously assumed.
- 3 of 9 RCTs where local anaesthetics were applied intranasally have been negative. These studies have claimed that the SPG was the target but this has not been proved.
- Further studies that assess the pharmacological and anatomical basis to support that a drug applied in the proximity of the sphenopalatine foramen, will actually reach the SPG by free diffusion, are warranted.

Abbreviations
CH: Cluster headache; CM: Chronic migraine; CT: Computerized tomography; INALA: Intranasal administration of local anaesthetics; LA: Local anesthetic; MRI: Magnetic resonance images; N/S: Not specified; NTG: Nitroglycerine; RCT: Randomized clinical trial; SPF: Sphenopalatine foramen; SPG: Sphenopalatine ganglion; TN: Trigeminal neuralgia

Acknowledgments
The authors want to thank Wenche M. Thorstensen and Arild Dalen for the acquisition of Fig. 3.

Funding
The study was funded by the Liaison Committee between the Central Norway Regional Health Authority (RHA) and the Norwegian University of Science and Technology (NTNU).

Authors' contributions
JC, DB and ET had the original idea for the manuscript. JC and DB analysed the data. JC reviewed the literature for the introduction and drafted the manuscript. KAJ, IA and MM revised the manuscript. DB, DD and ET: assistance for drafting the manuscript, revision of the text and approved the final manuscript. All authors read and approved the final manuscript.

Competing interests
The authors declare that they have no conflict of interest.

Author details
[1]Department of Neurology, St Olav's University Hospital, Edvards Grieg's gate 8, 7030 Trondheim, Norway. [2]Department of Neuromedicine and Movement Science, NTNU (University of Science and Technology), Trondheim, Norway. [3]Norwegian Advisory Unit on Headaches, Trondheim, Norway. [4]Department of Neurosurgery, St Olav's University Hospital, Trondheim, Norway. [5]Department of Neurology, Mayo Clinic, Phoenix, AZ, USA. [6]National Hospital of Neurology and Neurosurgery, London, UK. [7]Department of maxillofacial surgery, St Olav's University Hospital, Trondheim, Norway.

References
1. Sluder G (1908) The role of the sphenopalatine ganglion in nasal headaches. AR Elliott Publishing Company. N Y State J Med 27:8–13.
2. Robbins MS, Robertson CE, Kaplan E, Ailani J, Charleston L, Kuruvilla D et al (2016) The sphenopalatine ganglion: anatomy, pathophysiology, and therapeutic targeting in headache. Headache 56(2):240–258.
3. Androulakis XM, Krebs KA, Ashkenazi A (2016) Hemicrania continua may respond to repetitive sphenopalatine ganglion block: a case report. Headache 56(3):573–579.
4. Maizels M, Scott B, Cohen W, Chen W (1996) Intranasal lidocaine for treatment of migraine: a randomized, double-blind, controlled trial. JAMA 276(4):319–321.
5. Maizels M, Geiger AM (1999) Intranasal lidocaine for migraine: a randomized trial and open-label follow-up. Headache 39(8):543–551.
6. Marmura MJ, Silberstein SD, Schwedt TJ (2015) The acute treatment of migraine in adults: the american headache society evidence assessment of migraine pharmacotherapies. Headache 55(1):3–20.
7. Sluder G (1909) The anatomical and clinical relations of the sphenopalatine (Meckel's) ganglion to the nose and its accessory sinuses. N Y Med J 28: 293–298.
8. Bratbak DF, Folvik M, Nordgard S, Stovner LJ, Dodick DW, Matharu M, Tronvik, E (2017) Depicting the pterygopalatine ganglion on 3 Tesla magnetic resonance images. Surg Radiol Anat. https://doi.org/10.1007/s00276-017-1960-6
9. Keller H (1980) Über Die Hintere Pfortenregion Der Fossa Pterygopalatina Und Die Lage Des Ganglion Pterygopalatinum. Doctoral Dissertation, Julius-Maximilans-Universitäts Würburg.
10. Bratbak DF, Nordgard S, Stovner LJ, Linde M, Folvik M, Bugten V et al (2016) Pilot study of sphenopalatine injection of onabotulinumtoxinA for the treatment of intractable chronic cluster headache. Cephalalgia 36(6):503–509.
11. Bratbak DF, Nordgard S, Stovner LJ, Linde M, Dodick DW, Aschehoug I, Tronvik, E (2017) Pilot study of sphenopalatine injection of onabotulinumtoxinA for the treatment of intractable chronic migraine. Cephalalgia, 37(4):356-64
12. Kittrelle JP, Grouse DS, Seybold ME (1985) Cluster headache. Local anesthetic abortive agents. Arch Neurol 42(5):496–498.
13. Cady R, Saper J, Dexter K, Manley HR (2015) A double-blind, placebo-controlled study of repetitive transnasal sphenopalatine ganglion blockade with tx360((R)) as acute treatment for chronic migraine. Headache 55(1):101–116.
14. Penteshina, NA (1965) Morphology of the Pterygopalatine Ganglion. Zh Nevropat Psikhiat 65(9):1325–30.
15. Windsor RE, Jahnke S (2004) Sphenopalatine ganglion blockade: a review and proposed modification of the transnasal technique. Pain Physician 7(2): 283–286.
16. Ruskin AP (1979) Sphenopalatine (nasal) ganglion: remote effects including "psychosomatic" symptoms, rage reaction, pain, and spasm. Arch Phys Med Rehabil 60(8):353–359.
17. Berger JJ, Pyles ST, Saga-Rumley SA (1986) Does topical anesthesia of the sphenopalatine ganglion with cocaine or lidocaine relieve low back pain? Anesth Analg 65(6):700–702.
18. Rusu MC, Pop F, Curca GC, Podoleanu L, Voinea LM (2009) The pterygopalatine ganglion in humans: a morphological study. Ann Anat 191(2):196–202.
19. Gregoire A, Clair C, Delabrousse E, Aubry R, Boulahdour Z, Kastler B (2002) CT guided neurolysis of the sphenopalatine ganglion for management of refractory trigeminal neuralgia. J Radiol 83(9 Pt 1):1082–1084.
20. Barre F (1982) Cocaine as an abortive agent in cluster headache. Headache 22(2):69–73.
21. Alherabi A, Marglani O, Herzallah IR, Shaibah H, Alaidarous T, Alkaff H et al (2014) Endoscopic localization of the sphenopalatine foramen: do measurements matter? Eur Arch Otorhinolaryngol 271(9):2455–2460.
22. Scanavine AB, Navarro JA, Megale SR, Anselmo-Lima WT (2009) Anatomical study of the sphenopalatine foramen. Brazilian J Otorhinolaryngology 75(1):37–41.
23. Prades JM, Asanau A, Timoshenko AP, Faye MB, Martin C (2008) Surgical anatomy of the sphenopalatine foramen and its arterial content. Surgical Radiologic Anatomy : SRA 30(7):583–587.
24. Akerman S, Holland PR, Lasalandra MP, Goadsby PJ (2009) Oxygen inhibits neuronal activation in the trigeminocervical complex after stimulation of trigeminal autonomic reflex, but not during direct dural activation of trigeminal afferents. Headache 49(8):1131–1143.
25. Raskin, NH (1988) The Hypnic Headache Syndrome. Headache: the journal of head and face pain 28(8):534–36.
26. Robbins L (1995) Intranasal lidocaine for cluster headache. Headache 35(2): 83–84.
27. Hardebo JE, Elner A (1987) Nerves and vessels in the pterygopalatine fossa and symptoms of cluster headache. Headache 27(10):528–532.

28. Schueler M, Messlinger K, Dux M, Neuhuber WL, De Col R (2013) Extracranial projections of meningeal afferents and their impact on meningeal nociception and headache. Pain 154(9):1622–1631.
29. Blanda M, Rench T, Gerson LW, Weigand JV (2001) Intranasal lidocaine for the treatment of migraine headache: a randomized, controlled trial. Acad Emerg Med Off J Soc Acad Emerg Med 8(4):337–342.
30. Pfaffenrath V, Fenzl E, Bregman D, Farkkila M (2012) Intranasal ketorolac tromethamine (SPRIX(R)) containing 6% of lidocaine (ROX-828) for acute treatment of migraine: safety and efficacy data from a phase II clinical trial. Cephalalgia 32(10):766–777.
31. Schaffer JT, Hunter BR, Ball KM, Weaver CS (2015) Noninvasive sphenopalatine ganglion block for acute headache in the emergency department: a randomized placebo-controlled trial. Ann Emerg Med 65(5):503–510.
32. Cady RK, Saper J, Dexter K, Cady RJ, Manley HR (2015) Long-term efficacy of a double-blind, placebo-controlled, randomized study for repetitive sphenopalatine blockade with bupivacaine vs. saline with the Tx360 device for treatment of chronic migraine. Headache 55(4):529–542.
33. Saade E, Paige GB (1996) Patient-administered sphenopalatine ganglion block. Reg Anesth 21(1):68–70.
34. Costa A, Pucci E, Antonaci F, Sances G, Granella F, Broich G et al (2000) The effect of intranasal cocaine and lidocaine on nitroglycerin-induced attacks in cluster headache. Cephalalgia 20(2):85–91.
35. Raj PLL, Erdine S et al (2003) Radiographic imaging for regional anesthesia and pain management. Churchill Livingstone, New York, pp 66–71.
36. Levin M (2010) Nerve blocks in the treatment of headache. Neurotherapeutics 7(2):197–203.
37. Mohammadkarimi N, Jafari M, Mellat A, Kazemi E, Shirali A (2014) Evaluation of efficacy of intra-nasal lidocaine for headache relief in patients refer to emergency department. J Res Med Sci 19(4):331–335.
38. Kudrow L, Kudrow DB (1995) Intranasal lidocaine. Headache 35(9):565–566
39. Maizels M (1999) Intranasal lidocaine to prevent headache following migraine aura. Headache 39(6):439–442.
40. Saberski L, Ahmad M, Wiske P (1999) Sphenopalatine ganglion block for treatment of sinus arrest in postherpetic neuralgia. Headache 39(1):42–44
41. Chae HSJ, Nguyen M, Lee A (2006) The use of intranasal sphenopalatine ganglion blockade for the treatment of post-traumatic headache: a case series. Arch Phys Med Rehabil 87:E39.
42. Cohen S, Sakr A, Katyal S, Chopra D (2009) Sphenopalatine ganglion block for postdural puncture headache. Anaesthesia 64(5):574–575.
43. Bakbak B, Gedik S, Koktekir BE, Okka M (2012) Cluster headache with ptosis responsive to intranasal lidocaine application: a case report. J Med Case Rep 6:64.
44. Candido KD, Massey ST, Sauer R, Darabad RR, Knezevic NN (2013) A novel revision to the classical transnasal topical sphenopalatine ganglion block for the treatment of headache and facial pain. Pain Physician. 16(6):E769–E778.
45. Cohen S, Ramos D, Grubb W, Mellender S, Mohiuddin A, Chiricolo A (2014) Sphenopalatine ganglion block: a safer alternative to epidural blood patch for postdural puncture headache. Reg Anesth Pain Med 39(6):563.
46. Dance LAD, Schaefer C, Kaye R, Yonker M, Towbin, R (2017) Safety and efficacy of sphenopalatine ganglion blockade in children – initial experience. Journal of Vascular and Interventional Radiology 28:2(Supplement S8).

18

Effects of sildenafil and calcitonin gene-related peptide on brainstem glutamate levels: a pharmacological proton magnetic resonance spectroscopy study at 3.0 T

Samaira Younis[1], Anders Hougaard[1], Casper Emil Christensen[1], Mark Bitsch Vestergaard[2], Esben Thade Petersen[3], Olaf Bjarne Paulson[4], Henrik Bo Wiberg Larsson[2] and Messoud Ashina[1*]

Abstract

Background: Studies involving human pharmacological migraine models have predominantly focused on the vasoactive effects of headache-inducing drugs, including sildenafil and calcitonin gene-related peptide (CGRP). However, the role of possible glutamate level changes in the brainstem and thalamus is of emerging interest in the field of migraine research bringing forth the need for a novel, validated method to study the biochemical effects in these areas.

Methods: We applied an optimized in vivo human pharmacological proton (^{1}H) magnetic resonance spectroscopy (MRS) protocol (PRESS, repetition time 3000 ms, echo time 37.6–38.3 ms) at 3.0 T in combination with sildenafil and CGRP in a double-blind, placebo-controlled, randomized, double-dummy, three-way cross-over design. Seventeen healthy participants were scanned with the ^{1}H-MRS protocol at baseline and twice (at 40 min and 140 min) after drug administration to investigate the sildenafil- and CGRP-induced glutamate changes in both brainstem and thalamus.

Results: The glutamate levels increased transiently in the brainstem at 40–70 min after sildenafil administration compared to placebo (5.6%, $P = 0.039$). We found no sildenafil-induced glutamate changes in the thalamus, and no CGRP-induced glutamate changes in the brainstem or thalamus compared to placebo. Both sildenafil and CGRP induced headache in 53%–62% of participants. We found no interaction in the glutamate levels in the brainstem or thalamus between participants who developed sildenafil and/or CGRP-induced headache as compared to participants who did not.

Conclusions: The transient sildenafil-induced glutamate change in the brainstem possibly reflects increased excitability of the brainstem neurons. CGRP did not induce brainstem or thalamic glutamate changes, suggesting that it rather exerts its headache-inducing effects on the peripheral trigeminal pain pathways.

Keywords: MRS, Glutamate, Glx, Lactate, Migraine, Brainstem, Thalamus, CGRP, Sildenafil

Background

Human pharmacological migraine models have been used for the past two decades with great success to study migraine attack mechanisms using vasoactive drugs such as calcitonin gene-related peptide (CGRP) and sildenafil [1–7]. The models have been pivotal in the development of new anti-migraine therapy [8].

Human pathophysiological studies applying these models have predominantly focused on the cerebrovascular effects of the headache-inducing substances. However, emerging evidence suggests that metabolic changes, especially of brain glutamate levels [9, 10], in the brainstem [11–15] and thalamus [15] are key processes for the initiation of migraine headache attacks and thereby potentially important effects of the headache-inducing drugs. At present, methods for the study of pharmacologically induced biochemical effects on the brainstem glutamate levels have not been validated.

* Correspondence: ashina@dadlnet.dk
[1]Danish Headache Center, Department of Neurology, Rigshospitalet Glostrup, University of Copenhagen, Copenhagen, Denmark
Full list of author information is available at the end of the article

Pharmacological proton (^{1}H) magnetic resonance spectroscopy (MRS) provides the ability to non-invasively study drug-induced biochemical changes in the brain. Imaging of the deep brain structures, especially the brainstem by magnetic resonance imaging (MRI), is challenging due to the small size of the region of interest, location in areas of relatively high magnetic field inhomogeneity and potential physiological artifacts. Thus, it is essential to systematically investigate the quality and reproducibility of ^{1}H-MRS measurements in these areas before application of the method in patients. Only a few ^{1}H-MRS studies of the brainstem have previously been conducted. One such study, of patients with amyotrophic lateral sclerosis, did not report data on the reproducibility or variability of the glutamate measurements [16], while other ^{1}H-MRS brainstem studies did not measure the glutamate concentrations at all [17–20] .

The headache-inducing drugs, CGRP and sildenafil, were selected for the study based on their different modes of action. CGRP is generally considered to exert its primary effect outside of the central nervous system (CNS), in the meningeal vasculature and the first order trigeminal neurons [21, 22], while sildenafil, as a lipophilic molecule, readily crosses the blood-brain barrier [23].

Here, we conducted a double-blind, placebo-controlled, randomized, double-dummy, three-way cross-over pharmacological ^{1}H-MRS study to investigate the sildenafil- and CGRP-induced glutamate concentration changes in healthy participants. Our null-hypothesis was that the glutamate levels are not altered in the brainstem of healthy participants after administration of sildenafil and CGRP when compared to placebo. Additionally, we assessed the spectral quality and variability of the glutamate measurements over time in the brainstem based on our ^{1}H-MRS protocol.

Methods

Participants

Healthy volunteers were recruited through announcement on a Danish website for recruitment of participants to health research (www.forsoegsperson.dk). Inclusion criteria were: age 18–50 years and weight 50–100 kg. Exclusion criteria were: history of any primary headache disorders (except episodic tension-type headache for < 2 day per month during the last year) according to the diagnostic criteria of the beta version of the third International Classification of Headache Disorders (ICHD-3 beta) [24], first-degree family members with migraine or other primary headache disorders according to ICHD-3 beta (except episodic tension-type headache for < 6 days per month), daily intake of medication (except oral contraceptives), no usage of safe contraception, cardiovascular, cerebrovascular, or psychiatric disease, and drug abuse. Participants were excluded if there were any contraindications to MRI such as metal implants, pacemaker, insulin pump, claustrophobia and/or surgical

procedure during the last 6 weeks before inclusion. We also excluded participants with braces and teeth implants of metal, which are normally regarded MRI compatible, to avoid potential MR scan artifacts in the deep brain structures of interest.

Experimental design

All participants were randomly allocated to receive sildenafil, CGRP and placebo on three separate study days. On each study day, participants underwent an MRI scan protocol consisting of three scan sessions: a baseline MRI scan, followed by two additional post drug administration MRI scan sessions. The first post drug scan was initiated at 40 min (scan 1), and the second scan was initiated at 140 min (scan 2) after administration of sildenafil, CGRP or placebo (Fig. 1). MR spectra were obtained from brainstem and thalamus during each scan.

On the sildenafil day, the participants received sildenafil as two 50 mg tablets (STADA, Bad Vilbel, Germany) in two non-transparent capsules, combined with placebo isotonic saline infusion into the cubital vein for 20 min (Pressure tubes, Argon Medical Devices, The Hague, the Netherlands), at the time of infusion start. On the CGRP day, the participants received 1.5 µg/min human-alfa-CGRP (PolyPeptide, Strasbourg, France) via infusion for 20 min combined with placebo calcium in two non-transparent capsules. On the placebo day, the participants received placebo isotonic saline infusion for 20 min combined with placebo calcium in two non-transparent capsules. The sildenafil and CGRP dosages for the study were

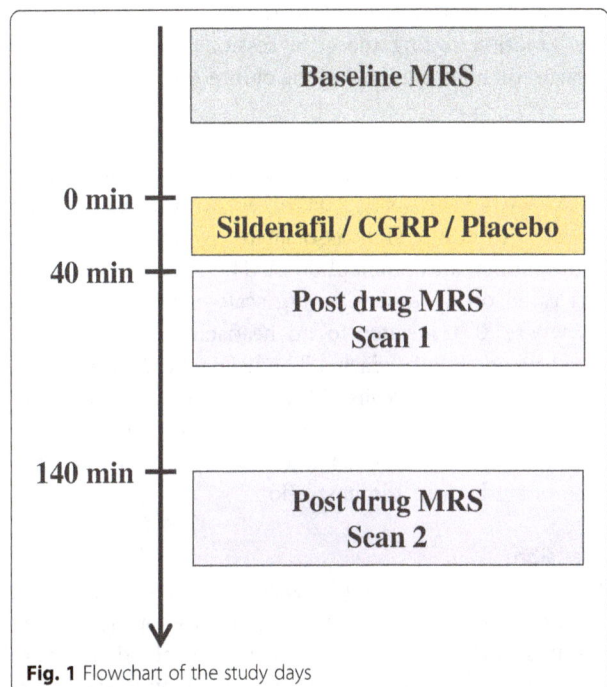

Fig. 1 Flowchart of the study days

determined based on findings of previous studies, which reported sildenafil- and CGRP-induced headache in healthy volunteers, and migraine-like attack in migraine patients [1–7]. The randomization was administered by the Hospital Pharmacy of the Capital Region of Denmark.

All participants were headache-free for at least 72 h before each study day. The participants were not allowed coffee, tea, cocoa, soft drinks, alcohol or tobacco for 12 h before study start on each study day, and fasted for all food and beverages (except for water), for 4 h before study start. Between scan 1 and scan 2, all participants were offered a standardized small meal consisting of soft bread with cheese, banana, and water. Other criteria for the study days were no intake of any medication four half-lives before the start of the study day, except for oral contraception. After insertion of a peripheral venous catheter (18G Vasofix® Safety, B.Braun, Melsungen, Germany) into a cubital vein, the participants were instructed to rest in a hospital bed for approximately 30 min before the baseline scans.

We aimed to initiate the scan sessions at the same time of the day on all three study days for each participant, allowing for a maximum time deviation of 1 h, to account for metabolite concentration variations due to the circadian rhythm [25, 26]. In addition, the timing of scan 1 and scan 2 was fixed according to the baseline scan. The ^{1}H-MRS sequences were part of a larger study (results of these will be presented elsewhere). Before and after each scan sequence it was ensured that participants remained awake, and data were excluded in case they fell asleep during the scans as this could affect the measurements [27]. Participants were instructed to remain still and avoid any head motion during the scan sessions to ensure stable measurements from the regions of interest.

Headache characteristics

Data on headache characteristics were acquired on each study day, i.e. intensity, quality, aggravation by physical activity, location and associated symptoms (nausea, photophobia, and phonophobia). The headache intensity was rated on a numeric rating scale ranging from 0 to 10, where '0' translated to no headache and '10' to the worst imaginable headache. The headache data were obtained between all scans. All participants were asked to register headache hourly in a standardized questionnaire after the last scan session until 24 h, starting from the time of study drug administration.

Vital signs

The vital variables were registered and monitored at baseline, and during the scan sessions after study drug administration. Systolic and diastolic blood pressure were measured with an interval of 10 min, and heart rate, blood oxygen saturation and nostril end-tidal CO_2 tension (water trap and gas sample line, Medrad, Warrendale, PA) (Veris Monitor, Medrad, Warrendale, PA) were monitored continuously.

Data acquisition and imaging protocol

All MRI scans were performed on a 3.0 T Philips Achieva MRI scanner (Philips Medical Systems, Best, The Netherlands) using a 32-channel phase array head coil.

Anatomical scan

High-resolution anatomical scans were obtained with a 3D T1-weighted turbo field echo sequence (field of view $240 \times 240 \times 170$ mm^3; voxel size $1.00 \times 1.08 \times 1.10$ mm^3; echo time 3.7 ms; repetition time 8.0 ms; flip angle 8°). The reconstruction software on the scanner was used to additionally obtain the axial and coronal anatomical views of the scan to ensure correct placement of the volumes-of-interest (VOIs) for brainstem and thalamus.

Magnetic resonance spectroscopy

We used proton (^{1}H) magnetic resonance spectroscopy (MRS) to measure the combined concentration of glutamate and glutamine (reported as 'glutamate'), lactate, N-Acetylaspartate (NAA) and the total concentration of creatine i.e. phosphocreatine and creatine. The water-suppressed point-resolved spectroscopy (PRESS) pulse sequence was used in brainstem (repetition time 3000 ms; echo time 38.3 ms, voxel size $10.5 \times 12.5 \times 22$ mm^3; 480 acquisitions; total duration 24 min) and thalamus (repetition time 3000 ms; echo time 37.6 ms; voxel size 16 mm $\times$ 12 mm $\times$ 12 mm; 192 acquisitions; total duration 9 min 36 s). High number of acquisitions was used to ensure sufficient signal-noise-ratio. Voxel size based shimming was performed using first-order pencil beam to reduce the inhomogeneity in the chosen VOIs. The protocol was thus optimized to precisely target small VOIs in deep brain structures and to avoid cerebrospinal fluid contributions and partial volume artifacts. The repetition time was 3000 ms to ensure sufficient relaxation. The unsuppressed water signal was measured from the VOIs and used as internal reference for quantification [28]. The first VOI was placed unilaterally in the right side of the brainstem, and the second VOI was placed in the left, contralateral thalamus, following the anatomical and functional trigeminal pain pathways.

Metabolite quantification and analysis

Post-processing and quantification of the spectral data were performed by LCModel (Version 6.3-1F, Toronto, Canada). Representative ^{1}H-MRS spectra obtained from brainstem and thalamus are illustrated in Fig. 2. Spectra were evaluated in a blinded manner and abnormal

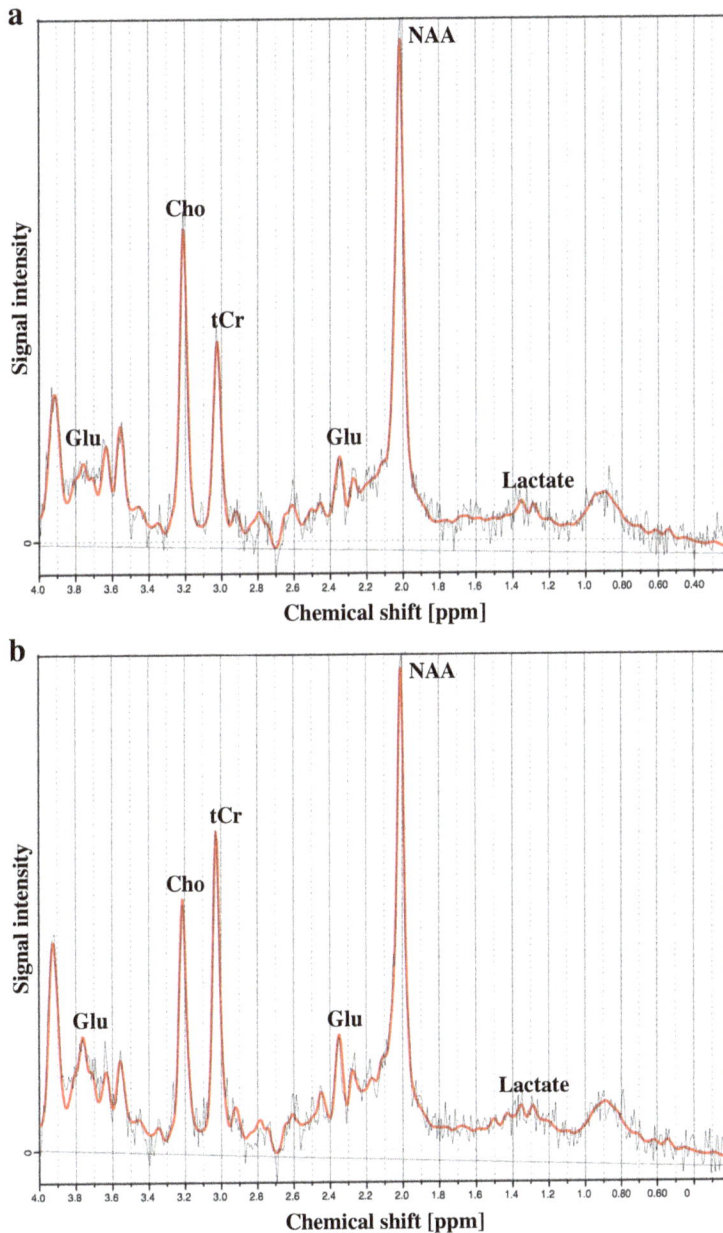

Fig. 2 MR spectra from brainstem and thalamus. Examples of (**a**) brainstem and (**b**) thalamus spectra are obtained at baseline with the point-resolved spectroscopy (PRESS) pulse sequence at 3.0 T. The spectra are acquired from LCModel. The red line represents the fit, and the horizontal linear line represents the baseline as estimated by LCModel. Cho: Choline, Glu: Glutamate, tCr: Total creatine, NAA: *N*-Acetylaspartate

spectra were excluded. The quality of the included spectra was estimated based on the signal-noise-ratio (SNR) and full-width of half-maximum (FWHM) of the spectra peaks as provided by LCModel. The means and standard deviations of the SNR and FWHM for the brainstem and thalamus spectra were calculated.

Statistical analysis

The primary endpoint was glutamate, lactate, NAA and total creatine concentration changes in brainstem and thalamus from baseline to after sildenafil and CGRP administration, compared to the corresponding placebo changes. A linear mixed model was used for each metabolite with interaction between scans (baseline, scan 1 and scan 2) and drug days (sildenafil, CGRP and placebo) and with subjects and study day (5 levels) nested within subjects as random effects. The placebo day baseline scan was set as the reference parameter in the model.

The secondary endpoint was changes in the metabolite concentrations in participants who developed pharmacologically induced headache during the scan sessions after sildenafil and CGRP, compared to participants who did not. A linear mixed model was used for each metabolite on the sildenafil and CGRP day with interaction between scans and headache and the random effects: subjects and study day nested within subjects. The data did not allow for correlation analyses between metabolite concentration and headache characteristics. The headache frequencies after sildenafil and CGRP were compared to placebo using McNemar's test.

For explorative vital parameter analyses, we included data from the following time points: 0, 20, 70, 120, and 170 min after infusion. Changes from baseline after sildenafil and CGRP were compared to placebo using a linear mixed model with interaction between drug days and the selected time points with subjects as random effects.

The variability structure of the glutamate measurements in the brainstem and thalamus was estimated in an explorative analysis based on baseline, scan 1, and scan 2 data acquired on the placebo day, and baseline data acquired on the sildenafil and CGRP day, using a linear mixed model with no fixed effects, and the random effects: subjects and study day (5 levels) nested within subjects.

All statistical analyses were performed using R (Version 3.4.2). P values were reported as two-tailed with a level of significance of 5%.

Results
Participants
Seventeen healthy volunteers participated in the study (10 women and 7 men) with mean age 22.9 (SD ± 3.4 and range 18–30 years) (Fig. 3). Vitals signs are presented in Fig. 4.

Alterations in metabolite concentration
Brainstem
The glutamate concentration significantly increased from baseline to scan 1 after sildenafil compared to the corresponding change after placebo ($P = 0.039$) (Table 1, Fig. 5). The lactate concentration decreased from baseline to scan 1 ($P = 0.017$), but not to scan 2 ($P = 0.156$) after sildenafil, compared to corresponding changes after placebo. In the brainstem, we did not detect changes in the metabolite concentrations from baseline to scan 1 or scan 2 after CGRP, compared to placebo.

Thalamus
We did not detect changes in the glutamate, lactate or NAA concentrations in the thalamus from baseline to scan 1 or scan 2 after sildenafil or CGRP, compared to placebo. The increase in the total creatine concentration from baseline to scan 2 after CGRP (3.3%, $P = 0.028$) was significant in comparison to placebo ($P = 0.004$).

Headache vs. no headache
The proportion of participants who developed headache during scan 1 and scan 2, and after the scan sessions and until 24 h from drug administration, is reported in Fig. 6. We found no interaction in the glutamate, lactate, NAA or total creatine concentrations in the brainstem or thalamus between participants who developed sildenafil- and/or CGRP-induced headaches as compared to participants who did not.

Quality of spectra
The brainstem spectra had mean SNR of 17.56 (± 2.33), and mean FWHM of 0.05 ppm (± 0.01) / 6.39 Hz (± 1.28). In thalamus, the mean SNR was 15.30 (± 1.86) and the mean FWHM was 0.04 ppm (± 0.01) / 5.11 Hz (± 1.28). In addition, the Cramér–Rao lower bound was < 12% for glutamate measurements in the brainstem and thalamus, except for 12–13% in four brainstem spectra and one thalamus spectrum in different subjects.

Glutamate variability in brainstem and thalamus
From the linear mixed model, we obtained separate brainstem glutamate concentration variations, where 6.9% was due to residual measurement error with additional 2.1% due to inter-subject variation, and 6.0% due to between day variations. The thalamic glutamate concentration variations were 6.8% due to residual measurement error with 2.7% inter-subject and 0% between day variations.

The mean time difference from day 1 to day 2 of the study days was 12.5 days (± 9.2) and 10.7 days (± 6.0) between day 2 and day 3. Participants were mainly scanned from afternoon time on all three scan days. The scans were initiated in the morning for three subjects, whereof one subject completed all three study days.

Discussion
The major outcome of the present study was an increase in the glutamate concentration in the brainstem after administration of sildenafil when compared to placebo. We did not detect any changes in the glutamate concentration in the brainstem after CGRP infusion.

Sildenafil-induced biochemical changes
Glutamate, as the major excitatory neurotransmitter in the brain, promotes neuronal depolarization [29]. Extracellular glutamate levels are directly correlated to levels of neuronal hyperexcitability and seizure intensity in animal models of epilepsy [30, 31]. Here, we evaluated the combined concentration of the glutamate and glutamine as these metabolites are not differentiable at 3.0 T ^{1}H-MRS. In healthy volunteers, the majority of the combined concentration consists of glutamate (~ 80%) [32] and 13%–22% of the glutamate concentration in the healthy brain is present in the

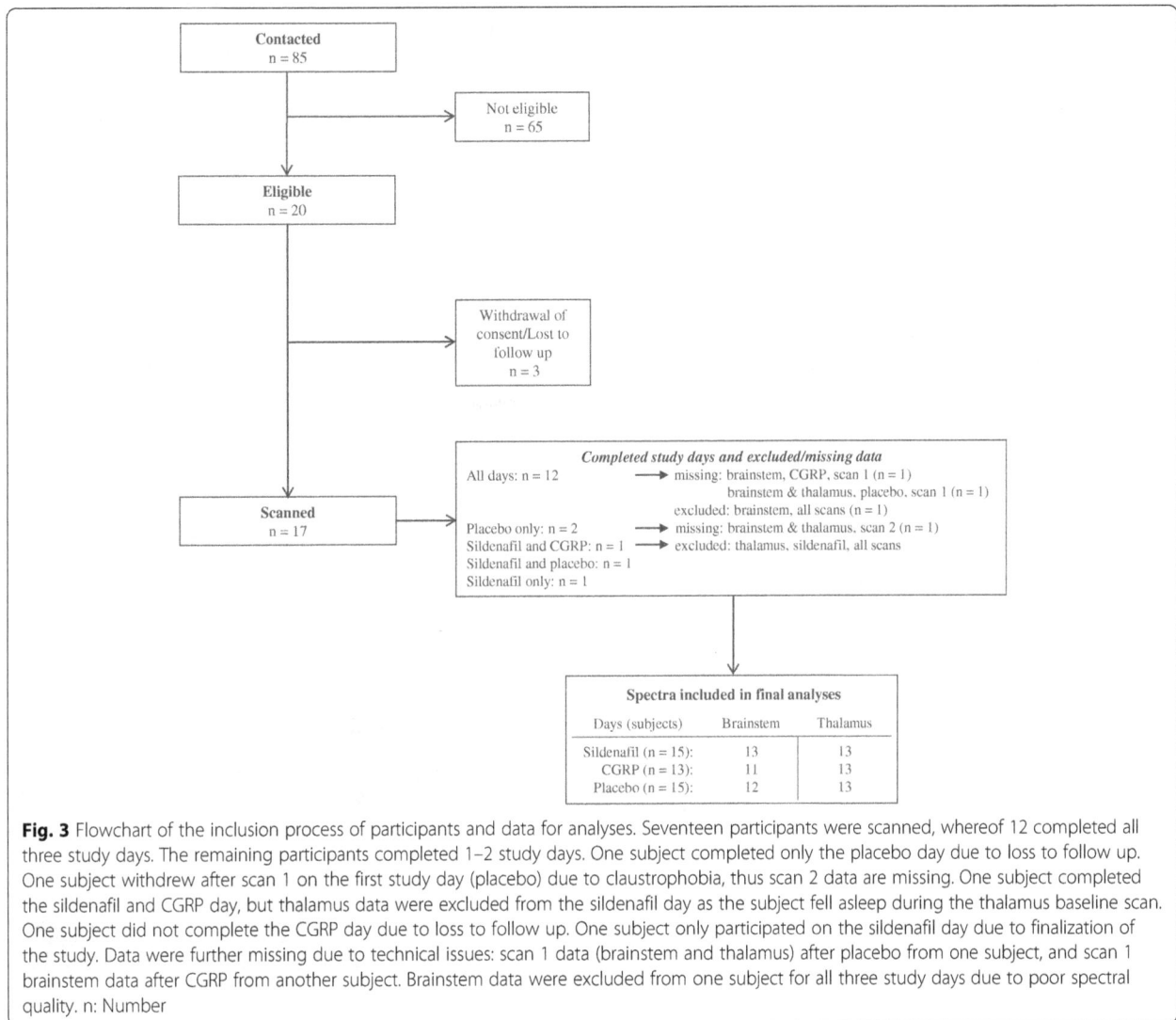

Fig. 3 Flowchart of the inclusion process of participants and data for analyses. Seventeen participants were scanned, whereof 12 completed all three study days. The remaining participants completed 1–2 study days. One subject completed only the placebo day due to loss to follow up. One subject withdrew after scan 1 on the first study day (placebo) due to claustrophobia, thus scan 2 data are missing. One subject completed the sildenafil and CGRP day, but thalamus data were excluded from the sildenafil day as the subject fell asleep during the thalamus baseline scan. One subject did not complete the CGRP day due to loss to follow up. One subject only participated on the sildenafil day due to finalization of the study. Data were further missing due to technical issues: scan 1 data (brainstem and thalamus) after placebo from one subject, and scan 1 brainstem data after CGRP from another subject. Brainstem data were excluded from one subject for all three study days due to poor spectral quality. n: Number

extracellular space [29]. Most likely, the glutamate concentrations measured by ^{1}H-MRS largely reflect the extracellular glutamate levels. In support of this, a ^{1}H-MRS study reported lower glutamate levels in amyotrophic lateral sclerosis patients treated with riluzole, a drug that increases glutamate uptake in central nervous system (CNS) neurons, compared to riluzole-naive amyotrophic lateral sclerosis patients and healthy controls [16]. The transient sildenafil-induced increase of glutamate in the brainstem in the present study thus likely reflects increased extracellular glutamate levels and possibly increased neuronal excitability. In support, sildenafil is able to cross the blood-brain barrier [23, 33] and some individuals report CNS side effects, such as dizziness and confusion [33–36]. Thus, sildenafil may be able to directly affect the neurons in deep brain structures such as the brainstem. In contrast, a functional MRI (fMRI) study of the visual cortex suggested that oral sildenafil intake did not change the neuronal activation threshold either at 1 or 2 h after administration [2]. The

plasma t_{max} of oral 100 mg sildenafil is about 1 h with a close to 4 h half-life in the fasting state [36]. Here, we detected an increased glutamate level at scan 1 (40–70 min after sildenafil), around the time of t_{max}, but not at scan 2 (140–170 min after sildenafil). Possibly, plasma concentrations of sildenafil above a certain level are needed to alter the glutamate levels. Another possibility is that the transient changes may be attributed to adaptation of sildenafil's effect at scan 2.

We detected no difference in the glutamate levels between groups of participants developing headache vs. no headache. It should be noted that the participants were healthy with no family history of migraine developing merely a mild to moderate non-migraine headache after the drug administration. Therefore, we speculate that a "healthy" trigeminonociceptive system would not be sufficiently activated to produce detectable changes in the glutamate level. This may also explain the lack of changes in the glutamate levels after CGRP as well as in the thalamus.

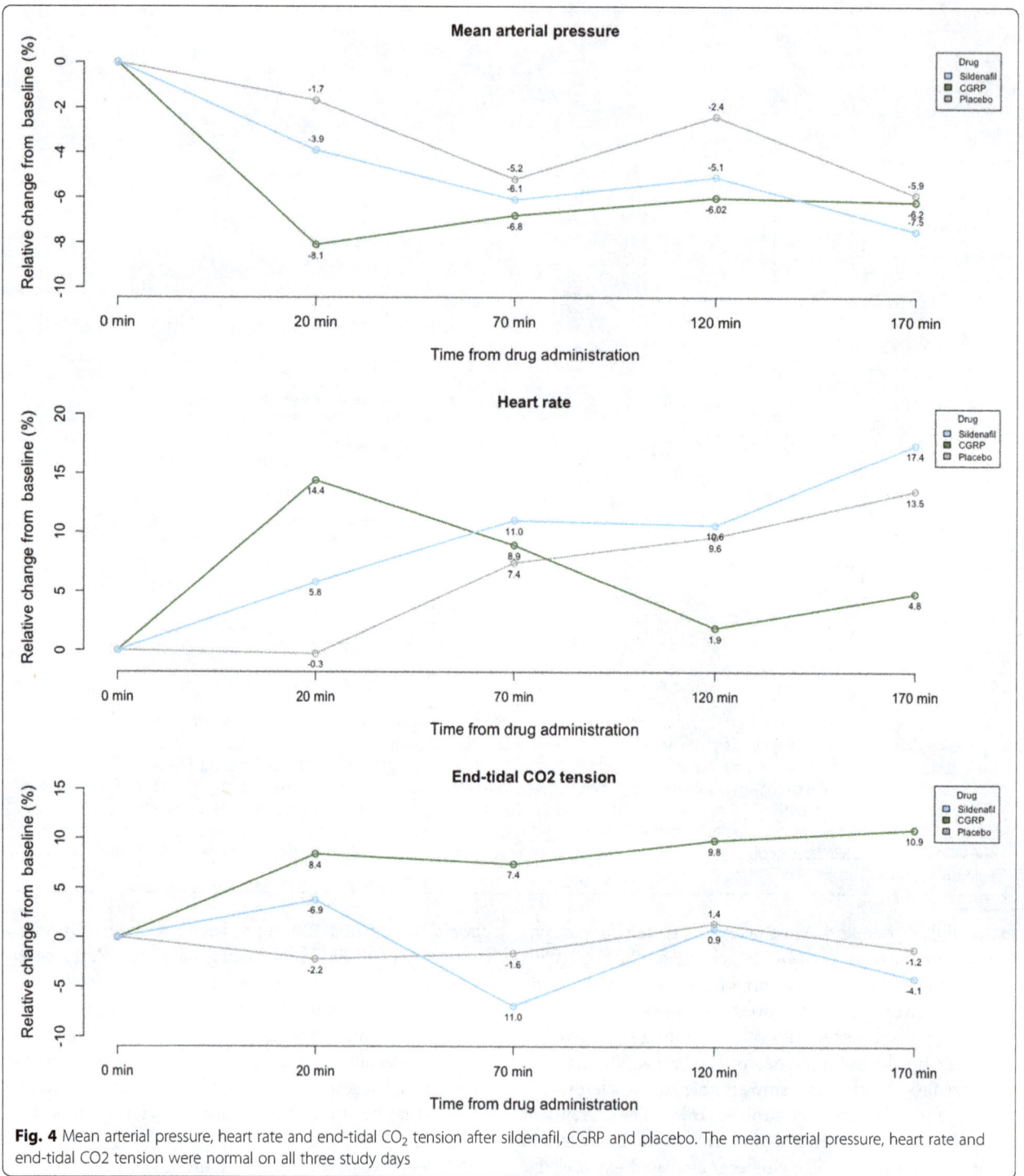

Fig. 4 Mean arterial pressure, heart rate and end-tidal CO_2 tension after sildenafil, CGRP and placebo. The mean arterial pressure, heart rate and end-tidal CO2 tension were normal on all three study days

Given the transient glutamate changes and lack of correlation to headache status, it is likely that the observed changes are related to the pharmacological effects of the drug rather than the headache per se.

The lactate concentration was decreased in the brainstem at scan 1 after sildenafil compared to the corresponding placebo change. This observation is very interesting since brain lactate levels under normal conditions increase during neuronal activation [37]. Therefore, we would expect the brainstem lactate levels to increase following sildenafil administration, along with the observed increase in glutamate. A possible explanation could be that the lactate decrease reflects a neuronal energy consumption via conversion to pyruvate [38]. The lactate concentration finding in the present study should be interpreted with caution due to the relatively large standard deviations. Also of note, the

Table 1 Summary of metabolite concentrations in brainstem after sildenafil, CGRP and placebo

	Baseline		Scan 1				Scan 2			
	Mean mmol/L	SD	Mean mmol/L	SD	% change from baseline	P	Mean mmol/L	SD	% change from baseline	P
Glutamate										
Sildenafil	7.77	0.65	8.21	0.53	5.6	0.039*	8.06	0.77	3.7	0.101
CGRP	7.92	1.11	7.49	0.88	−5.4	0.639	8.08	0.73	−2.0	0.228
Placebo	7.96	0.50	7.72	0.61	−3.0	−	7.70	0.65	−3.3	−
Lactate										
Sildenafil	0.90	0.21	0.45	0.41	−50.0	0.017*	0.43	0.33	− 51.9	0.156
CGRP	0.71	0.51	0.49	0.44	−30.9	0.151	0.42	0.41	−40.6	0.494
Placebo	0.75	0.65	0.89	0.68	21.6	−	0.62	0.42	−15.6	−
NAA										
Sildenafil	7.73	0.79	7.93	0.79	2.8	0.236	7.95	0.69	3.0	0.370
CGRP	7.58	0.72	7.56	0.68	−0.2	0.821	8.06	0.82	6.3	0.127
Placebo	7.61	0.63	7.64	0.58	0.4	−	7.73	0.72	1.6	−
Total creatine										
Sildenafil	4.25	0.35	4.33	0.32	1.0	0.978	4.23	0.28	−0.3	0.735
CGRP	4.38	0.38	4.39	0.53	0.03	0.562	4.50	0.33	2.7	0.170
Placebo	4.24	0.33	4.33	0.47	2.0	−	4.21	0.32	−0.7	−

*$P<0.05$. P values reported for delta change from baseline to scan 1 and 2 after sildenafil and CGRP, compared to the corresponding change from baseline after placebo
NAA N-Acetylaspartate, SD standard deviation

lactate concentration is very low in the healthy brain (below 1.0 mmol/L) [39]. This contributes to the risk of lactate signal loss in the spectrum due to chemical shift displacement or J-modulations deviations during the MRS measurements, which are known issues [39].

CGRP-induced biochemical changes

We detected no alterations in the glutamate levels after CGRP infusion in either brainstem or thalamus in healthy participants. This suggests that CGRP does *not* modify the neuronal excitability in these key CNS structures involved in pain processing in healthy subjects. The blood-brain barrier is believed to have no permeability to CGRP [4, 40],

and thus little or no direct effects on central brain regions, which our findings support.

In line with previous reports [3, 4], we found that participants developed more headache after CGRP, compared to placebo, demonstrating that CGRP is able to activate the trigeminal pain pathway. Given that systemic CGRP is unlikely to cross the blood-brain barrier, the present findings support the notion that CGRP acts on perivascular afferents [22] or the trigeminal ganglion [21, 41]. Interestingly, an fMRI study reported no change in the neuronal activation of the visual cortex of healthy volunteers after CGRP infusion [42]. Increased neuronal response to visual stimulation has previously been

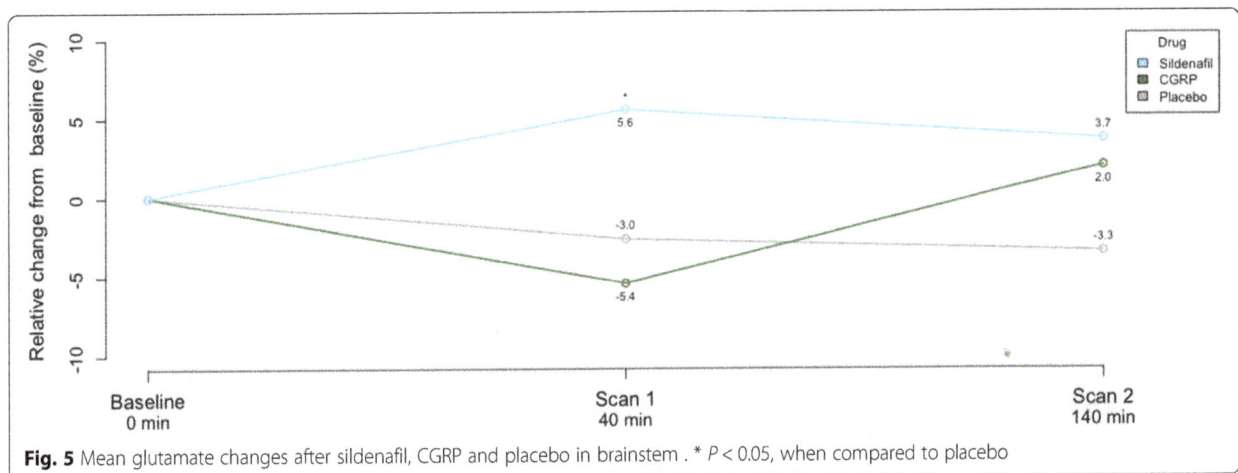

Fig. 5 Mean glutamate changes after sildenafil, CGRP and placebo in brainstem . * $P < 0.05$, when compared to placebo

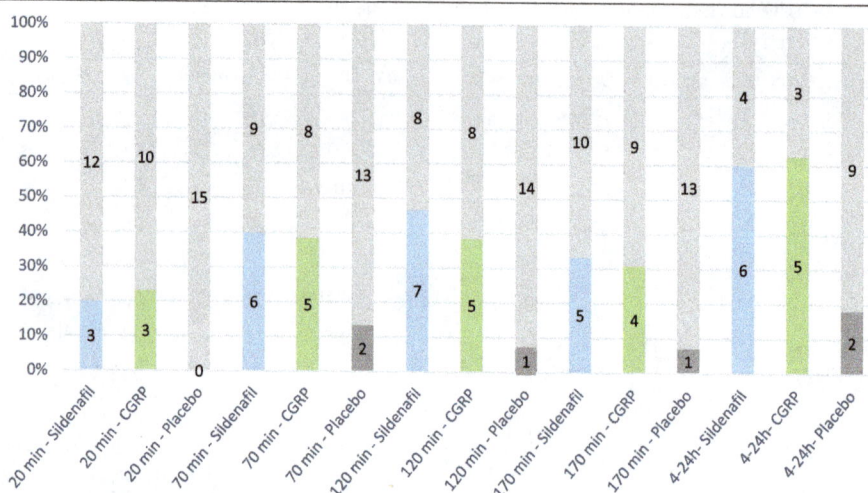

Fig. 6 Proportion of healthy participants who developed headache after sildenafil, CGRP and placebo. Blue, green and dark grey bars indicate headache. Light grey bars indicate no headache. During the scan sessions (0–4 h), 8 of 13 participants (62%) developed headache after CGRP (P = 0.041, compared to placebo), 8 of 15 (53%) developed headache after sildenafil (P = 0.131, compared to placebo), and 2 of 13 (13%) developed headache after placebo.

shown to be correlated with an increase in the glutamate levels [43, 44]. Another fMRI study involving application of heat pain to the forehead of healthy volunteers reported altered blood-oxygenation-level-dependent signal 40 min after administration of CGRP in pain associated brain regions, including the brainstem and thalamus, with no changes during placebo [45]. This observation suggests that CGRP may be capable of modulating the neuronal response indirectly (i.e. outside the CNS) given that the pain pathway is already activated [45].

Reliability of glutamate measurements

With our ^{1}H-MRS protocol, we obtained high quality spectra from the brainstem and thalamus with narrow line widths and relatively high SNR allowing for reliable quantification. A previous 3.0 T ^{1}H-MRS study measured glutamate changes in the brainstem without reporting the SNR or spectral line widths, but visual inspection of the brainstem spectrum reveals more noise compared to the brainstem spectra obtained in the present study [16]. Other ^{1}H-MRS brainstem studies reported relatively wider mean line widths of 8.1 Hz (± 0.9) [18], and 10.04 Hz (± 4.64) [17] at 3.0 T, and 7 Hz at 4.0 T [19] indicating spectra of lower quality. One of the studies reported the SNR as well, which was relatively high, 21(± 3), most likely due to the larger VOI used in the study [18]. None of the studies reported glutamate findings and the VOIs were larger than in the present study [17–19]. While large VOIs can improve the spectral quality, it also restricts the possibility of targeting a brain area with precision.

A previous 3.0 T ^{1}H-MRS study of thalamus used a larger VOI with fewer acquisitions, and reported a mean line width similar to the present study findings, but did not report the SNR value for comparison [17]. One 1.5 T ^{1}H-MRS thalamus study reported reduced mean line width of 3.2 Hz (± 0.5), however, the SNR of 3.9 (± 1.2) was much lower [46].

The brainstem ^{1}H-MRS spectra reveal a different metabolite composition compared to the conventional spectra obtained from e.g. the thalamus and occipital lope, as the choline peak is higher than the total creatine peak (Fig. 2), which is commonly reported [16, 17, 19].

To our knowledge, our study is the first ^{1}H-MRS study to provide information on the variability of glutamate levels in both brainstem and thalamus, based on repeated measurements, on the same day and on three separate days. In the present study, the overall variability of the glutamate measurements was low. For comparison, a previous 3.0 T ^{1}H-MRS study reported a higher inter-subject glutamate variability of 15.4%–16.3% in the deep brain area of the amygdala, based on two scans obtained 1 week apart [47]. Another 3.0 T ^{1}H-MRS study of repeated measurements on three consecutive days reported residual measurement error as the main contributor to the glutamate variability in a small hippocampus VOI [48]. Finally, one previous 7.0 T ^{1}H-MRS study reported higher glutamate variability of 11.48% (± 8.87) within day (based on two scans), and 6.56% (± 4.69) between day, measured in the visual cortical area of healthy subjects [49]. However, the study did not report a separate inter-subject and residual measurement error variability [49].

The present study has several major strengths to account for the measurement error variation, as all participants were scanned at fixed time points on each scan day, accounting for possible changes due to the metabolic circadian rhythm [25, 26]. In addition, we maintained identical and stable study conditions for all participants on all three study days, including detailed dietary restrictions before and during the scan sessions. All participants were carefully instructed to avoid any head motion during the scans. However, we cannot exclude the possibility of motion affecting our findings during the scan sessions. We estimated that the high acquisition number for the ^{1}H-MRS sequences was appropriate and feasible to obtain a sufficient signal noise ratio from the spectral VOIs. Additionally, as our primary aim was to investigate and compare relative changes from baseline within subjects, these issues were unlikely to affect our results.

Conclusion

Here we present a protocol for pharmacological ^{1}H-MRS at 3.0 T in the brainstem and thalamus, with good spectral quality, and overall low measurement variability. We demonstrated that sildenafil induces transiently increased glutamate levels in the brainstem, which suggest transiently increased excitability of the brainstem neurons. CGRP does not induce glutamate changes in the brainstem or thalamic neurons, suggesting that its headache-inducing effects are not mediated by biochemical changes in deep brain structures, but rather its effects on the peripheral trigeminal pain pathways.

Abbreviations

[1]H: proton; CGRP: calcitonin gene-related peptide; CNS: central nervous system; fMRI: functional magnetic resonance imaging; FWHM: full-width of half-maximum; ICHD-3 beta: The diagnostic criteria of the beta version of the third International Classification of Headache Disorders; MRI: magnetic resonance imaging; MRS: magnetic resonance spectroscopy; NAA: N-Acetylaspartate; PRESS: point-resolved spectroscopy pulse sequence; SNR: signal-noise-ratio; VOI: volume-of-interest

Funding

We thank the Lundbeck Foundation [grant number R155–2014-171] and the Research Foundation of Rigshospitalet [grant number E-23327-02]. Funding sources played no role in study design, data collection, analysis, interpretation, manuscript preparation, or submission.

Authors' contributions

SY drafted and revised the paper and contributed to study design, protocol development, participant enrolment, acquisition and processing of data, statistical analysis and interpretation of data. AH contributed to study design, protocol development, interpretation of data and revising manuscript for content. CEC contributed to protocol development, participant enrolment, acquisition of data, and revising manuscript for content. MBV contributed to study design, processing of data, statistical analysis, and revising manuscript for content. ETP and OBP contributed to study design and revising manuscript for content. HBWL contributed to study design, protocol development, statistical analysis, and revising manuscript for content. MA initiated the study and contributed to study design, protocol development, data interpretation, and revision of the manuscript. All authors read and approved the final manuscript.

Competing interests

MA reports personal fees from Alder BioPharmaceuticals, Allergan, Amgen, Alder, Eli Lilly, Novartis and Teva. MA participated in clinical trials as the principal investigator for Alder ALD403-CLIN-011 (Phase 3b), Amgen 20,120,178 (Phase 2), 20,120,295 (Phase 2), 20,130,255 (OLE), 20,120,297 (Phase 3), GM-11 gamma-Core-R trials, Novartis CAMG334a2301 (Phase 3b), Amgen PAC1 20,150,308 (Phase 2a), Teva TV48125-CNS-30068 (Phase 3). MA has no ownership interest and does not own stocks of any pharmaceutical company. MA serves as associated editor of Cephalalgia, co-editor of the Journal of Headache and Pain. MA is President-elect of the International Headache Society and General Secretary of the European Headache Federation. The remaining authors report no conflicts of interest.

Author details

[1]Danish Headache Center, Department of Neurology, Rigshospitalet Glostrup, University of Copenhagen, Copenhagen, Denmark. [2]Functional Imaging Unit, Department of Clinical Physiology, Nuclear Medicine and PET, Rigshospitalet Glostrup, University of Copenhagen, Copenhagen, Denmark. [3]Danish Research Centre for Magnetic Resonance, Centre for Functional and Diagnostic Imaging and research, Copenhagen University Hospital Hvidovre, Copenhagen, Denmark. [4]Neurobiology Research Unit, Department of Neurology, Rigshospitalet, University of Copenhagen, Copenhagen, Denmark.

References

1. Kruuse C, Thomsen LL, Jacobsen TB, Olesen J (2002) The phosphodiesterase 5 inhibitor sildenafil has no effect on cerebral blood flow or blood velocity, but nevertheless induces headache in healthy subjects. J Cereb Blood Flow Metab 22:1124–1131
2. Kruuse C, Hansen AE, Larsson HBW, Lauritzen M, Rostrup E (2009) Cerebral haemodynamic response or excitability is not affected by sildenafil. J Cereb Blood Flow Metab 29:830–839
3. Asghar MS, Hansen AE, Kapijimpanga T, van der Geest RJ, van der Koning P, Larsson HBW et al (2010) Dilation by CGRP of middle meningeal artery and reversal by sumatriptan in normal volunteers. Neurology 75:1520–1526
4. Petersen KA, Lassen LH, Birk S, Lesko L, Olesen J (2005) BIBN4096BS antagonizes human alpha-calcitonin gene related peptide-induced headache and extracerebral artery dilatation. Clin Pharmacol Ther 77:202–213
5. Kruuse C, Thomsen LL, Birk S, Olesen J (2003) Migraine can be induced by sildenafil without changes in middle cerebral artery diameter. Brain 126:241–247
6. Lassen LH, Haderslev PA, Jacobsen VB, Iversen HK, Sperling B, Olesen J (2002) CGRP may play a causative role in migraine. Cephalalgia 22:54–61
7. Asghar MS, Hansen AE, Amin FM, van der Geest RJ, Van Der KP, Larsson HBW et al (2011) Evidence for a vascular factor in migraine. Ann Neurol 69:635–645
8. Ashina M, Hansen JM, á Dunga BO, Olesen J (2017) Human models of migraine — short-term pain for long-term gain. Nat Rev Neurol 13:713–724
9. Hoffmann J, Charles A (2018) Glutamate and its receptors as therapeutic targets for migraine. Neurotherapeutics 15:361-370
10. Younis S, Hougaard A, Vestergaard MB, Larsson HBW, Ashina M (2017) Migraine and magnetic resonance spectroscopy : a systematic review. Curr Opin Neurol 30:246–262
11. Weiller C, May A, Limmroth V, Jüptner M, Kaube H, Schayck RV et al (1995) Brain stem activation in spontaneous human migraine attacks. Nat Med 1: 658–660
12. Afridi SK, Matharu MS, Lee L, Kaube H, Friston KJ, Frackowiak RSJ et al (2005) A PET study exploring the laterality of brainstem activation in migraine using glyceryl trinitrate. Brain 128:932–939
13. Stankewitz A, May A (2011) Increased limbic and brainstem activity during migraine attacks following olfactory stimulation. Neurology 77:476–482
14. Hougaard A, Amin FM, Christensen CE, Younis S, Wolfram F, Cramer SP et al (2017) Increased brainstem perfusion, but no blood- brain barrier disruption, during attacks of migraine with aura. Brain 140:1633–1642
15. Afridi SK, Giffin NJ, Kaube H, Friston KJ, Ward NS, Frackowiak RSJ et al (2005) A positron emission tomographic study in spontaneous migraine. Arch Neurol 62:1270–1275
16. Foerster BR, Pomper MG, Callaghan BC, Petrou M, Edden RAE, Mohamed MA et al (2013) An imbalance between excitatory and inhibitory

neurotransmitters in amyotrophic lateral sclerosis revealed by use of 3-T proton magnetic resonance spectroscopy. JAMA Neurol 70:1009–1016

17. Baker EH, Basso G, Barker PB, Smith MA, Bonekamp D, Horská A (2010) Regional apparent metabolite concentrations in young adult brain measured by 1H MR spectroscopy at 3 tesla. J Magn Reson Imaging 27: 489–499

18. Adanyeguh IM, Henry P-G, Nguyen TM, Rinaldi D, Jauffret C, Valabregue R et al (2015) In vivo neurometabolic profiling in patients with spinocerebellar ataxia types 1, 2, 3, and 7. Mov Disord 30:662–670

19. Öz G, Tkáč I (2011) Short-echo, single-shot, full-intensity proton magnetic resonance spectroscopy for neurochemical profiling at 4 T: validation in the cerebellum and brainstem. Magn Reson Med 65:901–910

20. Zielman R, Teeuwisse WM, Bakels F, Van der Grond J, Webb A, van Buchem MA et al (2014) Biochemical changes in the brain of hemiplegic migraine patients measured with 7 tesla 1H-MRS. Cephalalgia 34:959–967

21. Eftekhari S, Salvatore CA, Calamari A, Kane SA, Tajti J, Edvinsson L (2010) Differential distribution of calcitonin gene-related peptide and its receptor components in the human trigeminal ganglion. Neuroscience 169:683–696

22. Miller S, Liu H, Warfvinge K, Shi L, Dovlatyan M, Xu C et al (2016) Immunohistochemical localization of the calcitonin gene-related peptide binding site in the primate trigeminovascular system using functional antagonist antibodies. Neuroscience 328:165–183

23. Gómez-Vallejo V, Ugarte A, García-Barroso C, Cuadrado-Tejedor M, Szczupak B, Dopeso-Reyes IG et al (2016) Pharmacokinetic investigation of sildenafil using positron emission tomography and determination of its effect on cerebrospinal fluid cGMP levels. J Neurochem 136:403–415

24. Headache Classification Committee of the International Headache Society (IHS) (2013) The international classification of headache disorders, 3rd edition (beta version). Cephalalgia 33:629–808

25. Peng S-L, Dumas JA, Park DC, Liu P, Filbey FM, McAdams CJ et al (2014) Age-related increase of resting metabolic rate in the human brain. Neuroimage 98:176–183

26. Soreni N, Noseworthy MD, Cormier T, Oakden WK, Bells S, Schachar R (2006) Intraindividual variability of striatal 1H-MRS brain metabolite measurements at 3 T. Magn Reson Imaging 24:187–194

27. Lopez-Rodriguez F, Medina-Ceja L, Wilson CL, Jhung D, Morales-Villagran A (2007) Changes in extracellular glutamate levels in rat orbitofrontal cortex during sleep and wakefulness. Arch Med Res 38:52–55

28. Christiansen P, Henriksen O, Stubgaard M, Gideon P, Larsson HBW (1993) In vivo quantification of brain metabolites by 1H-MRS using water as an internal standard. Magn Reson Imaging 11:107–118

29. Danbolt NC (2001) Glutamate uptake. Prog Neurobiol 65:1–105

30. Hunsberger HC, Konat GW, Reed MN (2017) Peripheral viral challenge elevates extracellular glutamate in the hippocampus leading to seizure hypersusceptibility. J Neurochem 141:341–346

31. Hunsberger HC, Wang D, Petrisko TJ, Alhowail A, Setti SE, Suppiramaniam V et al (2016) Peripherally restricted viral challenge elevates extracellular glutamates and enhances synaptic transmission in the hippocampus. J Neurochem 138:307–316

32. Tkáč I, Öz G, Adriany G, Uğurbil K, Gruetter R (2009) In vivo 1H NMR spectroscopy of the human brain at high magnetic fields: metabolite quantification at 4T vs. 7T. Magn Reson Med 62:868–879

33. Milman HA, Arnold SB (2002) Neurologic, psychological, and aggressive disturbances with sildenafil. Ann Pharmacother 36:1129–1134

34. Moreira SG, Brannigan RE, Spitz A, Orejuela FJ, Lipshultz LI, Kim ED (2000) Side-effect profile of sildenafil citrate (Viagra) in clinical practice. Urology 4295:474–476

35. Schultheiss D, Müller SV, Nager W, Stief CG, Schlote N, Jonas U et al (2001) Central effects of sildenafil (Viagra) on auditory selective attention and verbal recognition memory in humans: a study with event-related brain potentials. World J Urol 19:46–50

36. Nichols DJ, Muirhead GJ, Harness JA (2002) Pharmacokinetics of sildenafil after single oral doses in healthy male subjects: absolute bioavailability, food effects and dose proportionality. Br J Clin Pharmacol 53:5S–12S

37. Mangia S, Giove F, Tkáč I, Logothetis NK, Henry P-G, Olman CA et al (2009) Metabolic and hemodynamic events after changes in neuronal activity: current hypotheses, theoretical predictions and in vivo NMR experimental findings. J Cereb Blood Flow Metab 29:441–463

38. Lemire J, Mailloux RJ, Appanna VD (2008) Mitochondrial lactate dehydrogenase is involved in oxidative-energy metabolism in human astrocytoma cells (CCF-STTG1). PLoS One 3:1–10

39. Lange T, Dydak U, Roberts TPL, Rowley HA, Bjeljac M, Boesiger P (2006) Pitfalls in lactate measurements at 3T. Am J Neuroradiol 27:895–901

40. Petersen KA, Birk S, Lassen LH, Kruuse C, Jonassen O, Lesko L et al (2005) The CGRP-antagonist, BIBN4096BS does not affect cerebral or systemic haemodynamics in healthy volunteers. Cephalalgia 25:139–147

41. Eftekhari S, Salvatore CA, Johansson S, Chen T, Zeng Z, Edvinsson L (2015) Localization of CGRP, CGRP receptor, PACAP and glutamate in trigeminal ganglion. Relation to the blood–brain barrier. Brain Res 1600:93–109

42. Asghar MS, Hansen AE, Larsson HBW, Olesen J, Ashina M (2012) Effect of CGRP and sumatriptan on the BOLD response in visual cortex. J Headache Pain 13:159–166

43. Bednařík P, Tkáč I, Giove F, DiNuzzo M, Deelchand DK, Emir UE et al (2015) Neurochemical and BOLD responses during neuronal activation measured in the human visual cortex at 7 tesla. J Cereb Blood Flow Metab 35:601–610

44. Schaller B, Xin L, O'Brien K, Magill AW, Gruetter R (2014) Are glutamate and lactate increases ubiquitous to physiological activation? A 1H functional MR spectroscopy study during motor activation in human brain at 7 tesla. Neuroimage 93:138–145

45. Asghar MS, Becerra L, Larsson HBW, Borsook D, Ashina M (2016) Calcitonin gene-related peptide modulates heat nociception in the human brain - an fMRI study in healthy volunteers. PLoS One 11:1–20

46. Helms G, Piringer A (2001) Restoration of motion-related signal loss and line-shape deterioration of proton MR spectra using the residual water as intrinsic reference. Magn Reson Med 46:395–400

47. Nacewicz BM, Angelos L, Dalton KM, Fischer R, Anderle MJ, Alexander AL et al (2012) Reliable non-invasive measurement of human neurochemistry using proton spectroscopy with an anatomically defined amygdala-specific voxel. Neuroimage 59:2548–2559

48. Allaïli N, Valabrègue R, Auerbach EJ, Guillemot V, Yahia-Cherif L, Bardinet E et al (2015) Single-voxel 1H spectroscopy in the human hippocampus at 3 T using the LASER sequence: characterization of neurochemical profile and reproducibility. NMR Biomed 28:1209–1217

49. Cai K, Nanga RPR, Lamprou L, Schinstine C, Elliott M, Hariharan H et al (2012) The impact of gabapentin administration on brain GABA and glutamate concentrations: a 7T 1H-MRS study. Neuropsychopharmacology 37:2764–2771

19

Disrupted default mode network connectivity in migraine without aura

Alessandro Tessitore[1*†], Antonio Russo[1,2†], Alfonso Giordano[1,2], Francesca Conte[1], Daniele Corbo[1], Manuela De Stefano[1], Sossio Cirillo[3], Mario Cirillo[3], Fabrizio Esposito[4,5] and Gioacchino Tedeschi[1,2]

Abstract

Background: Resting-state functional magnetic resonance imaging (RS-fMRI) has demonstrated disrupted default mode network (DMN) connectivity in a number of pain conditions, including migraine. However, the significance of altered resting-state brain functional connectivity in migraine is still unknown. The present study is aimed to explore DMN functional connectivity in patients with migraine without aura (MwoA) and investigate its clinical significance.

Methods: To calculate and compare the resting-state functional connectivity of the DMN in 20 patients with MwoA, during the interictal period, and 20 gender- and age-matched HC, Brain Voyager QX was used. Voxel-based morphometry was used to assess whether between-group differences in DMN functional connectivity were related to structural differences. Secondary analyses explored associations between DMN functional connectivity, clinical and neuropsychological features of migraineurs.

Results: In comparison to HC, patients with MwoA showed decreased connectivity in prefrontal and temporal regions of the DMN. Functional abnormalities were unrelated to detectable structural abnormalities or clinical and neuropsychological features of migraineurs.

Conclusions: Our study provides further evidence of disrupted DMN connectivity in patients with MwoA. We hypothesize that a DMN dysfunction may be related to behavioural processes such as a maladaptive response to stress which seems to characterize patients with migraine.

Keywords: Resting-state fMRI; Default mode network; Migraine

Background

Migraine is a common and disabling primary headache disorder clinically characterized by episodic attacks of throbbing headache with specific features and associated symptoms [1]. A great body of studies has been conducted on patients with migraine, however, its pathophysiology is not completely understood. Indeed, currently, no integrative model has been formulated that accounts for all the factors that may play a role in migraine pathophysiology such as spreading depression, neurogenic inflammation, excitatory/inhibitory balance, genetic background and disturbed energy metabolism [2,3]. More recently, converging evidence supports the role of a maladaptive stress

response in migraine mechanisms [4,5]. Resting-state fMRI (RS-fMRI) has allowed for the exploration of brain connectivity between functionally linked cortical regions, the so-called resting-state networks (RSNs) [6]. The most consistently reported RSN is the default mode network (DMN), which plays a relevant role in adaptive behavior other than in cognitive, emotional, and attention processes [7,8]. In the last years, several RS-fMRI studies have identified functional connectivity changes in patients with migraine without aura (MwoA) [9]. To our knowledge, only a few of them have focused on DMN integrity in patients with migraine, reporting inconsistent results [10-12]. For this reason, we investigated the DMN connectivity in patients with MwoA during the interictal period, by means of RS-fMRI using an independent component approach (ICA) to avoid any a priori hypothesis about the source of a possible functional disconnection [13]. In addition, we used Voxel Based Morphometry (VBM) to

* Correspondence: alessandro.tessitore@unina2.it
†Equal contributors
[1]Department of Neurology, Second University of Naples, Piazza Miraglia 2 - I-80138, Naples, Italy

assess whether any between-group differences in resting-state functional connectivity were dependent on structural abnormalities, recently described in patients with migraine [14]. We hypothesized that DMN connectivity could be decreased in patients with MwoA in comparison to healthy controls (HC), supporting the current view that migraine may be related to a maladaptive stress response.

Methods
Patients
Twenty-five consecutive patients with episodic MwoA, according to the International Headache Society criteria (Headache Classification Subcommittee of the International Headache Society, 2013) [15] were prospectively recruited from the migraine population referring to the outpatient headache clinic of the Department of Neurology at the Second University of Naples. Demographic data and the following clinical characteristics were obtained from the patients with MwoA: age of onset, disease duration, frequency (day/month), duration and mean pain intensity of migraine attacks and related disability. Mean pain intensity of migraine attacks was assessed using a visual analogic scale (VAS). To obtain an accurate assessment of patient's headache-related disability, all patients with MwoA completed the Migraine Disability Assessment Scale (MIDAS) and Headache Impact Test (HIT-6). Patients with hypertension, diabetes mellitus, heart disease, other chronic systemic diseases, stroke, cognitive impairment, substance abuse, chronic pain, as well as other neurological or psychiatric disorders were excluded. To avoid any possible migraine attack-related or pharmacologic interference with the RS-fMRI investigation, all patients with MwoA were both migraine-free and not taking attack medications for at least 3 days before scanning and were naïve for any commonly prescribed medications for migraine prevention. Moreover, all patients with MwoA were interviewed 7 days after scanning to ascertain if they were migraine-free also during the post-scan week. For this reason, five patients were excluded from the analyses herein, which focused on 20 right-handed patients (mean age ± SE: 28.15 ± 3.08 years, 10/10 males/females).

Healthy controls
Twenty age- and gender-matched, right-handed subjects (mean age ± SE: 28.90 ± 3.63 years, 10/10 females/males) with less than a few spontaneous non-throbbing headaches per year, with no family history of migraine, no hypertension, diabetes mellitus, heart disease, other chronic systemic diseases, stroke, cognitive impairment, substance abuse, chronic pain, as well as other neurological or psychiatric disorders were recruited as HC.

Standard protocol approvals, registrations, and patient consents
The study was approved by the Ethics Committee of Second University of Naples, and written informed consent was obtained from all subjects according to the Declaration of Helsinki.

Neuropsychological evaluation
To assess levels of depression and anxiety, patients with MwoA and HC completed the Hamilton Depression Rating Scale (HDRS) and the Hamilton Anxiety Rating Scale (HARS). An extensive neuropsychological evaluation was performed in patients with MwoA as previously described [16].

Imaging parameters
MRI was performed on a General Electric (Minneapolis, U.S.) Signa HDxt 3 Tesla whole-body scanner equipped with an 8-channel parallel head coil. RS-fMRI data consisted of 240 volumes of a repeated gradient-echo echo planar imaging T2*-weighted sequence (TR = 1508 ms, axial slices = 29, matrix = 64 × 64, field of view = 256 mm, thickness = 4 mm, interslice gap = 0 mm, 10 discarded scans at the beginning). During the functional scan, subjects were asked to simply stay motionless, awake, and relaxed, and to keep their eyes closed; no visual or auditory stimuli were presented at any time during functional scanning. Three-dimensional high-resolution T1-weighted sagittal images (GE sequence IR-FSPGR, TR = 6988 ms, TI = 1100 ms, TE = 3.9 ms, flip angle = 10, voxel size = 1 × 1 × 1.2 mm3) were acquired for registration and normalization of the functional images as well as for atrophy measures and VBM analysis.

Statistical analysis of clinical data
Demographic and clinical features of patients with MwoA and HC were compared by the t-test for independent samples or by $\chi2$, as appropriate.

RS-fMRI pre-processing and statistical analysis
Image data pre-processing and statistical analysis were performed with BrainVoyager QX (Brain Innovation BV, The Netherlands). Nuisance signals (global signal, white matter and cerebro-spinal fluid signals and motion parameters) were regressed out from each data set. Before statistical analyses, individual functional data were co-registered to their own anatomical data and spatially normalized to Talairach space. Single-subject and group-level ICA was carried out respectively with the fastICA and the self-organizing group ICA [sogICA] algorithms [13]. For each subject, 40 independent components (corresponding to one sixth of the number of time points, see, e.g., Grecius et al., 2007) [17] were extracted. All single-subject component maps were then "clustered"

at the group level, resulting in 40 single-group average maps that were visually inspected to recognize the main functional resting-state networks, and particularly, to select the DMN component. The sign-adjusted DMN components of all subjects were then submitted to a second-level multi-subject random effects analysis that treated the individual subject map values as random observations at each voxel. Single-group one-sample t-tests were used to analyze the whole-brain distribution of the DMN component in each group separately and the resulting t-maps were thresholded at $p = 0.05$ (Bonferroni corrected over the entire brain). An inclusive mask was also created from the union of the two single-group maps (patients with MwoA and HC) and used to define a new search volume for within-network between-group comparisons. The resulting statistical maps were overlaid on the standard "Colin-27" brain T1 template. To correct for multiple comparisons, regional effects were only accepted for clusters exceeding a minimum size determined with a non-parametric randomization approach. Namely, an initial voxel-level threshold was set to $p = 0.01$ (uncorrected) and a minimum cluster size was estimated after 1000 Montecarlo simulations that protected against false positive clusters up to 5%. Cluster-level correction is a very common and effective way to correct for multiple comparisons in fMRI statistical maps, including random-effects maps, obtained from RS-fMRI studies (see, e.g., Russo et al., 2012) [16]. Individual ICA z-scores for both groups were extracted from DMN clusters identified in the above analyses and used for linear correlation analyses with clinical parameters of disease severity and cognitive scores. ICA z-scores express the relative modulation of a given voxel by a specific ICA and hence reflect the amplitude of the correlated fluctuations within the corresponding functional connectivity network.

VBM

Data were processed and examined using SPM8 software (Wellcome Trust Centre for Neuroimaging, London, UK; http://www.fil.ion.ucl.ac.uk/spm). VBM was implemented in the VBM8 toolbox (http://dbm.neuro.uni-jena.de/vbm.html) with default parameters incorporating the DARTEL toolbox, which was used to obtain a high-dimensional normalization protocol [18]. Images were bias-corrected, tissue-classified, and registered using linear (12-parameter affine) and non-linear transformations (warping) within a unified model. Subsequently, the warped gray matter (GM) segments were affine-transformed into Montreal Neurological Institute (MNI) space and were scaled by the Jacobian determinants of the deformations to account for the local compression and stretching that occurs as a consequence of the warping and affine transformation (modulated GM volumes). Finally, the modulated volumes were smoothed with a Gaussian kernel of 8-mm full-width

at half maximum (FWHM). The GM volume maps were statistically analyzed using the general linear model based on Gaussian random field theory. Statistical analysis consisted of an analysis of covariance (ANCOVA) with total intracranial volume (TIV) and age as covariates of no interest. We assessed whole-brain regional differences, as well as differences over region of interest (ROI) based on the results of the whole-brain between groups RS-fMRI analysis. Statistical inference was performed at the voxel level, with both a family-wise error correction for multiple comparisons ($p < 0.05$) and an uncorrected threshold ($p < 0.001$; cluster size:100).

Results

Clinical and neuropsychological data

The groups (20 patients with MwoA and 20 HC) did not differ in age or male/female ratio (see Table 1 for further clinical details). Patients with MwoA and HC showed no significant differences in HDRS and HARS scores. Patients with MwoA did not show significant cognitive impairments as compared to published normative data (Table 2).

RS- fMRI and VBM

As illustrated in Figure 1, each group exhibited a DMN connectivity pattern consistent with prior reports, encompassing medial and inferior prefrontal cortices, temporal lobe areas, anterior and posterior cingulate cortices, precuneus and cerebellar areas [6-8]. The two-sample t-tests revealed significant group differences in the left superior prefrontal gyrus (l-SPFG) (Talairach coordinates x,y,z: -13, 43, 42; Brodmann area 8) and in the left temporal pole (l-TP) (Talairach coordinates x,y,z: -34, 10, -14; Brodmann area 38), indicating that these regions had reduced component time course-related activity in patients

Table 1 Clinical characteristics of patients with MwoA and HC

Parameter	Group	Mean ± SE	p-value
Gender	MwoA	10 M / 10 F	n.s.
	HC	10 M / 10 F	n.s.
Age (years)	MwoA	28.15 ± 3.08	0.49
	HC	28.90 ± 3.63	
Disease duration (years)	MwoA	8.22 ± 2.04	
Frequency (day/month)	MwoA	6 ± 2.04	
Side of attack	MwoA	10R / 10 L	n.s.
MIDAS	MwoA	17.64 ± 5.25	
HIT-6	MwoA	60.21 ± 7.98	
VAS of attack intensity	MwoA	8.0 ± 1.65	

MwoA = patients with migraine without aura; HC = healthy controls; M = male; F = female; R = right; L = left; MIDAS = Migraine Disability Assessment Scale; HIT-6 = Headache Impact Test; VAS = Visual Analogue Scale.

Table 2 Neuropsychological evaluation in patients with MwoA

	Mean ± SD	Cut-off*
Education (years)	12.26 ±3.52	
Global general cognition		
MMSE	28.50 ± 1.30	>26/30
Psychiatric symptoms		
HARS	4.65 ± 2.50	<14
HDRS	4 ± 3.45	<10
Neuropsychological test		
TMT A	35 ± 6.58	≤ 94
TMT B	74.02 ± 12.2	≤ 283
WCST categories	105 ± 0.47	≥ 5.04
WCST err. perseveration	0.20 ± 0.38	≤ 5.6
WCST err. n. perseveration	0.22 ± 0.52	≤ 8.52
PF	28.16 ± 9.17	≥17.35
FAB	17.34 ± 5.49	≥12.03
Raven PM 47	28.71 ± 2.43	≥18.96

MMSE: mini mental state examination; HARS: Hamilton anxiety rating scale; HDRS: Hamilton depression rating scale; TMT A: Trail Making Test Part A; TMT B: Trail Making Test Part B; WCST: Wisconsin Card Sorting Test; PF: phonemic fluency; FAB: frontal assessment battery; Raven PM 47: Raven Standard Progressive Matrices.
*Values are relative to published normative data (see references for further details).

with MwoA compared to HC (Figure 2A and 2B). Post-hoc correlation analyses revealed that individual ROI averaged ICA scores in the l-SPFG and l-TP were not correlated neither with clinical parameters of disease severity (i.e. duration, frequency, VAS, MIDAS and HIT-6 scores) nor with single cognitive tests scores. There were no differences in global GM, white matter (WM) or cerebro-spinal fluid (CSF) volumes between groups (GM: MwoA patients = 684.53 mm3 ± 77.80 mm3; HC = 688.32 mm3 ± 71.12 mm3; $p = 0.72$; WM: MwoA patients = 516.03 mm3 ± 59.60 mm3; HC = 451.33 mm3 ± 85.88 mm3; $p = 0.61$; CSF: MwoA patients = 203.67 mm3 ± 26.17 mm3; HC = 207.89 mm3 ± 48.31 mm3; $p = 0.64$; total atrophy: MwoA patients = 1419.11 mm3 ± 123.33 mm3; HC = 1347.08 mm3 ± 179.21 mm3; $p = 0.82$). Moreover, both whole-brain and ROI-based analyses of regional volumes did not reveal any significant differences in local GM between patients with MwoA and HC, using a significance level of $p \leq 0.05$, FWE-corrected for multiple comparisons.

Discussion

The present RS-fMRI study was designed to assess the functional integrity of DMN in patients with MwoA. Our findings demonstrate a reduced functional connectivity within the prefrontal and temporal cortices of the DMN in patients with MwoA during the interictal period. This altered functional connectivity was independent of

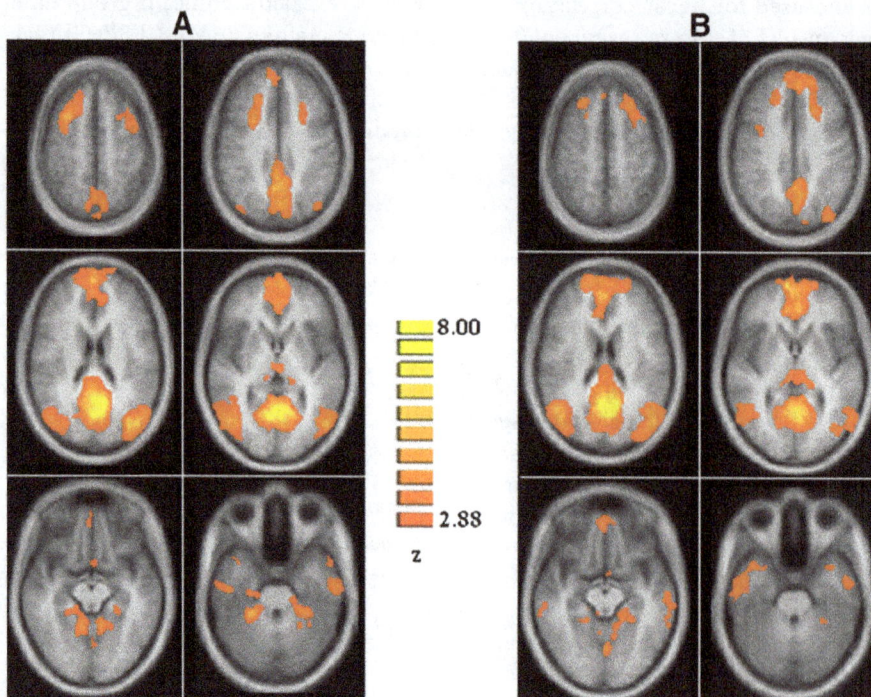

Figure 1 Group level DMN connectivity in HC (A) and patients with MwoA (B) ($p < 0.05$, cluster-level corrected) HC: healthy controls; MwoA: migraine without aura.

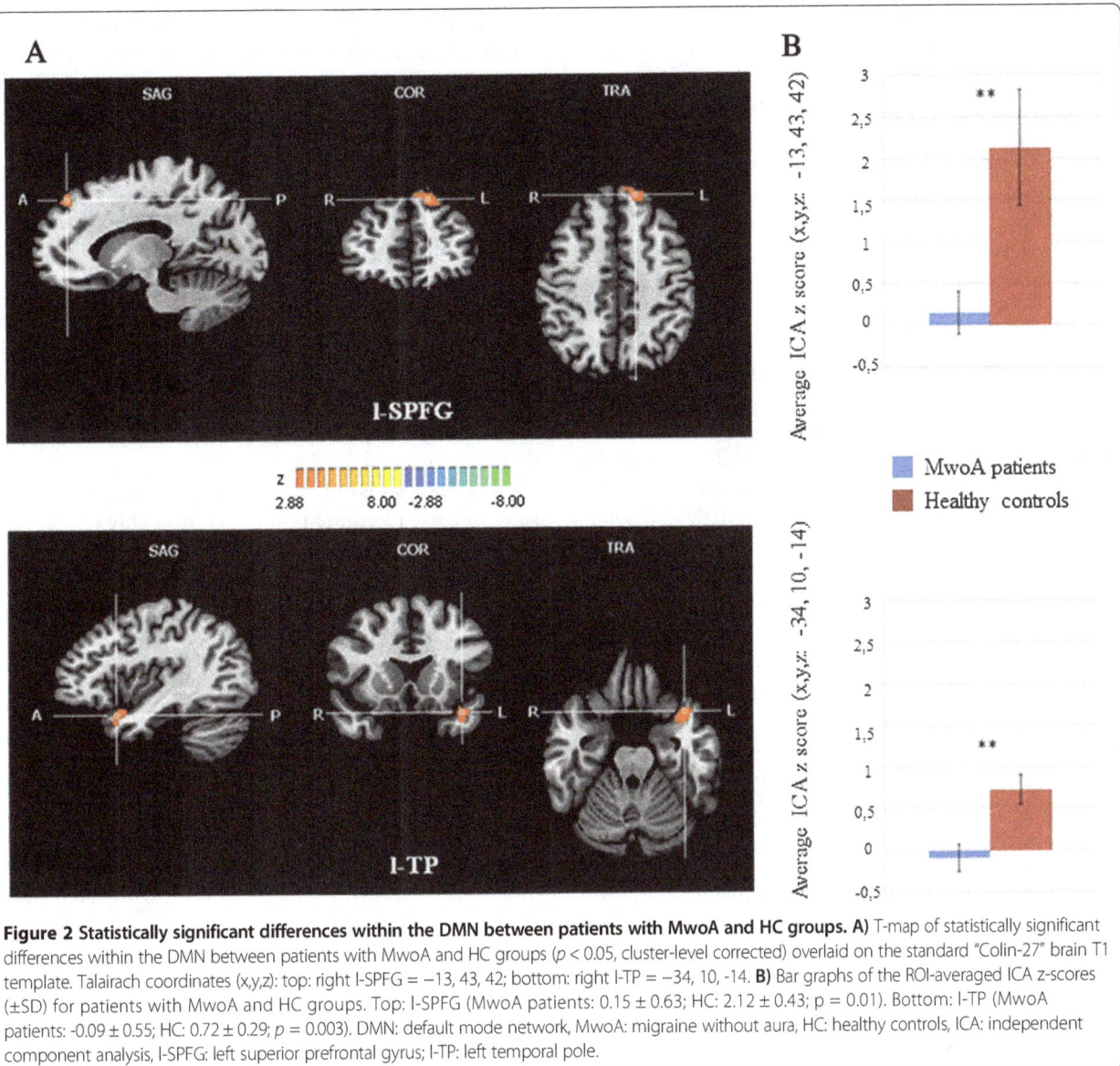

Figure 2 Statistically significant differences within the DMN between patients with MwoA and HC groups. A) T-map of statistically significant differences within the DMN between patients with MwoA and HC groups ($p < 0.05$, cluster-level corrected) overlaid on the standard "Colin-27" brain T1 template. Talairach coordinates (x,y,z): top: right l-SPFG = −13, 43, 42; bottom: right l-TP = −34, 10, -14. **B)** Bar graphs of the ROI-averaged ICA z-scores (±SD) for patients with MwoA and HC groups. Top: l-SPFG (MwoA patients: 0.15 ± 0.63; HC: 2.12 ± 0.43; p = 0.01). Bottom: l-TP (MwoA patients: -0.09 ± 0.55; HC: 0.72 ± 0.29; $p = 0.003$). DMN: default mode network, MwoA: migraine without aura, HC: healthy controls, ICA: independent component analysis, l-SPFG: left superior prefrontal gyrus; l-TP: left temporal pole.

structural abnormalities and not related to clinical or cognitive features of migraineurs. The DMN is a network highly relevant for cognitive processes and influences behavior in response to the environment in a predictive manner [7,8]. In other terms, DMN represents a neural network related to individual stressful experiences and coping strategies to promote adaptation (i.e. allostasis) [19,20]. This is done requiring most energy of brain baseline metabolic rate due to elevated levels of aerobic glycolysis required by the DMN [21]. Previous RS-fMRI studies investigating brain functional connectivity in patients suffering from different chronic pain conditions have already shown a dramatic alteration of DMN connectivity, suggesting that pain has a widespread impact on overall brain function, modifying brain dynamics beyond pain perception [22,23]. Although several RS-fMRI studies,

using different methodological approaches, have disclosed diffuse alterations in different brain areas and networks in patients with migraine [10-12,24,25], only a few of them have specifically investigated DMN integrity [10-12]. Xue and colleagues [10] have demonstrated an aberrant connectivity within the salience and executive networks in patients with MwoA; whereas DMN did not show any significant intra-network changes between patients with MwoA and HC. Nevertheless, an increased intrinsic DMN connectivity to brain regions outside the usual boundaries of this network (i.e. right insula) was reported. In another RS-fMRI study [11], the same group, using amplitude of low-frequency fluctuation and ROI-based functional connectivity analyses, has demonstrated a reduced DMN connectivity in left anterior cingulate cortex, bilateral prefrontal cortex and right thalamus. Furthermore, a significant decrease in regional homogeneity values has been observed in several brain areas involved in DMN in patients with MwoA [12]. DMN functional changes were negatively correlated only with disease duration [10-12]. These conflicting data may be explained by the small sample size, patients clinical heterogeneity, and lack of consistent methodological approach. Furthermore, it is noteworthy that in those studies the cognitive profile of patients with migraine was not investigated, then behavioral correlates of the observed functional abnormalities are still unclear. In the present study, to specifically address this issue, we have performed a correlation analysis between clinical, cognitive and functional data, and we did not find any significant association. This is not surprising, considering our previous study [16] showing no correlation between executive network changes and neuropsychological data in patients with MwoA. Thus, taken together, our findings may suggest a possible alternative behavioral correlation of resting-state connectivity changes. One possibility is that the observed DMN dysfunction could underlie or be related to a maladaptive brain response to repeated stress [19,20] which seems to characterize patients with migraine [4,5]. Indeed, according to recent studies, recurrent migraine attacks alter both functional and structural brain connectivity [14], and these changes may disrupt mechanisms of stress response [4,5]. When behavioral or physiological stressors are frequent or severe, allostatic responses can become maladaptive, leading, in a vicious cycle, to further allostatic load. Moreover, due to a high energetic demand, the observed DMN dysfunction may be associated with an impaired brain energy metabolism which has been demonstrated in previous MR spectroscopy studies in patients with migraine [26], likely due to an imbalance between ATP production and ATP use. In support of this notion, metabolic enhancers, such as riboflavin and coenzyme Q10 (both with a well-defined role in ATP generation), have shown effects in migraine prophylaxis [27]. In the present study, we identified two core regions of DMN [8], namely prefrontal and temporal areas, showing reduced functional connectivity in patients with MwoA. These areas have been demonstrated to be crucially involved in sensory-discriminative, cognitive and integrative pain functions within the so-called "neurolimbic pain network" [28]. In details, prefrontal cortex plays a specific role in mediating the attenuation of pain perception via cognitive control mechanisms [29,30] whereas temporal cortex is involved in affective response to pain experience and its activation has been demonstrated both during pain experience [31] and migraine attacks [32]. Moreover, recent studies have reported both cortical abnormalities and microstructural changes of these regions in migraineurs [33-35]. However, in the present study DMN connectivity disruption was detected in the absence of significant GM changes, possibly implying that functional changes may precede GM structural abnormalities. A few limitations of the current study should be considered. First, our methodological approach using ICA allows to evaluate functional interactions between brain areas but it does not provide information regarding causality and, consequently, it is still unclear whether functional changes are cause or consequence of repetitive migraine attacks. Second, we have studied a relatively small number of patients and further studies are needed to confirm our findings. Finally, the relationship between DMN functional changes and maladaptive brain response could be considered as a working hypothesis emerged from our work and future RS-fMRI studies are needed to further elucidate this potential correlation.

Conclusions

We believe that DMN connectivity changes may represent an early migraine biomarker, probably related to a maladaptive brain response. Future studies should examine other cortical resting-state networks and longitudinal studies are needed to evaluate the possibility that this modern neuroimaging approach can lead to the identification of different categories of patients or different timing of selective networks involvement.

Abbreviations

MwoA: Migraine without aura; HC: Healthy controls; RS: Resting-state; fMRI: Functional magnetic resonance; RSNs: Resting-state networks; ICA: Independent component approach; VBM: Voxel based morphometry; l-SPFG: Left superior prefrontal gyrus; l-TP: Left temporal pole; MIDAS: Migraine disability assessment scale; HIT-6: Headache impact test; VAS: Visual analogic scale; HDRS: Hamilton depression rating scale; HARS: Hamilton anxiety rating scale; MNI: Montreal neurological institute; FWHM: Full-width at half maximum; ANCOVA: Analysis of covariance; TIV: Total intracranial volume; TR: Repetition time; TI: Inversion time; TE: Echo time; ROI: Region of interest; GM: Gray matter; WM: White matter; CSF: Cerebro-spinal fluid; FWE: Familywise error rate; ATP: Adenosine triphosphate.

Competing interests

The authors confirm that there are no conflicts of interest.

Authors' contributions

AT: experimental design, image data analysis, results interpretation, manuscript drafting; AR: literature review, experimental design, results interpretation, manuscript drafting; AG: clinical data analysis, results interpretation and manuscript revision; FC: clinical data analysis, manuscript revision; DC: image data analysis, results interpretation; MDS: neuropsychological data acquisition, results interpretation; SC: image data analysis, results interpretation, manuscript revision; MC: image data acquisition, results interpretation; FE: image data analysis, results interpretation and manuscript drafting and revision; GT: experimental design, results interpretation, manuscript revision. All authors read and approved the final manuscript.

Author details

[1]Department of Neurology, Second University of Naples, Piazza Miraglia 2 - I-80138, Naples, Italy. [2]Institute for Diagnosis and Care "Hermitage Capodimonte", Naples, Italy. [3]Neuroradiology Service, Second University of Naples, Naples, Italy. [4]Department of Cognitive Neuroscience, Maastricht University, Maastricht, The Netherlands. [5]Department of Medicine and Surgery, University of Salerno, Salerno, Italy.

References

1. Silberstein SD (2004) Migraine. Lancet 363(9406):381–391
2. Pietrobon D, Moskowitz MA (2013) Pathophysiology of migraine. Annu Rev Physiol 75:365–391
3. Stuart S, Griffiths LR (2012) A possible role for mitochondrial dysfunction in migraine. Mol Genet Genomics 287(11–12):837–844
4. Maleki N, Becerra L, Borsook D (2012) Migraine: maladaptive brain responses to stress. Headache 52(2):102–106
5. Borsook D, Maleki N, Becerra L, McEwen B (2012) Understanding migraine through the lens of maladaptive stress responses: a model disease of allostatic load. Neuron 73(2):219–234
6. Mantini D, Perrucci MG, Del Gratta C, Romani GL, Corbetta M (2007) Electrophysiological signatures of resting state networks in the human brain. Proc Natl Acad Sci U S A 104(32):13170–13175
7. Raichle ME, Gusnard DA (2005) Intrinsic brain activity sets the stage for expression of motivated behavior. J Comp Neurol 493(1):167–176
8. Buckner RL, Andrews-Hanna JR, Schacter DL (2008) The brain's default network: anatomy, function, and relevance to disease. Ann N Y Acad Sci 1124:1–38
9. May A (2013) Pearls and pitfalls: neuroimaging in headache. Cephalalgia 33(8):554–565
10. Xue T, Yuan K, Zhao L, Yu D, Zhao L, Dong T, Cheng P, Von Deneen KM, Qin W, Tian J (2012) Intrinsic brain network abnormalities in migraines without aura revealed in resting-state fMRI. PLoS One 7(12):e52927
11. Xue T, Yuan K, Cheng P, Zhao L, Zhao L, Yu D, Dong T, Von Deneen KM, Gong Q, Qin W, Tian J (2013) Alterations of regional spontaneous neuronal activity and corresponding brain circuit changes during resting state in migraine without aura. NMR Biomed 26(9):1051–8
12. Yu D, Yuan K, Zhao L, Zhao L, Dong M, Liu P, Wang G, Liu J, Sun J, Zhou G, Von Deneen KM, Liang F, Qin W, Tian J (2012) Regional homogeneity abnormalities in patients with interictal Migraine without aura: A resting-state study. NMR Biomed 2:806–812
13. Esposito F, Aragri A, Pesaresi I, Cirillo S, Tedeschi G, Marciano E, Goebel R, Di Salle F (2008) Independent component model of the default-mode brain function: combining individual-level and population-level analyses in resting-state fMRI. Magn Reson Imaging 26(7):905–913
14. Ellerbrock I, Engel AK, May A (2013) Microstructural and network abnormalities in headache. Curr Opin Neurol 26(4):353–359
15. Headache Classification Committee of the International Headache Society (IHS) (2013) The International Classification of Headache Disorders, 3rd edition (beta version). Cephalalgia 33(9):629–808
16. Russo A, Tessitore A, Giordano A, Corbo D, Marcuccio L, De Stefano M, Salemi F, Conforti R, Esposito F, Tedeschi G (2012) Executive resting-state network connectivity in migraine without aura. Cephalalgia 32(14):1041–1048
17. Greicius MD, Flores BH, Menon V, Glover GH, Solvason HB, Kenna H, Reiss AL, Schatzberg AF (2007) Resting-state functional connectivity in major depression: abnormally increased contributions from subgenual cingulate cortex and thalamus. Biol Psychiatry 62(5):429–437
18. Ashburner J (2007) A fast diffeomorphic image registration algorithm. Neuroimage 38(1):95–113
19. McEwen BS, Gianaros PJ (2011) Stress- and allostasis-induced brain plasticity. Annu Rev Med 62:431–445
20. Soares JM, Sampaio A, Ferreira LM, Santos NC, Marques P, Marques F, Palha JA, Cerqueira JJ, Sousa N (2013) Stress Impact on Resting State Brain Networks. PLoS One 8(6):e66500
21. Clark DD, Sokoloff L (1999) Circulation and energy metabolism of the brain. In: Siegel GJ, Agranoff BW, Albers RW, Fisher SK, Uhler MD (eds) Basic neurochemistry. Molecular, cellular and medical aspects. Lippincott-Raven, Philadelphia, pp 637–670
22. Baliki MN, Geha PY, Apkarian AV, Chialvo DR (2008) Beyond feeling: chronic pain hurts the brain, disrupting the default-mode network dynamics. J Neurosci 28(6):1398–1403
23. Napadow V, LaCount L, Park K, As-Sanie S, Clauw DJ, Harris RE (2010) Intrinsic brain connectivity in fibromyalgia is associated with chronic pain intensity. Arthritis Rheum 62(8):2545–2555
24. Mainero C, Boshyan J, Hadjikhani N (2011) Altered functional magnetic resonance imaging resting-state connectivity in periaqueductal gray networks in migraine. Ann Neurol 70(5):838–845
25. Yuan K, Qin W, Liu P, Zhao L, Yu D, Zhao L, Dong M, Liu J, Yang X, Von Deneen KM, Liang F, Tian J (2012) Reduced fractional anisotropy of corpus callosum modulates inter-hemispheric resting state functional connectivity in migraine patients without aura. PLoS One 7(9):e45476
26. Reyngoudt H, Achten E, Paemeleire K (2012) Magnetic resonance spectroscopy in migraine: what have we learned so far? Cephalalgia 32(11):845–859
27. Markley HG (2012) CoEnzyme Q10 and riboflavin: the mitochondrial connection. Headache 52(Suppl 2):81–7
28. Maizels M, Aurora S, Heinricher M (2012) Beyond Neurovascular: Migraine as a Dysfunctional Neurolimbic Pain Network. Headache 52(10):1553–1565
29. Lorenz J, Minoshima S, Casey KL (2003) Keeping pain out of mind: the role of the dorsolateral prefrontal cortex in pain modulation. Brain 126(5):1079–1091
30. Aderjan D, Stankewitz A, May A (2010) Neuronal mechanisms during repetitive trigemino-nociceptive stimulation in migraine patients. Pain 151(1):97–103
31. Moulton EA, Becerra L, Maleki N, Pendse G, Tully S, Hargreaves R, Burstein R, Borsook D (2011) Painful heat reveals hyperexcitability of the temporal pole in interictal and ictal migraine states. Cereb Cortex 21(2):435–448
32. Afridi SK, Giffin NJ, Kaube H, Friston KJ, Ward NS, Frackowiak RS, Goadsby PJ (2005) A positron emission tomographic study in spontaneous migraine. Arch Neurol 62(8):1270–1275
33. Messina R, Rocca MA, Colombo B, Valsasina P, Horsfield MA, Copetti M, Falini A, Comi G, Filippi M (2013) Cortical abnormalities in patients with migraine: a surface-based analysis. Radiology 268(1):170–180
34. Rocca MA, Ceccarelli A, Falini A, Tortorella P, Colombo B, Pagani E, Comi G, Scotti G, Filippi M (2006) Diffusion tensor magnetic resonance imaging at 3.0 tesla shows subtle cerebral grey matter abnormalities in patients with migraine. J Neurol Neurosurg Psychiatry 77(5):686–689
35. Yu D, Yuan K, Qin W, Zhao L, Dong M, Liu P, Yang X, Liu J, Sun J, Zhou G, Von Deneen KM, Tian J (2013) Axonal loss of white matter in migraine without aura: a tract-based spatial statistics study. Cephalalgia 33(1):34–42

20

Alterations in regional homogeneity assessed by fMRI in patients with migraine without aura stratified by disease duration

Ling Zhao[1], Jixin Liu[2], Xilin Dong[1], Yulin Peng[1], Kai Yuan[2], Fumei Wu[1], Jinbo Sun[2], Qiyong Gong[3], Wei Qin[2*] and Fanrong Liang[1*]

Abstract

Background: Advanced neuroimaging approaches have been employed to prove that migraine was a central nervous system disorder. This study aims to examine resting-state abnormalities in migraine without aura (MWoA) patients stratified by disease duration, and to explore the neuroimaging markers for reflecting the disease duration.

Methods: 40 eligible MWoA patients and 20 matched healthy volunteers were included in the study. Regional homogeneity (ReHo) analysis was used to identify the local features of spontaneous brain activity in MWoA patients stratified by disease duration, and analysis was performed to investigate the correlation of overlapped brain dysfunction in MWoA patients with different disease duration (long-term and short-term) and course of disease.

Results: Compared with healthy controls, MWoA patients with long-term disease duration showed comprehensive neuronal dysfunction than patients with short-term disease duration. In addition, increased average ReHo values in the thalamus, brain stem, and temporal pole showed significantly positive correlations with the disease duration. On the contrary, ReHo values were negatively correlated with the duration of disease in the anterior cingulate cortex, insula, posterior cingulate cortex and superior occipital gyrus.

Conclusions: Our findings of progressive brain damage in relation to increasing disease duration suggest that migraine without aura is a progressive central nervous disease, and the length of the disease duration was one of the key reasons to cause brain dysfunction in MwoA patients. The repeated migraine attacks over time result in resting-state abnormalities of selective brain regions belonging to the pain processing and cognition. We predict that these brain regions are sensitive neuroimaging markers for reflecting the disease duration of migraine patients without aura.

Keywords: Migraine without aura; Functional MRI; Regional homogeneity; Resting state; Disease duration

Background

Migraine headache is a common neurological disorder which causes significant individual and societal burden due to pain and environmental sensitivities [1]. It was ranked the seventh highest among specific causes of disability globally. Migraine has two subtypes, and two thirds of migraine patients suffer from MWoA which is typically characterized as a unilateral and pulsating headache, and

an autonomic nervous system dysfunction [2]. The recurrent headache manifests in attacks lasting 4–72 hours and affects patients 1–14 times each month in the episodic form. It is aggravated by routine physical activity, and is accompanied by vomiting, nausea, photophobia or phonophobia. Migraine may result in substantial pain, a decreased overall quality of life, and cause higher risks for ischemic stroke, unstable angina, and affective disorders than people without migraine [3-6].

Advanced neuroimaging approaches have been employed to investigate structural and functional brain changes in migraineurs, and proved that migraine was a central nervous system disorder [1]. The insula, anterior cingulate

* Correspondence: chinwei@mail.xidian.edu.cn; acuresearch@126.com
[2]Life Sciences Research Center, School of Life Sciences and Technology, Xidian University, Xi'an, Shanxi 710071, China
[1]Acupuncture and Tuina School, Chengdu University of Traditional Chinese Medicine, Chengdu, Sichuan 610075, China

cortex (ACC), thalamus, prefrontal cortex (PFC), orbito-frontal cortex (OFC), parahippocampal cortex, periaque-ductal gray matter (PAG), inferior frontal gyrus (IFG), brainstem, precentral gyrus, and cerebellum have been reported to show structural and functional alterations [7-15]. Furthermore, gray matter reduction based on voxel-based morphometric (VBM) studies was correlated with attack frequency or headache duration in migraine patients [13,16-18]. Moreover, task-related functional magnetic resonance imaging (fMRI) studies revealed abnormal acti-vation of some brain regions associated with pain-related information processing in migraine patients, such as the ACC, the PFC, the OFC, insula and the supplementary motor area (SMA) [10,11,19]. Numerous findings have sup-ported that migraine may have cumulative effects on brain structure and function, and repeated attacks over time would result in secondary damage on several brain regions involved in central pain processing [14,17,20-22]. Moreover, some preliminary neuroimaging studies provided some evidence about increased risk of brain abnormalities with increasing attack frequency [5,17,21,23] and disease dur-ation [15,17,24] in migraineurs. However, few studies have evaluated the characteristic in the resting-state in MWoA patients stratified by disease duration.

In the current study, we performed a ReHo approach [25] to compare the blood oxygen level-dependent (BOLD) signals of the brains in MWoA patients along with healthy subjects during the resting-state. The ReHo method focuses on the similarities or coherence of the intraregional spontaneous low-frequency (<0.08 Hz) BOLD signal, which enables a novel perspective to understand the functional deficits in particular brain regions. An important advantage of using the ReHo method over other methods is that it can examine the regional activity characteristics of each voxel. It can also detect changes or modulations that are induced by differ-ent conditions across the whole brain in a voxel-by-voxel manner, without requiring any prior knowledge. Previ-ously, our group has employed the ReHo method only to find that MWoA patients showed a significant decrease in ReHo values in the right ACC, PFC, OFC and SMA [12]. In addition, the ReHo values were negatively correlated with the duration of disease in the right ACC and PFC [12]. In order to further assess and validate whether some brain abnormalities serve as markers for disease history in MWoA patients, we investigated the resting-state dif-ference between MWoA patients with long-term (LT) disease duration and MWoA patients with short-term (ST) disease duration. We hypothesized that, as compared with healthy controls, (1) MWoA patients with LT disease duration would display more neuronal dysfunction than patients with ST disease duration; (2) the overlapped brain dysfunction in LT and ST patients group may be asso-ciated with the course of disease in migraineurs.

Methods

Study participants

40 eligible MWoA patients were recruited from the neurology department of the Teaching Hospital of Chengdu University of Traditional Chinese Medicine. The diagnosis of MWoA was established according to the classification criteria of the International Headache Society (IHS) [26]. The inclusion criteria were as fol-lows:(1) all subjects were right-handed, and had 2 to 8 migraine attacks per month during the last 3 months and during the baseline period (4 weeks before enrol-ment); (2) all subjects were 18 to 55 years of age; in addition, start of headache should be before the age of 50 years; (3) had received education for more than 6 years and had completed a baseline headache diary; (4) MWoA patients were selected on the basis of disease duration >10 years (LT) or < 5 years (ST); (5) had no migraine 72 hours prior to the scan; (6) no habit of long-term analgesics consumption; (7) did not take any prophylactic migraine medication during the previous month; and (8) no contraindications for exposure to a high magnetic field. Healthy subjects were recruited from the local community and were screened by a neurologist specialized in headaches. 20 right-handed, age-matched and education-matched healthy subjects were enrolled. They either had no headache days per year or had family members who suffered regularly from a migraine or other headache.

Exclusion criteria for MWoA patients and healthy controls were: (1) existence of neurological diseases; (2) had hypertension, diabetes mellitus, hypercholesteremia, vascular/heart disease, and major systemic conditions; (3) pregnant or lactating women; (4) alcohol or drug abuse; (5) any neuroimaging research study participation during the last 6 months; and (6) inability to understand the doctor's instructions.

This study was approved by the ethics committee at the Teaching Hospital of Chengdu University of Traditional Chinese Medicine. All subjects gave written, informed consent after the experimental procedures had been fully explained.

Study design

All patients should have recorded headache diaries for 4 weeks (baseline phase) before enrolment to assess disease activity (disease duration, headache degree, and attack frequency). Patients meeting the inclusion criteria were assigned to two groups based on different disease duration after the baseline period.

The headache diary documented the migraine attack frequency and severity of headache according to the guidelines of the IHS for clinical trials for migraine [27]. The VAS score 0–10 measured the intensity of headache. fMRI scans were scheduled 2 weeks after enrolment. In addition, records in the headache diary were checked to insure every patient did not suffer from a migraine attack at least 72 hours prior to the brain scan.

Imaging data acquisition

The imaging data were carried out in a 3 Tesla Siemens MRI system (Allegra, Siemens Medical System, Erlangen, Germany) at the Huaxi MR Research Center, West China Hospital of Sichuan University, Chengdu, China. A standard eight-channel phase-array head coil was used, along with restraining foam pads to minimize head motion and to diminish scanner noise. Prior to the functional run, a high-resolution T1structural image for each subject was acquired using a three-dimensional MRI sequence with a voxel size of 1 mm^3 employing an axial fast spoiled gradient recalled sequence (TR = 1900 ms, TE = 2.26 ms, data matrix = 256 × 256, flip angle = 9°, FOV = 256 mm × 256 mm). The structural images were examined to exclude the possibility of clinically silent lesions for all of the participants by two expert radiologists. The resting-state functional images were obtained with echo-planar imaging (EPI) (30 continuous slices with a slice thickness = 5 mm, TR = 2000 ms, TE = 30 ms, flip angle = 90°, FOV = 240 mm × 240 mm, matrix = 64 × 64). During 6-min fMRI scanning, participants were instructed to keep their eyes closed, relax, move as little as possible, and stay awake. It needs to be emphasized that if there was an attack for migraine patients in the check reservation, they could not be scanned and the scan would be postponed to ensure they were scanned during the migraine interval.

Data preprocessing

In the functional image data preprocessing, the first five scans were discarded to eliminate nonequilibrium effects of magnetization and to allow participants to become familiar with the scanning circumstances. Data preprocessing was done using Statistical Parametric Mapping (SPM5, http://www.fil.ion.ucl.ac.uk/spm). The images were corrected for the acquisition delay between slices, aligned to the first image of each session for motion correction and spatially normalized to the standard Montreal Neurological Institute (MNI) template in SPM5. We calculated the maximum excursion movement values for each of the translation planes (x, y, and z) and each of the rotation planes (roll, pitch, and yaw) for every participant. None of them had head movements exceeding 1 mm on any axis and head rotation greater than 1° during the entire fMRI scan. Finally, a band-pass filter (0.01 Hz < f < 0.08 Hz) was applied to remove physiological and high-frequency noise.

Data analysis

Baseline and demographic data were analyzed by SPSS 14.0 statistical software (SPSS Inc., Chicago, IL, USA).

Baseline characteristics were summarized by descriptive statistics for each group and in the total study population. Two independent-sample t-tests were used to examine differences between groups (95% CI, 2-sided).

Kendall's coefficient of concordance (KCC) [28] was used to evaluate ReHo [25], which was performed using the Resting-State fMRI Data Analysis Toolkit (X.-W. Song et al., Beijing Normal University, Beijing, China, http://www.restfmri.net). Individual ReHo maps were generated by assigning each voxel a value corresponding to the KCC of its time series with its nearest 26 neighboring voxels [25]. Then, a mask (made from the MNI template to assure matching with the normalization step) was used to remove non-brain tissues and noise from the ReHo maps. Only the voxels within the mask were analyzed further. The individual ReHo maps were standardized by their own mean KCC within the mask. Then, a Gaussian kernel with a full-width at half-maximum of 4 mm was used to smooth the images in order to reduce noise and residual differences. Controlling for age, two independent-sample t-tests were used to compare the ReHo results between different groups. The false discovery rate (FDR) was used to correct the multiple comparisons. In addition, correlation analyses were performed in order to delineate possible correlations between average ReHo values of the overlapped brain dysfunctional regions in LT and ST groups and the disease duration.

Results

Participants

There were no significant differences in the demographics including age, gender, and education between MWoA patients and healthy subjects ($p > 0.05$) (Table 1). There were no significant differences in the demographics including sex, education, family history, migraine attack frequency, and visual analogue scale (VAS) score between ST group patients and LT group subjects ($p > 0.05$). Patients in the LT group were older and had longer disease duration compared with patients in the ST group ($p < 0.05$) (Table 2).

Table 1 Baseline and demographics for MWoA patients and healthy subjects

Items	MWoA patients (n = 40)	Healthy subjects (n = 20)	P value
Age (years) mean (SD)	30.5(10.8)	28.4(8.9)	0.4569
Gender (male/female)	12/28	5/15	0.4658
Education (years)	12.6(4.7)	14.2(6.4)	0.2764
Mean disease duration in years (SD)	10.15(7.01)	NA	

Notes: SD, Standard deviation.

Table 2 Baseline and demographics for MWoA patients

Items	ST group (n = 20)	LT group (n = 20)	P value
Age (years) mean (SD)	27.12 (8.18)	37.52 (12.2)	0.0009
Gender (male/female)	5/15	7/13	0.7311
Education (years)	13.2 (6.03)	13.8 (5.06)	0.7352
Family history (Y/N)	6/14	8/12	0.3705
Disease duration in years (SD)	4.05 (1.64)	16.25 (1.47)	0.0000
Affect frequency per month* (SD)	4.5 (3.5)	5.38 (5.8)	0.5647
VAS score*	5.37 (1.34)	5.0 (1.8)	0.4654

Notes: SD, Standard deviation; VAS, Visual Analogue Scale; Y, yes; N, no.
*measured for the 4 weeks before enrolment.

Neuroimaging results

Compared with healthy subjects, MWoA patients with ST disease duration showed significantly higher ReHo values in the bilateral thalamus, IFG (Brodmman area (BA) 47), middle occipital gyrus (MOG) (BA19), left insula (BA13), caudate, middle frontal gyrus (MFG) (BA8), middle temporal gyrus (MTG) (BA37), inferior occipital gyrus (IOG) (BA19), right ACC (BA32), medial frontal gyrus (MeFG) (BA25), and superior temporal gyrus (STG) (BA42). The results revealed MWoA patients with ST disease duration showed a significant decrease in ReHo values in the bilateral MFG (BA8, BA10), MTG (BA21), left lingual gyrus (BA17), right MOG (BA19), cerebellum, and brain stem (controlling for age, $p < 0.01$, FDR corrected) (Additional file 1, Figure 1a).

In this study, the MWoA patients with LT disease duration showed increased ReHo values in the bilateral ACC (BA24, BA32), amygdala, thalamus, caudate, lentiform nucleus, uncus, IFG (BA11, BA47), MFG (BA11), SFG (BA6, BA11), MTG (BA21), temporal pole (BA38), cerebellum, brain stem (including pons, medulla, and midbrain), and left hippocampus compared with healthy subjects. On the contrary, the results seemed decreased in the bilateral ACC (BA24), insula (BA13), IFG (BA45, BA47), MFG (BA6), MeFG (BA6, BA8), SFG (BA6), MTG (BA21, BA39), MOG (BA18, BA19), cuneus (BA18, BA19), lingual gyrus (BA18, BA19), inferior parietal lobule (IPL) (BA40), postcentral gyrus (BA6, BA43), and precuneus (BA19, BA31), left fusiform gyrus (BA19), and right posterior cingulate cortex (PCC) (BA31) (controlling for age, $p < 0.01$, FDR corrected) (Additional file 2, Figure 1b).

Correlation analysis results demonstrated that increased average ReHo values in the thalamus ($r = 0.5269$, $p = 0.0014$), brain stem ($r = 0.4180$, $p = 0.0139$), and temporal pole ($r = 0.4939$, $p = 0.0030$) showed significantly positive correlations with the disease duration (Figure 2). There were respectively significant negative correlations between the decreased average ReHo values of the ACC ($r = -0.5452$, $p = 8.5452*e-4$), insula ($r = -0.5891$, $p = 2.4653*e-4$), PCC ($r = -0.5800$, $p = 3.2389*e-4$), SOG ($r = -0.36$, $p = 0.049$) and the disease duration (Figure 2). The correlation between VAS score and attack frequency and resting-state properties were also checked, but no results exceeded the threshold.

Discussion

To our knowledge, this study is the first one to investigate characteristic of regional homogeneity in patients with episodic migraine without aura stratified by disease

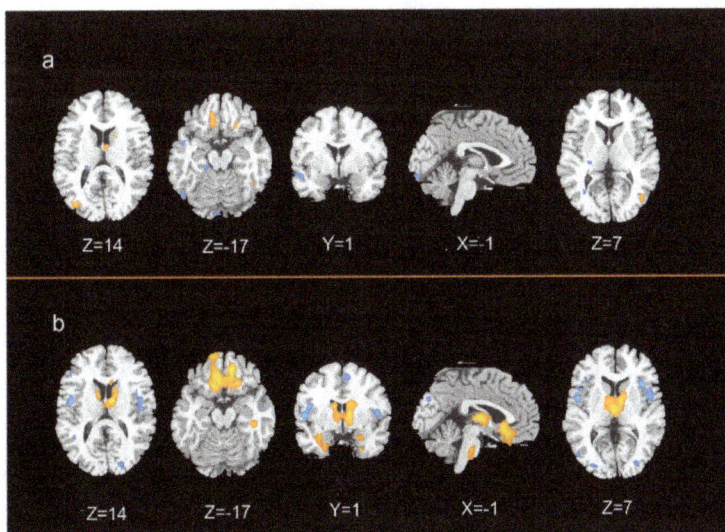

Figure 1 Differences between MWoA patients and healthy subjects in ReHo values. a. MWoA patients with ST disease duration; **b**. MWoA patients with LT disease duration; $p < 0.01$, FDR corrected; Warm colors indicate ReHo increases in MWoA patients; cool colors indicate ReHo decreases in MWoA patients.

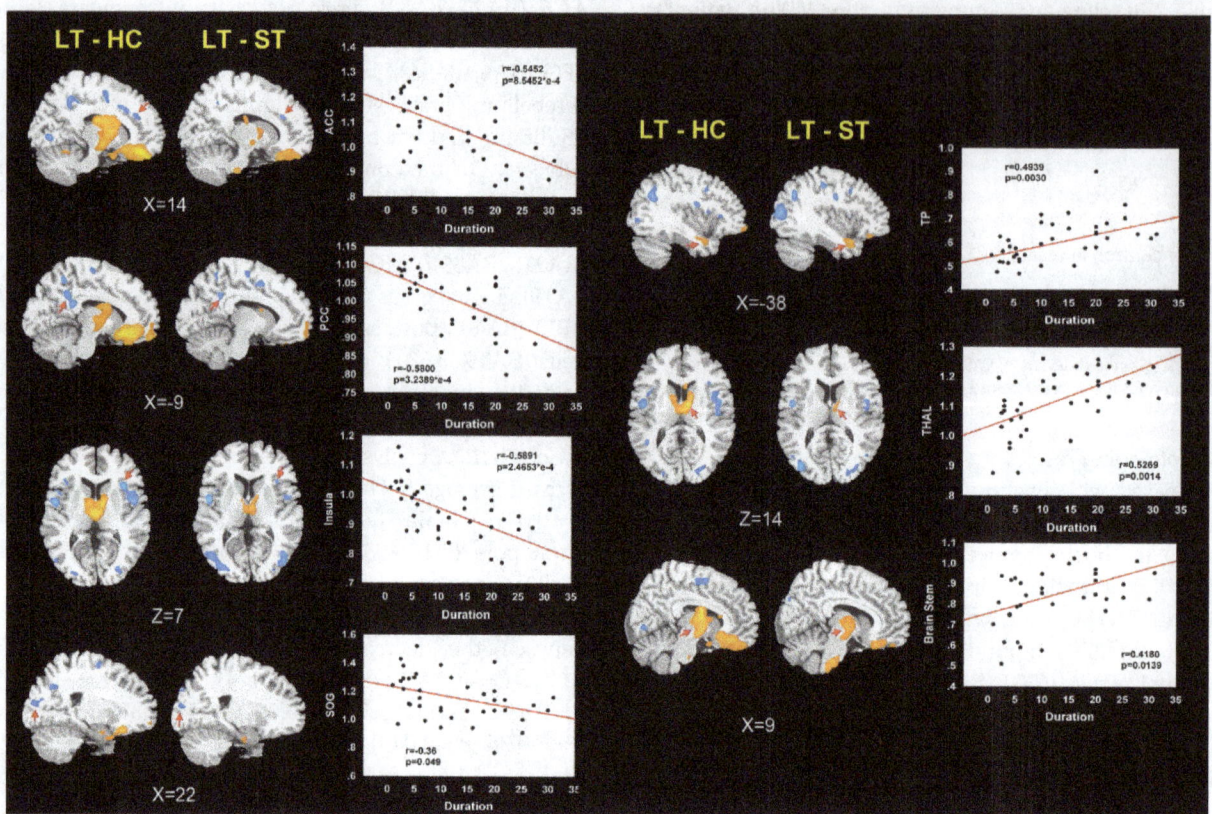

Figure 2 The correlation of average ReHo values of the overlapped brain dysfunction in LT *vs* HC and LT *vs* ST with the disease duration. Warm colors indicate ReHo increases in MWoA patients; cool colors indicate ReHo decreases in MWoA patients; ACC, anterior cingulate cortex; THAL, thalamus; TP, temporal pole; PCC, posterior cingulate cortex; SOG, superior occipital gyrus; LT, MWoA patients with long-term disease duration; ST, MWoA patients with short-term disease duration; HC, healthy controls.

duration. ReHo hypothesizes that a given voxel is temporally similar to that of its neighbors [25]. It is calculated by using Kendall's coefficient of concordance, which could obtain reliable results in a resting-state fMRI data analysis [29]. Therefore, ReHo reflects the temporal homogeneity of the regional BOLD signal rather than its density. Compared with healthy controls, several common brain regions showed abnormalities in MWoA patients with ST and LT disease duration during the resting-state, including IFG, MFG, MTG, ACC, thalamus, and basal ganglia. These results were mainly involved in pain-related processing, and were similar to previous reports in migraineur studies which focused on structural [16,17,30,31], task-related [11,19,21], and resting-state [12-15,24] abnormalities. Furthermore, compared with healthy controls, MWoA patients with LT disease duration might display comprehensive neuronal dysfunction than patients with ST disease duration. PCC, lentiform nucleus, uncus, temporal pole, MOG, cuneus, fusiform gyrus, inferior parietal lobule, postcentral gyrus, precuneus, and brain stem were only found in MWoA patients with LT disease duration. In the current study, abnormal ReHo in MwoA patients was relevant to the

changes of temporal aspects of neural activity in the brain regions. Increased or decreased ReHo suggests that neural function in local regions is more or less synchronous during resting-state. The results demonstrated that the long history of disease might contribute to accumulating brain damage due to the repetitive occurrence of pain-related processes.

We were interested in whether brain abnormalities would progressively influence individuals as the result of migraine attack history. To explore which brain regions might relate to the course of disease, a correlation analysis was performed. The results showed that the average ReHo value of the thalamus, brain stem, and temporal pole were positively related to the disease duration. The ReHo value of the ACC, insula, PCC and SOG were negatively correlated with the history of MWoA. Therefore, the ReHo increase in the thalamus, brain stem, and temporal pole in MwoA patients may reflect a dynamic compensation for the disorder signals from the brain, whereas the decreased hemodynamic synchronization in the ACC, insula, PCC, and SOG could be explained by MwoA -related dysfunction. Additionally, we speculated these ReHo changes might reflect not only as a consequence of repeated painful attacks in a pain disorder, but also as indicators specific to migraine without aura.

As we all know, the ACC, insula, and thalamus are the key regions composed of the "pain matrix". Recent neuroimaging evidence supported that the ACC and insula were the common "brain signature" structures in chronic pain diseases, such as fibromyalgia [32], irritable bowel syndrome [33], chronic tension type headache [34], and migraine [16,35,36]. ACC has a close interconnection with the insula, thalamus, prefrontal cortex, and other subcortical structures, and is considered to be implicated in both affective and cognitive-attentional dimensions of pain and plays a deterministic role in pain modulation and analgesia [37]. In the current study, ACC demonstrated negative correlation with disease duration, which was consistent with previous correlation analysis reports separately on regional metabolism [35] and average ReHo values [12] of the ACC. The insula is a complex, multisensory integration area that is involved in processing many aspects involved with the conscious experience of pain such as affect, autonomic activity and interoception. A recent study strongly suggested that if the full pain experience involves the pain matrix network, a part of the insula seems to play a leading role in the triggering of this network and the resulting emergence of the subjective pain experience [38]. Functional imaging experiments have revealed that the insula is a major site for emotional processing, and it also processes sensory-discriminative aspects of pain perception [39]. Coghill et al., reported the insula cortex plays reciprocal role in pain, emotions and pain-related emotions, due to its anatomic connections [40]. We found that the progressive dysfunction of the insula showed a significant correlation with disease history, and did not detect a significant relationship between the insula and headache degree or attack frequency. The thalamus was also found to have a dysfunction in migraine patients in previous documents [41-43], but few studies have evaluated the correlation between the abnormality of the thalamus and clinical parameters. The thalamus is the "relay center" of the brain, and it is involved in the formation of the lateral and medial pain system. The lateral nuclei of the thalamus deal with discriminative sensory pain transmission, and the medial nuclei of the thalamus are involved in emotional and somatic responses to pain [44]. In the current study, increased ReHo values of the thalamus were positively correlated with disease duration, suggesting that this cumulative alteration was mainly due to migraine, and not only the secondary effect of having migraine headaches. Our results demonstrated that the ACC, insula, and thalamus were not only related to central pain processing for migraine without aura, but also involved in expressing the relationship between brain dysfunction and disease history.

Moreover, several independent functional imaging studies have reinforced the fact that the pathogenesis of migraine is related to the dysfunction of the brain stem. A series of positron emission tomographic (PET) studies consistently observed an increase in regional cerebral blood flow in the brain stem during migraine attacks [41,45-47], and the brain stem was also found to be activated in migraine patients with some stimulus detected by fMRI [48-50]. Dysfunction of the brain stem is involved in antinociception, extracerebral and intracerebral vascular control and sensory gating provides an explanation for many of the facets of migraine. In this study, increased ReHo values in the brain stem were related with disease duration during the resting-state facilitation that the brain stem has a crucial role in migraine, and may serve as an indicator to reflect the progress of migraine.

PCC participates in the composition of the default mode network (DMN), and it seldom detected significant abnormal findings in migraine patients checked by neuroimaging. It is not the traditional pain-processing area, but recently, Loggia et al. reported that some DMN subregions (such as the PCC) respond in a perception-related manner to pain, suggesting closer linkage between the DMN and pain processing than previously thought [51]. Furthermore, the PCC is recognized that subjects with cognitive impairment showed reduced cerebral blood flow in the PCC, and some clinical evidence indicated that migraine patients had deficits in cognitive function relative to healthy controls [52-54]. Our findings of progressive ReHo changes in the PCC in relation to increasing disease duration suggest that repeated migraine attacks over time may lead to resting-state abnormalities of selective brain regions belonging to pain perception and cognitive control. The temporal pole was found to have an increase in the fMRI BOLD response during the interictal period in migraineurs in response to a thermal stimulus [11], and also showed significantly higher activation during odor stimulation by $H_2^{15}O$-PET [55]. The role of the temporal pole in pain processing is not well understood, but it is an associative multisensory area and plays a role in assigning affective tone to short-term memories relating to pain, which may be related to reports of impaired memory in migraine patients during the interictal period [11]. We found the ReHo properties of the temporal pole were positively correlated with the duration of disease, which suggests that temporal pole excitability as sensitization during both the resting-state and stimulation may contribute to repeated migraine attack. Lesions in the occipital lobe result in visual disturbance, memory deficits and motion perception disorders. Occipital lobes had bilateral hypoperfusion in a patient with spontaneous migraine without aura as detected by PET [56,57], and an fMRI study found that the occipital cortex showed structural deficits in MWoA patients [13]. In the current study, our results showed decreased ReHo values in the SOG which were negatively correlated with the disease duration. Therefore, we inferred that the observed PCC, temporal pole and SOG dysfunction in MWoA patients may provide a potential neurobiological mechanism for cognitive deficits in migraineurs.

There are some limitations in the present study. Firstly, disease duration was used to classify the MWoA patients with ST and LT, not including the MWoA patients with moderate-term disease duration (between 5 years and 10 years). Further studies need to recruit a large number of MWoA patients and stratify the detailed data, and give more evidence to strengthen our findings. Secondly, in order to test the reproducibility of our results and to verify the consequences of brain damage in migraineurs, further neuroimaging investigations have to quantify brain abnormalities in a longitudinal design. Lastly, we will plan to assess cerebral structural changes in MwoA patients by using DTI, VBM, or surface-based techniques in the future work, and help us to better understand the pathophysiology of migraine.

Conclusion

In conclusion, the current study employed the ReHo method to investigate the difference in resting-state properties between MWoA patients stratified with different disease duration and healthy controls, as well as the correlation of abnormal cerebral activity in MWoA patients and disease duration. Our findings of progressive abnormal ReHo values in relation to increasing disease duration suggest that migraine without aura is a progressive central nervous disease, and the length of the disease duration was one of the key reasons to cause brain dysfunction in MwoA patients. The repeated migraine attacks over time result in resting-state abnormalities of selective brain regions belonging to the pain processing and cognition. Our results provided more scientific and sensitive neuroimaging markers for reflecting the disease duration of migraine patients without aura, and helped to identify indicators of predilection sites for possible progressive brain damage in migraineurs. It is expected that these findings may be advance the understanding of the pathology of migraine without aura and helpful to the diagnosis and therapy for MwoA patients. For example, take the appropriate individual treatment program depending on the different length of dur-

ation of disease, and increase some special assessment in brain function for migraine patients with long disease duration.

Abbreviations
ACC: Anterior cingulate cortex; PFC: Prefrontal cortex; OFC: Orbitofrontal cortex; PAG,: Periaqueductal gray matter; IFG: Inferior frontal gyrus; VBM: Voxel-based morphometric; fMRI: Functional MRI; SMA: Supplementary motor area; ReHo: Regional homogeneity; BOLD: Blood oxygen level-dependent; IHS: International Headache Society; VAS: Visual analogue scale; KCC: Kendall's coefficient of concordance; FDR: False discovery rate; MOG: Middle occipital gyrus; MFG: Middle frontal gyrus; MTG: Middle temporal gyrus; IOG: Inferior occipital gyrus; SOG: Superior occipital gyrus; MeFG: Medial frontal gyrus; STG: Superior temporal gyrus; DMN: Default mode network.

Competing interests
The authors declare that they have no conflicts of interest or financial disclosures.

Authors' contributions
LZ: conceived, designed, performed the experiment, and drafted the manuscript. JXL: analyzed the data and drafted the manuscript. XLD, YLP, and FMW: performed the experiments. KY and JBS: contributed to the acquisition of fMRI data and analyzed them. QYG: revised the manuscript. WQ and FRL: conceived, designed the experiments and revised the manuscript critically for important intellectual content. All authors read and approved the final manuscript. Ling Zhao and Jixin Liu contributed equally to this article.

Acknowledgements
This study was supported by the National Basic Research Program of China (973 Program, No. 2012CB518501), National Natural Science Foundation of China (Nos. 30930112, 30901900, 81001483), the Project of Administration of Traditional Chinese Medicine of Sichuan Province (No.2012-E-038).

Author details
[1]Acupuncture and Tuina School, Chengdu University of Traditional Chinese Medicine, Chengdu, Sichuan 610075, China. [2]Life Sciences Research Center, School of Life Sciences and Technology, Xidian University, Xi'an, Shanxi 710071, China. [3]Department of Radiology, The Center for Medical Imaging, Huaxi MR Research Center, West China Hospital of Sichuan University, Chengdu, 610041 Sichuan, China.

References
1. Schwedt TJ, Dodick DW (2009) Advanced neuroimaging of migraine. Lancet Neurol 8(6):560–568. doi:S1474-4422(09)70107-3
2. Van DeVen RC, Kaja S, Plomp JJ, Frants RR, Van Den Maagdenberg AM (2007) Ferrari MD (2007) Genetic models of migraine. Arch Neurol 64(5):643–646. doi:64/5/643
3. Raggi A, Leonardi M, Bussone G, D'Amico D (2011) Value and utility of disease-specific and generic instruments for assessing disability in patients with migraine, and their relationships with health-related quality of life. Neurol Sci 32(3):387–392. doi:10.1007/s10072-010-0466-3
4. Velentgas P, Cole JA, Mo J, Sikes CR, Walker AM (2004) Severe vascular events in migraine patients. Headache 44(7):642–651. doi:10.1111/j.1526-4610.2004.04122.x HED04122
5. Kruit MC, van Buchem MA, Hofman PA, Bakkers JT, Terwindt GM, Ferrari MD, Launer LJ (2004) Migraine as a risk factor for subclinical brain lesions. Jama 291(4):427–434. doi:10.1001/jama.291.4.427 291/4/427
6. Hung CI, Liu CY, Cheng YT, Wang SJ (2009) Migraine: a missing link between somatic symptoms and major depressive disorder. J Affect Disord 117(1–2):108–115. doi:10.1016/j.jad.2008.12.015 S0165-0327(08)00490

7. Chiapparini L, Ferraro S, Grazzi L, Bussone G (2010) Neuroimaging in chronic migraine. Neurol Sci 31(Suppl 1):S19–22. doi:10.1007/s10072-010-0266-9

8. May A (2009) New insights into headache: an update on functional and structural imaging findings. Nat Rev Neurol 5(4):199–209. doi:10.1038/nrneurol.2009.28 nrneurol.2009.28

9. Sanchez Del Rio M, Alvarez Linera J (2004) Functional neuroimaging of headaches. Lancet Neurol 3(11):645–651. doi:S1474442204009044 10.1016/S1474-4422(04)00904-4

10. Aderjan D, Stankewitz A, May A (2010) Neuronal mechanisms during repetitive trigemino-nociceptive stimulation in migraine patients. Pain 151(1):97–103. doi:S0304-3959(10)00386-6 10.1016/j.pain.2010.06.024

11. Moulton EA, Becerra L, Maleki N, Pendse G, Tully S, Hargreaves R, Burstein R, Borsook D (2011) Painful heat reveals hyperexcitability of the temporal pole in interictal and ictal migraine States. Cereb Cortex 21(2):435–448. doi:bhq109 10.1093/cercor/bhq109

12. Yu D, Yuan K, Zhao L, Dong M, Liu P, Wang G, Liu J, Sun J, Zhou G, von Deneen KM, Liang F, Qin W, Tian J (2012) Regional homogeneity abnormalities in patients with interictal migraine without aura: a resting-state study. NMR Biomed 25(5):806–812. doi:10.1002/nbm.1796

13. Jin C, Yuan K, Zhao L, Yu D, von Deneen KM, Zhang M, Qin W, Sun W, Tian J (2012) Structural and functional abnormalities in migraine patients without aura. NMR Biomed. doi:10.1002/nbm.2819

14. Mainero C, Boshyan J, Hadjikhani N (2011) Altered functional magnetic resonance imaging resting-state connectivity in periaqueductal gray networks in migraine. Ann Neurol 70(5):838–845. doi:10.1002/ana.22537

15. Liu J, Zhao L, Li G, Xiong S, Nan J, Li J, Yuan K, von Deneen KM, Liang F, Qin W, Tian J (2012) Hierarchical alteration of brain structural and functional networks in female migraine sufferers. PLoS One 7(12):e51250. doi:10.1371/journal.pone.0051250 PONE-D-12-16392

16. Valfre W, Rainero I, Bergui M, Pinessi L (2008) Voxel-based morphometry reveals gray matter abnormalities in migraine. Headache 48(1):109–117. doi:HED723 10.1111/j.1526-4610.2007.00723.x

17. Schmitz N, Admiraal Behloul F, Arkink EB, Kruit MC, Schoonman GG, Ferrari MD, Van Buchem MA (2008) Attack frequency and disease duration as indicators for brain damage in migraine. Headache 48(7):1044–1055. doi:HED1133 10.1111/j.1526-4610.2008.01133.x

18. Rocca MA, Ceccarelli A, Falini A, Colombo B, Tortorella P, Bernasconi L, Comi G, Scotti G, Filippi M (2006) Brain gray matter changes in migraine patients with T2-visible lesions: a 3-T MRI study. Stroke 37(7):1765–1770. doi:01.STR.0000226589.00599.4d 10.1161/01.STR.0000226589.00599.4d

19. Eck J, Richter M, Straube T, Miltner WH, Weiss T (2011) Affective brain regions are activated during the processing of pain-related words in migraine patients. Pain 152(5):1104–1113. doi:S0304-3959(11)00033-9 10.1016/j.pain.2011.01.026

20. Peyron R, Laurent B, Garcia Larrea L (2000) Functional imaging of brain responses to pain. A review and meta-analysis. Neurophysiol Clin 30(5):263–288. doi:S0987-7053(00)00227-6

21. Maleki N, Becerra L, Nutile L, Pendse G, Brawn J, Bigal M, Burstein R, Borsook D (2011) Migraine attacks the Basal Ganglia. Mol Pain 7:71. doi:1744-8069-7-71 10.1186/1744-8069-7-71

22. Lipton RB, Pan J (2004) Is migraine a progressive brain disease? Jama 291(4):493–494. doi:10.1001/jama.291.4.493 291/4/493

23. Kruit MC, Van Buchem MA, Launer LJ, Terwindt GM, Ferrari MD (2010) Migraine is associated with an increased risk of deep white matter lesions, subclinical posterior circulation infarcts and brain iron accumulation: the population-based MRI CAMERA study. Cephalalgia 30(2):129–136. doi:CHA1904 10.1111/j.1468-2982.2009.01904.x

24. Xue T, Yuan K, Zhao L, Yu D, Dong T, Cheng P, von Deneen KM, Qin W, Tian J (2012) Intrinsic Brain Network Abnormalities in Migraines without Aura Revealed in Resting-State fMRI. PLoS One 7(12):e52927. doi:10.1371/journal.pone.0052927 PONE-D-12-26054

25. Zang Y, Jiang T, Lu Y, He Y, Tian L (2004) Regional homogeneity approach to fMRI data analysis. Neuroimage 22(1):394–400. doi:10.1016/j.neuroimage.2003.12.030 S1053811904000035

26. Headache Classification Subcommittee of the international Headache Society (2004) The International Classification of Headache Disorders: 2nd edition. Cephalalgia 1(24):9–160

27. Tfelt Hansen P, Block G, Dahlof C, Diener HC, Ferrari MD, Goadsby PJ, Guidetti V, Jones B, Lipton RB, Massiou H, Meinert C, Sandrini G, Steiner T, Winter PB (2000) Guidelines for controlled trials of drugs in migraine: second edition. Cephalalgia 20(9):765–786. doi:cha117

28. Kendall M, Gibbons J (1990) Rank Correlation Methods. Oxford University Press, Oxford

29. Zuo XN, Xu T, Jiang L, Yang Z, Cao XY, He Y, Zang YF, Castellanos FX, Milham MP (2013) Toward reliable characterization of functional homogeneity in the human brain: preprocessing, scan duration, imaging resolution and computational space. Neuroimage 65:374–386. doi:10.1016/j.neuroimage.2012.10.017 S1053-8119(12)01020-8

30. Kim JH, Suh SI, Seol HY, Oh K, Seo WK, Yu SW, Park KW, Koh SB (2008) Regional grey matter changes in patients with migraine: a voxel-based morphometry study. Cephalalgia 28(6):598–604. doi:CHA1550 10.1111/j.1468-2982.2008.01550.x

31. Schmidt Wilcke T, Ganssbauer S, Neuner T, Bogdahn U, May A (2008) Subtle grey matter changes between migraine patients and healthy controls. Cephalalgia 28(1):1–4. doi:CHA1428 10.1111/j.1468-2982.2007.01428.x

32. Kuchinad A, Schweinhardt P, Seminowicz DA, Wood PB, Chizh BA, Bushnell MC (2007) Accelerated brain gray matter loss in fibromyalgia patients: premature aging of the brain. J Neurosci 27(15):4004–4007. doi:27/15/4004 10.1523/JNEUROSCI.0098-07.2007

33. Davis KD, Pope G, Chen J, Kwan CL, Crawley AP, Diamant NE (2008) Cortical thinning in IBS: implications for homeostatic, attention, and pain processing. Neurology 70(2):153–154. doi:01.wnl.0000295509.30630.10 10.1212/01.wnl.0000295509.30630.10

34. Schmidt Wilcke T, Leinisch E, Straube A, Kampfe N, Draganski B, Diener HC, Bogdahn U, May A (2005) Gray matter decrease in patients with chronic tension type headache. Neurology 65(9):1483–1486. doi:65/9/1483 10.1212/01.wnl.0000183067.94400.80

35. Kim JH, Kim S, Suh SI, Koh SB, Park KW, Oh K (2010) Interictal metabolic changes in episodic migraine: a voxel-based FDG-PET study. Cephalalgia 30(1):53–61. doi:30/1/53 10.1111/j.1468-2982.2009.01890.x

36. Prescot A, Becerra L, Pendse G, Tully S, Jensen E, Hargreaves R, Renshaw P, Burstein R, Borsook D (2009) Excitatory neurotransmitters in brain regions in interictal migraine patients. Mol Pain 5:34. doi:1744-8069-5-34 10.1186/1744-8069-5-34

37. May A (2008) Chronic pain may change the structure of the brain. Pain 137(1):7–15. doi:S0304-3959(08)00128-0 10.1016/j.pain.2008.02.034

38. Isnard J, Magnin M, Jung J, Mauguiere F, Garcia-Larrea L (2011) Does the insula tell our brain that we are in pain? Pain 152(4):946–951. doi:10.1016/j.pain.2010.12.025 S0304-3959(10)00775-X

39. Duerden EG, Albanese MC (2011) Localization of pain-related brain activation: A meta-analysis of neuroimaging data. Hum Brain Mapp. doi:10.1002/hbm.21416

40. Coghill RC, Sang CN, Maisog JM, Iadarola MJ (1999) Pain intensity processing within the human brain: a bilateral, distributed mechanism. J Neurophysiol 82(4):1934–1943

41. Afridi SK, Giffin NJ, Kaube H, Friston KJ, Ward NS, Frackowiak RS, Goadsby PJ (2005) A positron emission tomographic study in spontaneous migraine. Arch Neurol 62(8):1270–1275. doi:62/8/1270 10.1001/archneur.62.8.1270

42. Kobari M, Meyer JS, Ichijo M, Imai A, Oravez WT (1989) Hyperperfusion of cerebral cortex, thalamus and basal ganglia during spontaneously occurring migraine headaches. Headache 29(5):282–289

43. Gu T, Ma XX, Xu YH, Xiu JJ, Li CF (2008) Metabolite concentration ratios in thalami of patients with migraine and trigeminal neuralgia measured with 1H-MRS. Neurol Res 30(3):229–233. doi:10.1179/016164107X235473

44. May A (2007) Neuroimaging: visualising the brain in pain. Neurol Sci 28 (Suppl 2):S101–107. doi:10.1007/s10072-007-0760-x

45. Weiller C, May A, Limmroth V, Juptner M, Kaube H, Schayck RV, Coenen HH, Diener HC (1995) Brain stem activation in spontaneous human migraine attacks. Nat Med 1(7):658–660

46. Bahra A, Matharu MS, Buchel C, Frackowiak RS, Goadsby PJ (2001) Brainstem activation specific to migraine headache. Lancet 357(9261):1016–1017. doi:S0140673600042501

47. Afridi SK, Matharu MS, Lee L, Kaube H, Friston KJ, Frackowiak RS, Goadsby PJ (2005) A PET study exploring the laterality of brainstem activation in migraine using glyceryl trinitrate. Brain 128(Pt 4):932–939. doi:awh416 10.1093/brain/awh416

48. Moulton EA, Burstein R, Tully S, Hargreaves R, Becerra L, Borsook D (2008) Interictal dysfunction of a brainstem descending modulatory center in migraine patients. PLoS One 3(11):e3799. doi:10.1371/journal.pone.0003799

49. Cao Y, Aurora SK, Nagesh V, Patel SC, Welch KM (2002) Functional MRI-BOLD of brainstem structures during visually triggered migraine. Neurology 59(1):72–78

50. Stankewitz A, May A (2011) Increased limbic and brainstem activity during migraine attacks following olfactory stimulation. Neurology 77(5):476–482. doi:WNL.0b013e318227e4a8 10.1212/WNL.0b013e318227e4a8

51. Loggia ML, Edwards RR, Kim J, Vangel MG, Wasan AD, Gollub RL, Harris RE, Park K, Napadow V (2012) Disentangling linear and nonlinear brain responses to evoked deep tissue pain. Pain 153(10):2140–2151. doi:10.1016/j.pain.2012.07.014 S0304-3959(12)00425-3

52. Calandre EP, Bembibre J, Arnedo ML, Becerra D (2002) Cognitive disturbances and regional cerebral blood flow abnormalities in migraine patients: their relationship with the clinical manifestations of the illness. Cephalalgia 22(4):291–302. doi:370

53. Suhr JA, Seng EK (2012) Neuropsychological functioning in migraine: clinical and research implications. Cephalalgia 32(1):39–54. doi:0333102411430265 10.1177/0333102411430265

54. Koppen H, Palm Meinders I, Kruit M, Lim V, Nugroho A, Westhof I, Terwindt G, Van Buchem M, Ferrari M, Hommel B (2011) The impact of a migraine attack and its after-effects on perceptual organization, attention, and working memory. Cephalalgia 31(14):141–1427. doi:0333102411417900 10.1177/0333102411417900

55. Demarquay G, Royet JP, Mick G, Ryvlin P (2008) Olfactory hypersensitivity in migraineurs: a H(2)(15)O-PET study. Cephalalgia 28(10):1069. doi:CHA1672 10.1111/j.1468-2982.2008.01672.x

56. Denuelle M, Fabre N, Payoux P, Chollet F, Geraud G (2008) Posterior cerebral hypoperfusion in migraine without aura. Cephalalgia 28(8):856–862. doi:10.1111/j.1468-2982.2008.01623.x CHA1623

57. Woods RP, Iacoboni M, Mazziotta JC (1994) Brief report: bilateral spreading cerebral hypoperfusion during spontaneous migraine headache. N Engl J Med 331(25):1689–1692. doi:10.1056/NEJM199412223312505

21

New daily persistent headache with a thunderclap headache onset and complete response to Nimodipine (A new distinct subtype of NDPH)

Todd D Rozen[*] and Jennifer L Beams

Abstract

At present new daily persistent headache is just a group of conditions that are connected based on the temporal profile of their mode of onset. If new daily persistent headache is a true distinct syndrome like migraine then we need to start to define subtypes that have specific effective treatments such has been noted for migraine sub-forms. We present what we believe is the first recognized subtype of new daily persistent headache that which starts with a thunderclap headache onset. A patient presented with a 13 month history of a daily headache from onset which initiated as a thunderclap headache along with persistent acalculia. All neuroimaging studies for secondary causes were negative. Nimodipine rapidly and completely alleviated her headache and associated neurologic symptoms. We propose that this subtype of new daily persistent headache is caused by a very rapid increase in CSF tumor necrosis factor alpha levels leading to cerebral artery vasospasm with a subsequent thunderclap headache, then continuous or near continuous cerebral artery vasospasm leading to a persistent daily headache. Nimodipine which not only inhibits cerebral artery vasospasm but also tumor necrosis factor alpha production appears to be a specific treatment for this distinct subtype of new daily persistent headache.

Keywords: New daily persistent headache; Thunderclap headache; Vasospasm; Nimodipine; Reversible cerebral vasoconstriction syndrome; Acalculia

Background

The lack of consensus on a clear definition of new daily persistent headache (NDPH) and the fact that we are still searching for adequate therapy reflects on how little we know about this syndrome [1]. Is NDPH a group of conditions that just happen to all start daily from onset and have little else in common including no shared underlying pathogenesis or is there some distinct cortical change that causes a daily headache from onset in all patients with NDPH although the mechanism by which this cortical phenomena is triggered may be different for individual patients (post-infectious, post-surgical for example)? If NDPH is a distinct all-encompassing syndrome like migraine then we need to define sub-forms that may have specific effective treatments such has been noted for migraine with aura for example [2]. The end result of this will be improved patient satisfaction.

The presented case appears to be the first documented distinct subtype of NDPH: NDPH with a thunderclap headache onset. The treatment for this distinct case of NDPH is nimodipine.

Case presentation

A 46-year-old woman presented with a daily headache from onset that began 13 months prior. The daily headache started as a thunderclap headache. She was playing bingo and she suddenly developed the worst headache of her life which peaked immediately to 10/10 in intensity without latency. This was associated with vomiting and dizziness. The peak headache lasted for approximately 24 hours and thereafter she was left with a persistent lower grade headache which never waned. She denied having any further thunderclap headaches. With the original thunderclap headache she did not seek emergency attention. She saw her PCP the following day and had a brain MRI with and without gadolinium within 7 days which was reportedly normal with no evidence

* Correspondence: tdrozmigraine@yahoo.com
Department of Neurology, Geisinger Health System, Geisinger Headache Clinic, MC 37-32, 1000 East Mountain Blvd, Wilkes-Barre, PA 18711, USA

of subarachnoid blood. No lumbar puncture was ever completed. Her persistent daily headache was typically of moderate severity (4-5/10 VAS) and was localized to the right occipito-nuchal region. There was never any pain free time and she experienced intermittent associated symptoms including nausea and photophobia. She never experienced any cranial autonomic associated symptoms. The patient denied any headache triggering or alleviating maneuvers. She could not identify any precipitating event just prior to the onset of her daily persistent headache including no viral infection, stressful life event and she had not had any surgical procedures. She was on citalopram at the time of headache onset although she denied the use of marijuana, ecstasy or pseudoephedrine. In addition to head pain the patient also complained of having issues with numbers including doing simple addition and subtraction, recognizing the order of numbers and even recognizing certain numbers. She had to change her pin number multiple times because she could not place the numbers in the correct order on a keypad. She was even unable to copy down telephone numbers. She worked as a pharmacist and was actually very proficient in mathematics so the issue with numbers and calculations was very troubling to her and she was at risk of losing her job. Her acalculia (part spatial, part anarithmetria) started the same day as her daily headache. Her neurologic examination on presentation to the headache clinic was intact including a normal neurovascular examination, normal language examination, normal ability to read and write, but on serial 7 s testing she could not get below 93 when starting at 100. She also could not copy numbers in a correct order when they were presented to her verbally. In addition she had right greater occipital notch and occiput based pain to palpation although she stated this palpable tenderness was not her true pain which was "deep" to the skull. As the patient already had brain neuroimaging, cerebral vessel imaging was ordered to complete the evaluation for thunderclap headache and this included CT angiography of the head and neck vessels as well as brain venography and all studies were negative including no evidence for aneurysms, vessel dissection, vasospasm or thrombosis. An EEG was also completed and this was a normal study. Prior failed therapies which were minimal before coming to the dedicated headache clinic included near daily over the counter analgesics which were minimally effective, topiramate which lowered daily headache intensity but did not provide any pain free time and did not alter calculation issues, and oral prednisone which reduced but did not eliminate her headache (of note sedimentation rate and c-reactive protein were normal). The patient was given a diagnosis of NDPH as she met ICHD-3 beta criteria [3] which began as a thunderclap headache. Her headache did not meet criteria for hemicrania continua although it was one-sided.

She also had persistent acalculia. As nothing was noted on imaging the authors surmised that this may be a syndrome of persistent vasospasm and possibly even reversible cerebral vasoconstriction syndrome (RCVS) induced by citalopram and the acalculia was caused by persistent oligemia to the cortex. Citalopram was discontinued. Nimodipine was started for preventive therapy at a dose of 30 mg PO BID and within 4 days of starting therapy the patient became headache free. After 3 weeks on nimodipine her acalculia resolved. On re-evaluation two months after her initial visit she remained pain free. After 4 months on medication the patient decided to taper off her nimodipine and her daily headaches returned almost immediately although the calculation issues remained resolved. Nimodipine was restarted at 30 mg bid and within 3 days her headaches again ceased. This verified that the nimodipine had cured her headaches and it was not just being off citalopram. Over time she has been able to reduce the dose to 30 mg one time per day and still she remains headache free. She is hesitant to come off the medication in fear the pain will return. She has been followed for almost one year.

Conclusions

The question arises does this patient have a distinct subtype of NDPH and if so was it caused by continuous vasospasm and did the vasospasm lead to oligemia to specific regions of the cortex which led to acalculia? Based on the patient's response to nimodipine (a known inhibitor of cerebral artery vasoconstriction) this is a distinct possibility. Isolated acalculia without agraphia or alexia has been attributed to lesions mainly involving the dominant parieto-temporal cortex but has also been associated with injury to the medial frontal cortex, caudate nucleus, internal capsule, putamen and can also involve the non-dominant hemisphere when there is impairment with spatial organization of numbers which this patient displayed [4]. No ischemia was noted on this patient's brain MRI but that does not mean that one or more of these cortical regions was not altered from persistent oligemia; it just means that changes could not be seen by conventional neuroimaging. We wanted to do SPECT or PET imaging to better asses for changes in cortical blood flow, but her medical insurance denied coverage for this testing.

If vasospasm is the probable cause of NDPH with a thunderclap headache onset then one needs to then question if this subtype of NDPH is a prolonged subform of RCVS and thus an overlap disorder that could be placed under two ICHD sub-headings? In most instances RCVS is a self-limited syndrome of individual thunderclap headaches that by ICHD-3 beta criteria [3] does not last longer than one month in duration [4]. However, Hastriter et al. [5] in a Mayo Clinic series identified 16 patients with RCVS of whom six patients developed chronic daily headache when followed over and average of 99 weeks. The number of these patients who had a presentation of daily persistent headache after their initial thunderclap headache was not stated in the published abstract, although five patients were documented to have a continuous headache in between their thunderclap headaches, thus a possible NDPH type picture. Treatment for these patients was also not reported. In the Hastriter et al. [5] population there was documented resolution of vasoconstriction around 20 weeks after symptom onset, thus the cause of the patient's chronic headaches was not felt to be from vasospasm and thus not known. It is possible our patient was an outlier case of prolonged RCVS and the result of persistent cerebral artery vasospasm that lasted for more than one year's duration, which was not picked up on CT angiography, did not cause ischemia on MRI, but did cause enough oligemia leading to acalculia and head pain and nimodipine alleviated the vasospasm and thus headache and neurologic symptoms; but this can only be hypothesized. Conventional angiography would have been helpful as it could have better identified vasospasm but it was not completed as the patient so quickly responded to treatment and we did not want to subject her to another test which conceivably had a stroke risk as a potential complication. What possibly goes against the hypothesis of very prolonged vasospasm for our patient is the data of Hastriter et al. [5] which showed self-limited vasoconstriction even in those RCVS patients who developed chronic daily headache. What also is atypical for a diagnosis of RCVS is the fact that our patient only experienced a single thunderclap headache while most patients with RCVS have recurrent quick peaking headaches. If indeed our patient had a daily persistent headache secondary to RCVS or a sequela of some other underlying phenomenon but the testing for secondary causes is all negative then classification of this disorder as a primary headache syndrome demonstrates some of the limitations of the current ICHD criteria [3]. This patient's headache did indeed meet the ICHD-3 beta criteria [3] for primary NDPH as no secondary cause was found on neuroimaging but with response to nimodipine there is high clinical suspect the headache was at least partially secondary to cerebral artery vasospasm. The duration of time from onset of symptoms to when the patient was seen at a dedicated headache clinic also complicates issues with classification, as secondary causes which may have been noted on imaging or other testing if ordered properly at the onset of symptoms, may not be present when ordered many months later, thus a correct secondary diagnosis cannot be made at the time when a patient is evaluated by a headache specialist. For NDPH in particular where the underlying pathogenesis has not been elucidated and in which most patients have

negative studies, classifying any form as primary NDPH is actually difficult if not impossible, when all cases may have a secondary underlying cause like the proposed cerebral artery vasospastic issue in our case patient.

Nimodipine has shown very little effect in preventive migraine studies [6]. Nimodipine has however shown efficacy in the treatment of non-migrainous vascular headaches in individuals with chronic brain ischemia especially those with more significant headache intensity [7]. The proposed mechanism of action for headache control was inhibition of cerebral vasoconstriction. Nimodipine has not previously been documented to have been tried in NDPH [1]. There is recent animal data indicating that nimodipine can decrease the expression of CGRP in the trigeminal nucleus caudalis of rats [8]. As CGRP is a known trigger of migraine attacks it conceivably may also have a role in the pathogenesis of NDPH, another trigeminal based pain syndrome [9]. Why nimodipine however would be more effective for NDPH than for migraine would be hard to understand if its effect was solely by modulating CGRP expression. Nimodipine has also been shown to inhibit glial activation and tumor necrosis factor (TNF) alpha production in several animal models and this could be one mechanism by which it may work in NDPH [10,11]. One of the authors (TDR) has previously shown that patients with NDPH had elevation of CSF TNF alpha levels and thus TNF alpha was a probable inciting cytokine in the pathogenesis of this syndrome, most likely thru its ability to produce CNS inflammation [12]. TNF alpha also is a vasoconstrictive cytokine and thus could have a distinct triggering potential in NDPH with a thunderclap headache onset [13]. In mice TNF alpha is able to evoke a direct vasoconstrictor effect on isolated cerebral vessels through Rac-1 activation [13]. In humans there is anecdotal evidence that TNF alpha plays a role in cerebral artery vasospasm as demonstrated by peak elevations of CSF TNF alpha levels on the days corresponding to peak vasospasm time in patients who have had a subarachnoid hemorrhage and in those showing elevated flow velocities on transcranial doppler after a subarachnoid bleed [14]. We can thus hypothesize that the syndrome of NDPH with a thunderclap headache onset is caused by a very rapid increase in CSF TNF alpha levels leading to cerebral artery vasospasm with a subsequent thunderclap headache, then continuous or near continuous cerebral artery vasospasm leading to a persistent daily headache and possibly other neurologic sequelae. To prove this hypothesis a csf analysis would need to be completed at the time of NDPH and thunderclap headache onset and it would need to demonstrate TNF alpha levels higher than that noted in the author's prior csf study in typical NDPH without a thunderclap headache onset. This could not be done in this patient as we met her 13 months after symptom onset. Nimodipine theoretically works in this specific subtype of NDPH in a dual fashion by directly inhibiting cerebral artery vasospasm (calcium channel effect) and also by inhibiting TNF alpha production which not only prevents cerebral artery vasospasm, but in addition blocks the TNF alpha cytokine inflammatory response a proposed trigger of NDPH pain.

As NDPH is recognized as one of the most treatment refractory of all chronic headache conditions, documenting treatment responsive subtypes will be beneficial to both patients and providers. How rare is the subtype of NDPH with a thunderclap headache onset is unknown at present. The authors can state that in their practice which has a certain bias for NDPH patients, that this is the only patient who has fit this exact clinical presentation over the past year. Two other patients had a similar presentation of daily headache after a thunderclap headache onset with complete relief of their syndrome with nimodipine, but both had multiple thunderclap headaches during the first month of onset of their NDPH and thus were felt to be more consistent with a variant of RCVS and in line with the Hastriter et al. [5] reported patients, while our above reported case subject had only a single thunderclap headache at the outset of her daily persistent headache with no other recurrent thunderclaps, which distinguished her clinical presentation and placed it more in line in our opinion with an NDPH variant. It is certainly important when taking an NDPH history to ascertain what was the presentation of the original headache because if it was thunderclap then the provider should not only do the proper secondary work-up (neuroimaging should include MR angiography of the head and neck vessels, MR venography, MRI brain with and without gadolinium and a lumbar puncture if the patient is seen in the acute headache setting) but they should now think of nimodipine as a possible treatment option, which at present has not been part of the typical NDPH treatment protocol. There are two other case reports in the literature that should be mentioned which have some similarities to the present case report. A case of juvenile myoclonic epilepsy published by one of the authors (TDR) in which treatment of an associated neurologic condition in this case epilepsy with lamotrigine led to alleviation of NDPH which mimics our present case in which treatment of probable under-lying vasospasm and TNF alpha elevation with nimodipine alleviated co-associated NDPH [15]. A second case report where NDPH was preceded by an acute clinical event also known to be associated with an elevation of TNF alpha, in this case heat stroke, and with no other secondary medical issues noted [16]. In conclusion the hope is that this present case will stimulate others to publish cases of NDPH with a thunderclap headache onset to determine how rare or common this presentation of NDPH truly is.

Abbreviations
(NDPH): New daily persistent headache; (RCVS): Reversible cerebral vasoconstriction syndrome; (TNF): Tumor necrosis factor.

Competing interests
The authors declare that they have no competing interests.

Authors' contributions
Both authors equally prepared in the drafting and finalizing of this manuscript. Both authors read and approved the final manuscript.

References
1. Rozen TD (2011) New daily persistent headache: a clinical perspective. Headache 51:641–649
2. Holland PR, Akerman S, Andreou AP, Karsan N, Wemmie JA, Goadsby PJ (2012) Acid-sensing ion channel 1: a novel therapeutic target for migraine with aura. Ann Neurol 72:559–563
3. Headache classification committee of the international headache society (IHS) (2013) The international classification of headache disorders, 3rd edition (beta version). Cephalalgia 33:1–808
4. (2007) The localization of lesions affecting the cerebral hemispheres. In: Brazis PW, Masdeu JC, Biller J (eds) Localization in Clinical Neurology, 5th edn. Lippincott Williams and Wilkins, Philadelphia, PA
5. Hastriter EV, Halker R, Vargas B, Dodick D (2011) Headache prognosis in reversible cerebral vasoconstriction syndrome (RCVS). Neurology 76(supl 4):266
6. Toda N, Tfelt-Hansen P (2006) Calcium antagonists in migraine prophylaxis. In: Olesen J, Goadsby PJ, Ramadan NM, Tflelt-Hansen P, Welch KMA (eds) The Headaches, 3rd edn. Lippincott Williams and Wilkins, Philadelphia, PA
7. Hadjiev D, Velcheva I, Ivanova L (1986) Nimodipine in the treatment of headache in chronic cerebral ischemia. Cephalalgia 6:131–134
8. Vijayan L, Bansal D, Ray SB (2012) Nimodipine down-regulates CGRP expression in the rat trigeminal nucleus caudalis. Indian J Exp Biol 50:320–324
9. Hansen JM, Hauge AW, Olesen J, Ashina M (2010) Calcitonin gene-related peptide triggers migraine-like attacks in patients with migraine with aura. Cephalalgia 30:1179–1186
10. Li Y, Hu X, Liu Y, Bao Y, An L (2009) Nimodipine protects dopaminergic neurons against inflammation-mediated degeneration through inhibition of microglial activation. Neuropharmacology 56:580–589
11. Zhang XL, Zheng SL, Dong FR, Wang ZM (2012) Nimodipine improves regional cerebral blood flow and suppresses inflammatory factors in the hippocampus of rats with vascular dementia. J Int Med Res 40:1036–1045
12. Rozen TD, Swidan S (2007) Elevation of CSF Tumor Necrosis Factor Alpha Levels In New Daily Persistent Headache and Treatment Refractory Chronic Daily Migraine. Headache 47:1050–1055
13. Vecchione C, Frati A, di Pardo A et al (2009) Tumor necrosis factor-alpha mediates hemolysis-induced vasoconstriction and the cerebral vasospasm evoked by subarachnoid hemorrhage. Hypertension 54:150–156
14. Hanafy KA, Stuart RM, Khandji AG et al (2010) Relationship between brain interstitial fluid tumor necrosis factor-α and cerebral vasospasm after aneurysmal subarachnoid hemorrhage. J Clin Neurosci 17:853–856
15. Rozen TD (2011) Juvenile Myoclonic Epilepsy Presenting as a New Daily Persistent-Like Headache. J Headache Pain 12:645–647
16. di Lorenzo C, Ambrosini A, Coppola G, Pierelli F (2008) Heat stress disorders and headache: a case of new daily persistent headache secondary to heat stroke. J Neurol Neurosurg Psychiatry 79:610–611

22

Carotid dissection mimicking a new attack of cluster headache

Elisa Candeloro[1*], Isabella Canavero[1], Maurizia Maurelli[1], Anna Cavallini[1], Natascia Ghiotto[2], Paolo Vitali[3] and Giuseppe Micieli[1]

Abstract

Background: Symptomatic cluster headache (CH) secondary to internal carotid artery dissection (ICAD) has been frequently reported, however, as far as we know, the coexistence of episodic CH and acute symptomatic CH secondary to ICAD has not.

Case report: A 39 year-old man, affected by episodic CH since the age of 19, presented an atypical headache associated with his usual autonomic symptoms. After a series of negative tests, MRA eventually revealed dissection of the right distal internal carotid artery.

Discussion and conclusions: The coexistence of episodic CH and acute CH symptomatic of ICAD in our patient suggests that, at least in some cases, CH and ICAD may be different expressions of a common underlying cause: hidden vessel wall damage. When risk factors and the change - though partial - of clinical features suggest symptomatic cases, CH patients have to be strictly monitored over time. Given the lack of a *gold standard* investigation for dynamic diseases such as dissections, these patients require multimodal diagnostic investigation over time, even in cases where exams are normal at onset.

Keywords: Carotid dissection; Cluster headache; Dissection mimics

Background

It is widely recognized that carotid dissection could simulate a cluster headache (CH) attack. In fact, many cases of symptomatic CH secondary to internal carotid artery dissection (ICAD) have been reported [1-5]. However, to our knowledge, the occurrence of acute symptomatic CH secondary to ICAD in a patient affected by episodic CH has never been reported. We speculate about a pathogenetic connection between the two conditions in our patient. The peculiarity of the case also offers an example of a challenging differential diagnosis in the emergency department setting.

Case presentation

On 8th March 2012, a 39 year-old man presented to the emergency department 12 hours after the onset of right orbital, enduring, pressing pain. Neurological examination revealed miosis and ptosis in the right eye.

From the age of 19 the patient had suffered from episodic cluster headache, with attacks of right-orbital boring pain, lasting about 30 minutes, with conjunctival injection, rhinorrea, miosis and ptosis in the right eye. The condition was responsive to sumatriptan and verapamil. His last cluster attack had occurred in May 2011. In previous years he had undergone several neuroimaging examinations (computed tomography, magnetic resonance imaging, magnetic resonance angiography), showing no pathological findings. Past medical history also revealed a childhood post-traumatic fracture of the right petrous apex; MTHFR C677T homozygosis. The patient was practicing sport intensively, including the use of fitness equipment that implied the repetitive flexion-extension of the neck.

The atypically enduring pain led us to exclude secondary forms of cluster headache. An urgent brain computed tomography (CT) with computed tomography angiography (CTA) of intra-extracranial vessels was performed in the emergency department. CTA showed

* Correspondence: elisa.candeloro@mondino.it
[1]Cerebrovascular Diseases and Stroke Unit, Department of Emergency Neurology, IRCCS National Institute of Neurology Foundation Casimiro Mondino, Pavia, Italy
Full list of author information is available at the end of the article

only a subtle asymmetry of the internal carotid lumen filling by contrast (Figure 1A, 1B) and was reported as negative for artery dissection.

Due to persisting pain and Horner's syndrome, the man was admitted to the neurology department for further investigations. On 9th March he underwent a Duplex sonography of the supra-aortic vessels and a transcranial Doppler; the findings were normal (complete filling of the ICA lumen with normal Pulse Repetition Frequency [Figure 2A] and a normal waveform [Figure 2C]). A few hours later, a brain magnetic resonance imaging (MRI) with an extra-intracranial magnetic resonance angiography (MRA) demonstrated an intramural hematoma of the right distal internal carotid (about one centimeter before the intracranial segment), without stenosis of the vessel (Figure 3A, 3B). He was immediately anti-coagulated with heparin in order to prevent a stroke.

During hospitalization, the patient developed arterial hypertension, bradycardia and transient paresthesias of the right hemiface. For this reason, on the 5th day Duplex sonography was performed and disclosed a steno-occlusive distal process: the investigation disclosed the complete filling of the lumen with Pulse Repetition Frequency (Figure 2B) and a waveform with a very low amplitude, high-resistance and no diastolic flow (Figure 2D); the increased pulsatility and notable reduction in blood flow amplitude and velocity were consistent with the development of a stenosis downstream and suggested a possible worsening of carotid dissection. An extra-intracranial MRA showed apparent carotid occlusion (Figure 3C) and DWI sequences on MRI and ruled out the occurrence of a stroke. On the 10th day

subtotal carotid recanalization was documented by MRA (Figure 3D). At the six-month follow up, neurological examination was normal and neuroimaging showed stable partial recanalization.

Discussion

To our knowledge, a coexistence of episodic CH and acute symptomatic CH secondary to ICAD has never been previously reported.

CH and ICAD could present with unilateral orbital pain in association with ipsilateral miosis and ptosis due to sympathetic dysfunction. Either in CH or in ICAD, rarely, it could be found also unilateral tearing, conjunctival injection and rhinorrhea due to parasympathetic dysfunction [4,5].

In both CH and ICAD, the pericarotid plexus is involved in autonomic symptoms and trigeminal fibers in pain and parasympathetic symptoms [1,4].

According to some authors, in CH the simultaneity of pain and autonomic symptoms is due to a "pathophysiologic focus" in the superior pericarotid cavernous sinus plexus [6], where the fibers of the trigeminal nerve, superior cervical ganglion and sphenopalatine ganglion take connection [1-7]. Evidence for such a "peripheral" origin of symptoms comes from the observation that clinical features of symptomatic forms secondary to the involvement of these structures are almost indistinguishable from those in primary CH [8].

In ICAD, local signs and symptoms are thought to derive from the involvement of the adjacent structures. Autonomic symptoms could derive from the stretching and disruption of the pericarotid sympathetic nerve

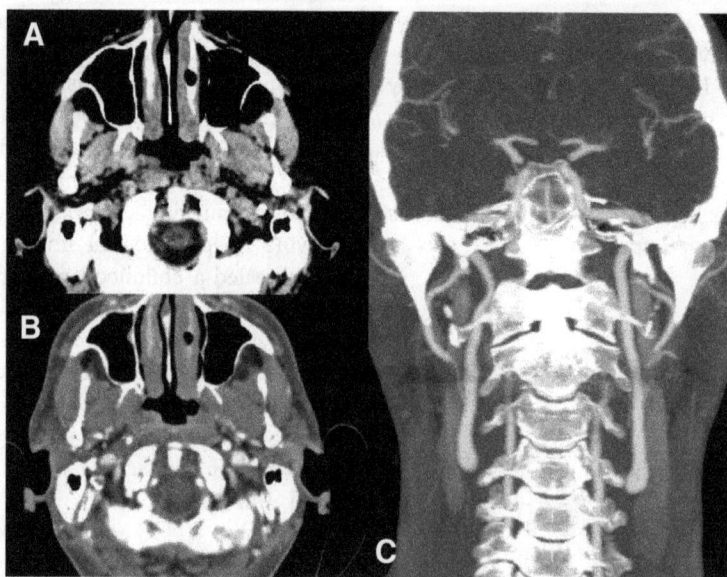

Figure 1 CT findings (performed in emergency department). A. Non-contrast axial CT shows normal findings. **B**. Axial CTA shows only a subtle asymmetry of the internal carotid lumen filling by contrast and was reported as negative for artery dissection. **C**. Coronal CTA shows normal findings.

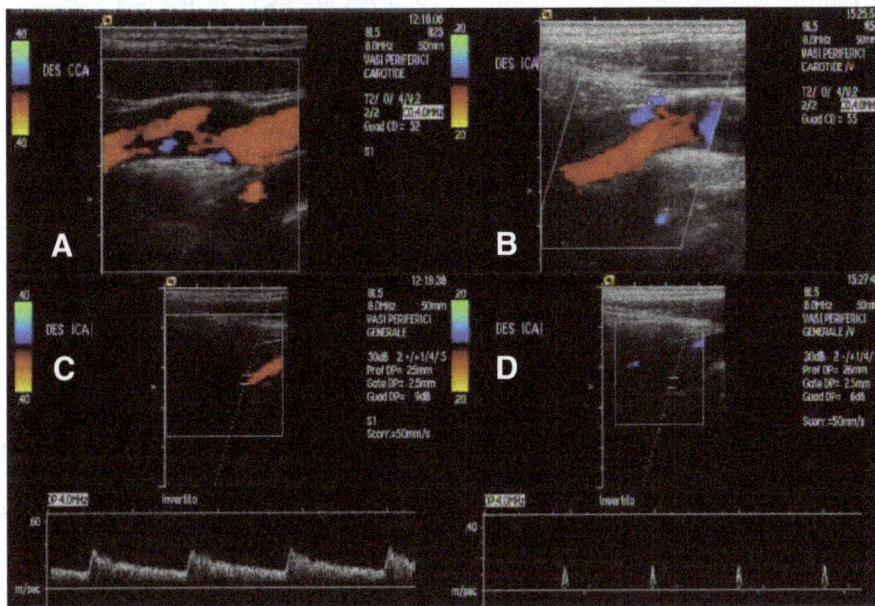

Figure 2 Duplex sonography findings. A. B-mode image performed on 9th March: complete filling of the right ICA lumen with normal PRF. **B**. B-mode image performed on 14th March: complete filling of the right ICA lumen with normal PRF. **C**. Doppler flow measurement performed on 9th March: normal waveform. **D**. Doppler flow measurement performed on 14th March: a waveform with a very low amplitude, high-resistance and no diastolic flow.

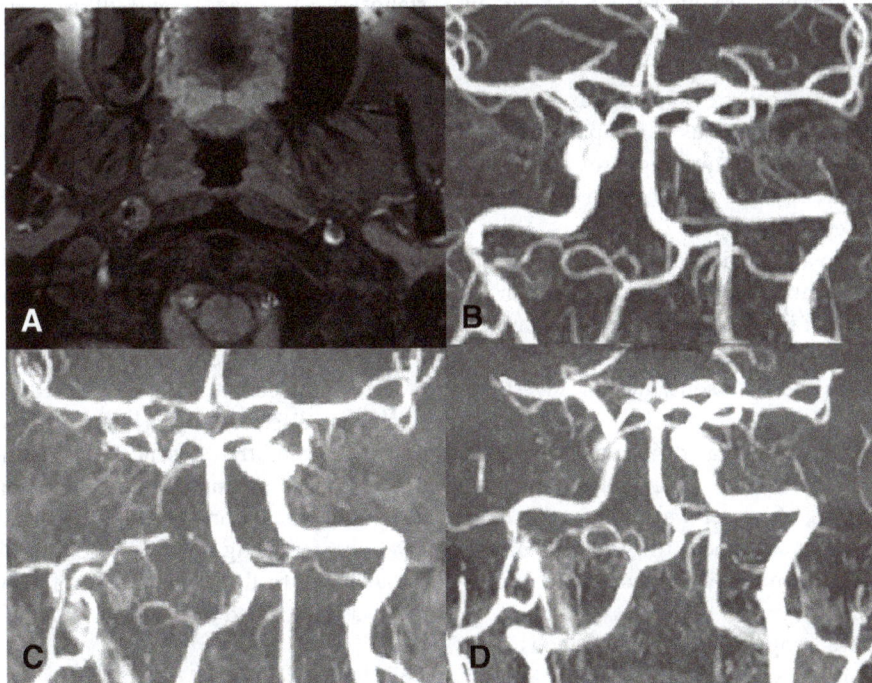

Figure 3 MR findings. A. Axial T1 fat-sat image (performed on 9th March) shows the typical semilunar image of the intramural hematoma in the right ICA. **B**. Time-of-flight (TOF) MRA (performed on 9th March) shows a focal "minus" image at the extra-intracranial passage in the right ICA. **C**. On 14th March MRA shows extension of contrastographic defect in the right ICA, due to the cranio-caudal extension of the intramural hematoma. **D**. On 19th March MRA shows a subtotal re-canalisation of the right ICA.

fibers, due to the enlargement of the vessel by intramural hematoma [9]. Pain could be determined by stimulation of the trigemino-vascular system [3]. An enlarged vessel can also determine the compression of other contiguous structures such as the carotid sinus and the trigeminal nerve. In our patient, the compression of these structures resulted in "baroceptor failure syndrome", with hypertension and bradycardia, and transient parestesias in the right hemiface.

In ICAD pathogenesis, it has been hypothesized that an interaction between genetic (e.g. MTHFR C677T homozygosis) and environmental factors (e.g. craniocervical traumas, mechanical stresses during sports activity and chiropractic manipulation) may lead to the initial vessel wall damage [10].

Therefore, in our case, the presence of several of these risk factors (the post-traumatic petrous apex fracture, MTHFR C677T homozygosis and repeated mechanical stress during sports activity), the coexistence of CH and ICAD with overlapping clinical features and the inferable involvement of the same afore-mentioned anatomical structures, suggest that the two diseases could share a common "pathophysiologic focus": probably hidden vessel wall damage.

A clinical differential diagnosis between CH and ICAD is influenced by the similarity of the symptoms, even more so if the two conditions co-exist. In ICAD pain is often associated with ipsilateral Horner syndrome, while other autonomic symptoms are unusual. However, in literature it has been described a case of ICAD whose CH-like symptoms were Horner syndrome, tearing and rhinorrhea [4]. The time course of pain was the only feature to be distinctive from CH, as in our patient.

Clinical observation and monitoring are crucial in order to note every new, atypical feature of symptoms such as, in our case, enduring pain.

However, anamnestic and clinical data could be unable to support the differential diagnosis, as reported by Godeiro-Junior et al. [5]: in their report ICAD presented with CH-like pain, Horner syndrome and other autonomic symptoms. For these reasons, further investigations are mandatory.

Nevertheless, even instrumental differential diagnosis is hindered by some factors: the heterogeneous anatomopathological features of vessel wall injury, the high dynamicity of dissections, and the intrinsic limits of the available instrumental techniques (especially in emergency departments).

Some Authors have proposed that spontaneous cervical artery dissections affect primarily the outer arterial layers, taking origin from a degenerative process at the medial-adventitial border. This may lead to the formation of a neoangiogenetic network and, subsequently, intramural hematomas [11]. The direction of expansion of the intramural hematoma determines the successive steps: if it is towards the lumen, stenosis or occlusion of the vessel could occur, with, though not necessarily, the formation of a double-lumen and an intimal flap; if it is towards the surrounding tissues, it could produce dilatation of the vessel and cause compressive local signs. Intimal flap, double lumen, pseudoaneurysm are considered pathognomonic of arterial dissection, but not invariably found. Their absence does not exclude the diagnosis. Further, it is difficult to predict if dissection will evolve into arterial steno-occlusion or recanalization; the timing of these changes could be even harder to predict [12]. It follows that the assumption that there is a correspondence between the time of the onset of dissection and the time of the onset of symptoms and signs may not be true in all cases [13], as the incidental finding of asymptomatic cases demonstrates.

The high anatomical heterogeneity and the unpredictable natural course of ICAD hinder instrumental diagnoses, especially in the absence of a *gold standard* test [13]. The available techniques are able to evaluate different aspects of the disease. CTA investigates mainly the lumen; it has a good sensitivity for stenosis, intimal flap and pseudoaneurysm but poor sensitivity for isolated intramural hematoma [14]. Owing to the mostly distal location of ICAD, often only indirect signs are detectable with Duplex sonography. This technique assesses a reduction of blood flow with good sensitivity only with stenosis > 50% downstream; ultrasound investigation has poor sensitivity in non-stroke patients with isolated Horner syndrome [15]. B-mode images visualize the arterial wall and the surrounding tissue: they may identify the double lumen but with poor sensitivity and only when located in the proximal extracranial carotid segment [16]. MRA evaluates the vessel wall and is able to detect intramural hematoma despite vessel occlusion: axial MRA T1-weighted imaging with fat suppression allows an optimal discrimination between intramural hematoma and perivascular tissue [17].

At the onset of symptoms in our patient the only sign of artery dissection was an isolated intramural hematoma, as disclosed by MRA; CTA was reported as normal given the absence of stenosis/intimal flap/ pseudoaneurysm and Duplex sonography was normal due to the distal non-stenosing localization of the injury. Over the following days, ultrasounds showed abnormal findings due to the development of a significant stenosis that was confirmed by MRA.

Conclusions

Our case suggests that, in some cases, episodic CH and symptomatic CH in ICAD could share a common etiopathogenetic mechanism. This being, to our knowledge, the first case of association between CH and

ICAD, and considering the available current literature [8,13], we believe that this hypothesis deserves attention and requires further studies to be confirmed.

From this report we could infer that patients with typical CH attacks [18], in the presence of risk factors for vessel wall damage, should undergo a careful clinical-instrumental follow up, paying particular attention to the development of atypical clinical features, such as pain.

This case highlights the need to combine different investigations and repeat them over time in CH patients who develop new atypical symptoms suggestive of ICAD. In fact, a negative initial investigation does not rule out the diagnosis of dissection.

Abbreviations

CH: Cluster headache; ICA: Internal carotid artery; ICAD: Internal carotid artery dissection; MRI: Magnetic resonance imaging; MRA: Magnetic resonance angiography; CT: Computed tomography; CTA: Computed tomography angiography; PRF: Pulse repetition frequency.

Competing interests

The authors declare that they have no competing interests.

Authors' contributions

CE conceived of the study, participated in clinical management of the patient, reviewed the literature on the item and drafted the manuscript. CI participated in the design of the paper, in reviewing the literature and drafting the manuscript. MM had the first approach with the patient at the ER, made the correct diagnosis and participated in his clinical management. CA has contributed in the clinical management of the patient and revised the manuscript. GN performed the neurosonological investigation and reviewed the literature concerning the technique. VP performed the neuroradiological investigation and reviewed the literature concerning the technique. MG has contributed in the clinical management of the patient and revised the manuscript. All authors read and approved the final manuscript.

Author details

[1]Cerebrovascular Diseases and Stroke Unit, Department of Emergency Neurology, IRCCS National Institute of Neurology Foundation Casimiro Mondino, Pavia, Italy. [2]Neurosonology Unit, Department of Neuropathophysiology, IRCCS National Institute of Neurology Foundation Casimiro Mondino, Pavia, Italy. [3]Department of Neuroradiology, IRCCS National Institute of Neurology Foundation Casimiro Mondino, Pavia, Italy.

References

1. Hannerz J, Arnardottir S, Bro Skejø HP, Lilja JA, Ericson K (2005) Peripheral postganglionic sympathicoplegia mimicking cluster headache attacks. Headache 45(1):84–86
2. Frigerio S, Bühler R, Hess CW, Sturzenegger M (2003) Symptomatic cluster headache in internal carotid artery dissection--consider anhidrosis. Headache 43(8):896–900
3. Biousse V, D'Anglejan-Chatillon J, Massiou H, Bousser MG (1994) Head pain in non-traumatic carotid artery dissection: a series of 65 patients. Cephalalgia 14(1):33–36
4. Tsivgoulis G, Mantatzis M, Vadikolias K, Heliopoulos I, Charalampopoulos K, Mitsoglou A, Georgiadisa GS, Giannopoulos S, Piperidou C (2013) Internal carotid artery dissection presenting as new-onset cluster headache. Neurol Sci 34(7):1251–1252
5. Godeiro-Junior C, Kuster GW, Felicio AC, Porto PP Jr, Pieri A, Coelho FM (2008) Internal carotid artery dissection presenting as cluster headache. Arq Neuropsiquiatr 66(3):763–764
6. Moskowitz MA (1988) Cluster headache: evidence for a pathophysiologic focus in the superior pericarotid cavernous sinus plexus. Headache 28(9):584–586
7. Gentile S, Fontanella M, Giudice RL, Rainero I, Rubino E, Pinessi L (2006) Resolution of cluster headache after closure of an anterior communicating artery aneurysm: the role of pericarotid sympathetic fibres. Clin Neurol Neurosurg 108(2):195–198
8. Leone M, Bussone G (2009) Pathophysiology of trigeminal autonomic cephalalgias. Lancet Neurol 8(8):755–764
9. Sturzenegger M, Huber P (1993) Cranial nerve palsies in spontaneous carotid artery dissection. J Neurol Neurosurg Psychiatry 56(11):1191–1199
10. Debette S, Grond-Ginsbach C, Bodenant M, Kloss M, Engelter S, Metso T, Pezzini A, Brandt T, Caso V, Touzé E, Metso A, Canaple S, Abboud S, Giacalone G, Lyrer P, Del Zotto E, Giroud M, Samson Y, Dallongeville J, Tatlisumak T, Leys D, Martin JJ, Cervical Artery Dissection Ischemic Stroke Patients (CADISP) Group (2011) Differential features of carotid and vertebral artery dissections: the CADISP study. Neurology 77(12):1174–81
11. Völker W, Dittrich R, Grewe S, Nassenstein I, Csiba L, Herczeg L, Borsay BA, Robenek H, Kuhlenbäumer G, Ringelstein EB (2011) The outer arterial wall layers are primarily affected in spontaneous cervical artery dissection. Neurology Apr 76:1463–1471
12. Sengelhoff C, Nebelsieck J, Nassenstein I, Maintz D, Nabavi DG, Kuhlenbaeumer G, Ringelstein EB, Dittrich R (2008) Neurosonographical follow-up in patients with spontaneous cervical artery dissection. Neurol Res 30(7):687–689
13. Provenzale JM, Sarikaya B (2009) Comparison of test performance characteristics of MRI, MR angiography, and CT angiography in the diagnosis of carotid and vertebral artery dissection: a review of the medical literature. AJR Am J Roentgenol 193(4):1167–1174
14. Goyal MS, Derdeyn CP (2009) The diagnosis and management of supraaortic arterial dissections. Curr Opin Neurol 22(1):80–89
15. Arnold M, Baumgartner RW, Stapf C, Nedeltchev K, Buffon F, Benninger D, Georgiadis D, Sturzenegger M, Mattle HP, Bousser MG (2008) Ultrasound diagnosis of spontaneous carotid dissection with isolated Horner syndrome. Stroke 39(1):82–86
16. Benninger DH, Baumgartner RW (2006) Ultrasound diagnosis of cervical artery dissection. Front Neurol Neurosci 21:70–84
17. Ozdoba C, Sturzenegger M, Schroth G (1996) Internal carotid artery dissection: MR imaging features and clinical-radiologic correlation. Radiology 199(1):191–198
18. Headache Classification Committee of the International Headache Society (IHS) (2013) The International Classification of Headache Disorders, 3rd edition (beta version). Cephalalgia 33(9):629–808

23

Migraine misdiagnosis as a sinusitis, a delay that can last for many years

Jasem Y Al-Hashel[1,2], Samar Farouk Ahmed[1,3*], Raed Alroughani[4,5] and Peter J Goadsby[6]

Abstract

Background: Sinusitis is the most frequent misdiagnosis given to patients with migraine. Therefore we decided to estimate the frequency of misdiagnosis of sinusitis among migraine patients.

Methods: The study included migraine patients with a past history of sinusitis. All included cases fulfilled the International Classification of Headache Disorders, 3rd edition (ICHD-III- beta) criteria. We excluded patients with evidence of sinusitis within the past 6 months of evaluation. Demographic data, headache history, medical consultation, and medication intake for headache and effectiveness of therapy before and after diagnosis were collected.

Results: A total of 130 migraine patients were recruited. Of these patients 106 (81.5%) were misdiagnosed as sinusitis. The mean time delay of migraine diagnosis was (7.75 ± 6.29, range 1 to 38 years). Chronic migraine was significantly higher ($p < 0.02$) in misdiagnosed patients than in patients with proper diagnosis. Medication overuse headache (MOH) was reported only in patients misdiagnosed as sinusitis. The misdiagnosed patients were treated either medically 87.7%, or surgically12.3% without relieve of their symptoms in 84.9% and 76.9% respectively. However, migraine headache improved in 68.9% after proper diagnosis and treatment.

Conclusions: Many migraine patients were misdiagnosed as sinusitis. Strict adherence to the diagnostic criteria will prevent the delay in migraine diagnosis and help to prevent chronification of the headache and possible MOH.

Keywords: Migraine misdiagnosis; Sinus headache

Background

Migraine continues being an underdiagnosed condition [1] because it can be accompanied by symptoms commonly associated with other causes of facial pain [2,3]. Many patients visit their general practitioner because of their headache and, in many cases, a proper diagnosis and treatment may take years [4,5].

"Sinusitis" may constitute one of the most commonly confusing clinical presentation of migraine [6], probably because cranial autonomic symptoms are common in migraine [7] based on activation of the trigeminal-autonomic reflex [8]. Headaches located in the frontal, supraorbital, or infraorbital region are sinus headaches [9]. These headaches are usually recurrent, non-seasonal, and unassociated with fever, localized tenderness, or erythema [10].

Migraine-associated alterations in trigeminal and/or autonomic activity may explain nasal and ocular symptoms in migraine. For example, "sinus" symptoms in migraine have been hypothesized to arise from activation of the trigeminal-autonomic reflex, which is mediated by a circuit of trigeminal afferents and parasympathetic efferent that innervate the lacrimal glands and the nasal mucosa [11].

This study aimed to estimate the frequency of misdiagnosis of sinusitis among patients with migraine headache who fulfilled the diagnostic criteria according to the International Classification of Headache Disorders, 3rd edition (ICHD-III- beta) criteria [12].

Methods

This retrospective study included 130 male and female migraine patients aged above 12 years with history of sinusitis. Every headache was assigned a diagnosis based ICHD-III-beta [12].

* Correspondence: samerelshayb@hotmail.com
[1]Department of Neurology, Ibn Sina Hospital, P.O. Box 25427, Safat 13115 Kuwait City, Kuwait
[3]Department of Neurology and Psychiatry, Al-Minia University, Minia, Egypt

Exclusion criteria included radiographic evidence of sinus infection, the occurrence of fever, or purulent nasal discharge associated with their headaches within the past six months of evaluation. Patients who were unable to give reliable information about their medical history and headache characteristics or have incomplete medical files were excluded from the study (n = 17).

Patient identification

The data were collected from a hospital-based cohort of headache patients referred to both Mubarak and Ibn Sina Hospitals, Kuwait. We examined the medical files of all patients diagnosed with headache who were registered between 2010 and 2012. The records were examined and standardized data collection forms were completed retrospectively by the study group.

Clinical data

The diagnosis of migraine was made during face to face interview with headache specialist. Demographic characteristics, headache frequency, duration, and associated headache symptoms were recorded for each patient. Patients were asked about the onset of their headache, how long it took them to receive a correct diagnosis (latency of diagnosis) and what different physicians they had consulted prior to the current consultation. Results of previous diagnostic investigation including brain and sinus imaging were retrieved also.

Patients were asked about their use of medical and surgical treatments for headache before migraine diagnosis and to rate the effectiveness of each treatment before and after diagnosis on a 4-point scale: [13]

1. Very effective – complete and long-lasting relief
2. Effective –partial and/or short-lasting relief
3. Ineffective
4. Headache worsened.

Data analysis

All analyses were performed using SPSS 19 for Windows. Simple descriptive statistical tests (Mean and Standard deviation) were used to describe the numerical values of the sample. Frequency and percentage were used to describe the non-numerical values of the sample. The significance of the differences between the patients with proper and misdiagnosis was determined using a chi-squared test for non- numerical variables. $P < 0.05$ was defined as statistically significant.

The study received the approval of the local ethic committee, and all the patients signed the appropriate informed consents.

Results

Table 1 describes the demographic and characteristic data of 130 migraine patients.

Symptoms

The symptoms referred to the sinus areas were: sinus pain (76.2%), sinus pressure (60%) and nasal congestion (55.4%). Most of our patients had at least one investigation looking at the sinuses. Thirteen patients (10%) showed thickened sinus mucosa in CT sinuses. Many patients had at least one performed neuroimaging test and all of them were normal (Table 1).

Headache diagnosis

We found that 106 (81.5%) of our patients had been misdiagnosed as sinusitis. Chronic migraine was significantly higher ($p < 0.0001$) in misdiagnosed patients and medication over use headache (MOH) reported only in patients misdiagnosed as sinusitis (Table 2).

Misdiagnosis results

The mean duration of headache in misdiagnosed patients was 11.15 ± 7.85 (range 2 to 40 years) and the mean time between the first attack of headache and the diagnosis of migraine was 7.75 ± 6.29 (range 1 to 38 years). 59/106 (56.6%) of them had consulted a primary care physician, and 47/106 patients (43.4%) assessed by otorhinolaryngology specialist before the diagnosis of migraine was made.

Thirteen patients (12.3%) of them had prior "sinus surgery" based on suspected lesions on CT sinuses and 93

Table 1 Demographic data and characteristic of all migraine patients (n = 130) according to ICHD-III-beta

Variable	Mean ± SD/no. (%)
Age	35.88 ± 9.87
Duration of headache	10.22 ± 7.60
Sex	
Male	30 (23.1%)
Female	100 (76.9%)
Symptoms referred to sinus area	
Sinus pain	99 (76.2%)
Sinus congestion	78 (60%)
Nasal congestion	72 (55.4%)
Investigations looking at the sinuses	
Sinus x ray	58 (44.6%)
Sinus CT	21 (16.2%)
Endoscopy	3 (2.3%)
Neuroimaging	
MRI brain	44 (33.8%)
CT brain	6 (4.6%)
MRI cervical spine	2 (1.5%)

Table 2 Comparison of headache profiles according to ICHD-III between migraine patients with proper diagnosis and those with misdiagnosis

Type of headache	Migraine patients with proper diagnosis (n = 24)	Migraine patients misdiagnosed as sinusitis (n = 106)	P value
Migraine without aura [1.1]	13 (54.2%)	43 (40.6%)	0.2
Migraine with aura [1.2]	8 (33.3%)	22 (20.8%)	0.1
Chronic migraine [1.3]	3 (12.5%)	30 (28.3%)	0.02*
Medication over use headache [8.2]	0	11 (11.4%)	

*Significant.

(87.7%) received medical treatment for sinusitis. Both surgical and medical treatment were ineffective in most of the patients. Of those who received ineffective medical or surgical treatment, 73 (69%) were more satisfied in 2–4 months after initiating anti-migraine treatment (topiramate, propranolol, amitriptyline or sodium valproate) after their proper diagnosis (Table 3).

Discussion

Our study included 130 patients with migraine-type headache according to 3rd edition (ICHD-III-beta). We found that 81.5% of them were misdiagnosed and managed as sinusitis. The similarity of sinusitis symptoms and migraine complicates the diagnostic evaluation process. Although both historical and new data show that nasal symptoms frequently accompany a migraine, these symptoms are not required by the ICHD-III-beta diagnostic criteria for a migraine.

Our data are in agreement with the study of Schreiber and colleagues [6] which included approximately 3000

Table 3 Effective of management prior and after migraine diagnosis

Variable	No. (%)
Effective of management prior migraine diagnosis	
Surgical (no = 13)	
Very effective – complete and long-lasting relief	0/13
Effective –partial and/or short-lasting relief	3/13 (22.1%)
Ineffective	9/13 (69.2%)
Headache worsened	1/13 (7.7%)
Medical (no = 93)	
Very effective – complete and long-lasting relief	0/93
Effective –partial and/or short-lasting relief	14/93 (15.1%)
Ineffective	65/93 (69.8%)
Headache worsened	14/93 (15.1%)
Effective of treatment after migraine diagnosis (no = 106)	
Very effective – complete and long-lasting relief	73/106 (68.9%)
Effective –partial and/or short-lasting relief	22/106 (20.8%)
Ineffective	8/106 (7.5%)
Headache worsened	3/106 (2.8%)

patients with a history of self-described or physician-diagnosed "sinus" headache and they determined that 80% of patients met ICHD criteria for migraine. Our data are also in agreement with the other previous studies [3,9,14,15] which reported that "sinus headache" is one of the most commonly reported terms used in combination with a migraine diagnosis and most patients presenting with a "sinus headache" may not actually have a rhino sinusitis associated headache.

Migraine can be mistaken for rhinosinusitis because of similarity in location of the headache and the commonly accompanying nasal autonomic symptoms. The presence or absence of purulent nasal discharge and/or other features diagnostic of acute rhinosinusitis help to differentiate these conditions [12]. In order to properly establish a diagnosis of migraine, it is essential to know the ICHD criteria and apply these criteria in clinical practice.

We demonstrated that chronic migraine was significantly higher in patients misdiagnosed with sinusitis. MOH was reported only in those patients. A delay in the diagnosis of migraine led to chronification of the headache and transformation, in some cases, into MOH.

We found that the diagnosis of migraine was delayed in more than 80% of our cohort up to 38 years. Eross and colleagues [15] similarly found that their patients waited 25.3 years (longest of 62 years) prior to the correct diagnosis. Previous studies showed this as well [4,5]. The diagnostic delay in our cohort could be explained by the presence of sinus pain, sinus congestion and nasal discharge during headache attacks. These symptoms have been reported with previous studies which concluded that presence of autonomic symptoms during migraine attacks often leads to confusion and incorrect diagnosis of sinusitis [16,17]. The ICHD criteria do not highlight the presence of cranial autonomic symptoms in the disorder, or perhaps more usefully comment upon them. This may help general practitioner and otorhinolaryngology specialist to be aware of the phenotyping overlap.

The majority of our patients had at least one investigation looking at the sinuses which were all normal. This result is similar to previous results which demonstrated that patients with "sinus headache" did not have findings suggestive of sinusitis on endoscopy or CT scan [14] and over 50% of them were diagnosed with migraine later [18].

These unnecessary investigations increase time delay to obtain the correct diagnosis and management [19].

We demonstrated that 56% of the misdiagnosed patients had consulted a primary care physician and 44% of them an otorhinolaryngology specialist before the diagnosis of migraine was made. We are in agreement with Foroughipour and colleagues [17] who studied 58 patients with the diagnosis of sinusitis made by a primary care physician. After comprehensive otorhinolaryngologic and neurologic evaluation, the final diagnoses was migraine in 68% of the patients. Furthermore, our study demonstrated that the misdiagnosed patient received either medical in 87.7%, or surgical treatment in 12.3% of them without relieve of their symptoms in 84.9% and 76.9% respectively. However, migraine headache improved in 68.9% after proper diagnosis and treatment. These results are similar to that of Foroughipour and colleagues [17] who reported that recurrent antibiotic therapy was received by 66% patients and therapeutic nasal septoplasty was performed in 16% of the patients with a final diagnosis of migraine.

An appropriate recognition of migraine in patients who complain about sinus headaches may help to minimize the suffering and unnecessary interventions, start migraine directed therapy [20] and improve quality of life [9].

Conclusion

In conclusion, symptoms suggestive of sinusitis are frequently seen in migraine patients and may lead to delayed diagnosis and treatment of migraine. General practitioner and otorhinolaryngology specialist should be aware of the diagnostic criteria for migraine and consider it in their differential diagnosis of patients suffering from "sinusitis". Going forward it is important to consider how best to draw attention to cranial autonomic symptoms in migraine and their place in diagnostic criteria.

Competing interest
The authors declare that there are no conflicts of interest.

Authors' contributions
JAH designed the study, collected the data and revised the manuscript, SFA collected, and analyzed the data, and wrote the manuscript, RA and PJG revised the manuscript. All authors read and approved the final manuscript.

Funding
This research received no specific grant from any funding agency in the public, commercial, or not-for-profit sectors.

Author details
[1]Department of Neurology, Ibn Sina Hospital, P.O. Box 25427, Safat 13115 Kuwait City, Kuwait. [2]Department of Medicine, Faculty of Medicine, Health Sciences Centre, Kuwait University, Kuwait City, Kuwait. [3]Department of Neurology and Psychiatry, Al-Minia University, Minia, Egypt. [4]Division of Neurology, Amiri Hospital, P.O. Box 1661, Qurtoba 73767 Kuwait City, Kuwait. [5]Division of Neurology, Dasman Diabetes Institute, P.O. Box 1180, Dasman 15462 Kuwait City, Kuwait. [6]Wellcome Trust Clinical Research Facility, Kings College Hospital, London, UK.

References
1. Stewart WF, Simon D, Shechter A, Lipton RB (1995) Population variation in migraine prevalence: a meta-analysis. J Clin Epidemiol 48:269–80
2. Cady RK, Schreiber CP (2002) Sinus headache or migraine? considerations in making a differential diagnosis. Neurology 58(suppl 6):S10–S14
3. Diamond ML (2002) The role of concomitant headache types and non-headache comorbidities in the underdiagnosis of migraine. Neurology 58(suppl 6):S3–S9
4. De Diego EV, Lanteri-Minet M (2005) Recognition and management of migraine in primary care: influence of functional impact measured by the headache impact test (HIT). Cephalalgia 25(3):184–90
5. Ryan RE, Jr, Pearlman SH (2004) Common headache misdiagnoses. Prim Care Clin Office Pract 31:395–405
6. BCPS; Powers C, Schreiber CP, Hutchinson S, Webster CJ, Ames M, Richardson MS, Pharm D (2004) Prevalence of migraine in patients with a history of self-reported or physician-diagnosed "Sinus" headache. Arch Intern Med 164:1769–1772
7. Peter JG (2009) Lacrimation, conjunctival injection, nasal symptoms…cluster headache, migraine and cranial autonomic symptoms in primary headache disorders- what's new? J Neurol Neursurg Psychiatry 80:1057–1058
8. May A, Goadsby PJ (1999) The trigeminovascular system in humans: pathophysiological implications for primary headache syndromes of the neural influences on the cerebral circulation. J Cereb Blood Flow Metab 19:115–127
9. Dadgarnia MH, Atighechi S, Baradaranfar MH (2010) The response to sodium valproate of patients with sinus headaches with normal endoscopic and CT Findings. Eur Arch Otorhinolaryngol 267:375–379
10. Levine HL, Setzen M, Cady RK, et al. (2006) An otolaryngology, neurology, allergy and primary care consensus on diagnosis and treatment of sinus headache. A literature review. Otolaryngol Head Neck Surg 134:516–523
11. Akerman S, Holland P, Goadsby PJ (2011) Diencephalic and brainstem mechanisms in migraine. Nat Rev Neurosci 12:570–584
12. Headache Classification Committee of the International Headache Society (2013) The International Classification of Headache Disorders, 3rd edition (beta version). Cephalalgia 33:629–808
13. Rossi P, Faroni J, Tassorelli C, Nappi G (2009) Diagnostic delay and suboptimal management in a referral population with hemicrania continua. Headache 49:227–234
14. Mehle ME, Kremer PS (2008) Sinus CT scan findings in "Sinus Headache" migraineurs. Headache 48:67–71
15. Eross E, Dodick D, Eross M (2007) The Sinus, Allergy and Migraine Study (SAMS). Headache 47:213–224
16. Barbanti P, Fabbrini G, Pesare M, et al. (2002) Unilateral cranial autonomic symptoms in migraine. Cephalalgia 22:256–259
17. Foroughipour M, Sharifian SM, Shoeibi A, Ebdali Barabad N, Bakhshaee M (2011) Causes of headache in patients with a primary diagnosis of sinus headache. Eur Arch Otorhinolaryngol 268(11):1593–6
18. Perry BF, Login IS, Kountakis SE (2004) Nonrhinologic headache in a tertiary rhinology practice. Otolaryngol Head Neck Surg 130:449–452
19. Viticchi G, Silvestrini M, Falsetti L, Lanciotti C, Cerqua R, Luzzi S, Provinciali L, Bartolini M (2011) The role of instrumental examinations in delayed migraine diagnosis. Neurol Sci 32(Suppl 1):S143–4
20. Patel ZM, Kennedy DW, Setzen M, Poetker DM, Delgaudio JM (2013) "Sinus headache": rhinogenic headache or migraine? An evidence-based guide to diagnosis and treatment. Int Forum Allergy Rhinol 3:221–230

24

Electrophysiological correlates of episodic migraine chronification: evidence for thalamic involvement

Gianluca Coppola[1]*[†], Elisa Iacovelli[2†], Martina Bracaglia[2], Mariano Serrao[2], Cherubino Di Lorenzo[3] and Francesco Pierelli[4]

Abstract

Background: Episodic migraine is characterized by decreased high-frequency somatosensory oscillations (HFOs), reflecting thalamo-cortical activity, and deficient habituation of low-frequency (LF-) somatosensory evoked potentials (SSEPs) to repetitive sensory stimulation between attacks. Here, we study conventional LF-SSEPs and HFOs in episodic migraineurs who developed chronic migraine (CM).

Methods: Thirty-four episodic (15 interictally [MOii], 19 ictally [MOi]) and 19 CM patients underwent right median nerve SSEPs. The patient groups were compared to a group of 20 healthy volunteers (HV) of comparable age and gender distribution. We measured the N20-P25 LF-SSEP 1st amplitude block and habituation, and, after applying a band-pass filter (450–750 Hz), maximal peak-to-peak latency and the amplitudes of the early and late HFOs.

Results: Reduced early HFOs, lower 1st block LF-SSEPs and deficient habituation characterize MOii. Initially higher SSEP amplitudes and late normal habituation characterize both CM and MOi patients. After the digital filtration, both patient groups showed shortened latency peaks and normalization of early HFO amplitudes with increased late HFOs. When data of MO and CM patients were combined, the monthly number of days with headache negatively correlated with the LF-SSEP slope (r = −0.385, p = 0.006), which in turn negatively correlated with the 1st amplitude block (r = 0.568, p < 0.001).

Conclusions: Our results show abnormalities in chronic migraine that are also reported during attacks in episodic migraineurs, namely early response sensitization and late habituation. The HFO analysis suggests that this sensory sensitization may be explained by an increase in the strength of the connections between the thalamus and cortex compared to episodic migraine between attacks. Whether this electro-functional behaviour is primary or secondary to daily headache, thus reflecting an electrophysiological fingerprint of the somatosensory system central sensitization process, remains to be determined.

Keywords: Chronic migraine; Thalamus; Somatosensory evoked potentials; Central sensitization; Habituation

Background

Migraine is one of the most prevalent and disabling neurological disorders [1,2]. It is characterized by recurrent attacks of headache widely variable in duration and intensity, usually accompanied by nausea/vomiting and/or photo-/phono- phobia. In some cases, migraine patients experience a progressive increase in the frequency of the attacks, leading to headache chronification. This clinical

condition is defined as 15 or more headache days with 8 or more migraine attacks per month [3]. The exact pathophysiological mechanisms underlying chronic migraine are still under intense scrutiny. Possible culprits for pain chronification include central sensitization and defective central pain control systems [4,5].

During the last decades, clinical neurophysiology methods have allowed in vivo measurements of the migraineur's electrocortical responses to various sensory stimuli. Altered thalamo-cortical connections [6,7], with cortical dysexcitability [8] and lack of habituation in response to various sensory stimuli, characterize episodic migraineurs' brains [9]. This abnormal information

* Correspondence: gianluca.coppola@gmail.com
[†]Equal contributors
[1]G.B. Bietti Foundation IRCCS, Department of Neurophysiology of Vision and Neurophthalmology G.B. Bietti Foundation-IRCCS, Via Livenza 3, Rome 00198, Italy
Full list of author information is available at the end of the article

processing increases during the pain-free days, reaching its maximum just before the attack onset, and disappears in the ictal phase [6,10-16]. Less is known about how mechanisms underlying headache chronification alter this electro-functional profile in episodic patients experiencing a conversion to CM [17].

Evidence has been recently found in favour of persistent somatosensory system central sensitization in chronic headache secondary to medication overuse (medication overuse headache, MOH) by recording cortical somatosensory evoked potentials (SSEPs) [10,18]. To the best of our knowledge, no study has investigated simultaneously SSEP habituation as well as thalamo-cortical connections in episodic migraine patients who developed chronic migraine without the confounding factor of medication overuse. Having this information may contribute to shed more light on the mechanisms underlying headache transformation.

With this specific purpose, we designed the present study to explore whether the sensory cortical response pattern differs between CM patients and patients with episodic migraine without aura recorded both during and between attacks. To do so we recorded low-frequency (LF) SSEP in order to assess habituation/sensitization phenomena. Thereafter, we studied high-frequency oscillations (HFOs) embedded in the common SSEPs in order to identify two bursts of HFOs: an early component thought to be generated by pre-synaptic thalamo-cortical afferents, and a late component reflecting post-synaptic cortical activation [19-21]. We also sought possible correlations between the electrophysiological pattern and clinical features including the number of days with headache and the duration of the chronification phase.

Methods

Subjects - Among consecutive patients attending our headache clinic, 53 patients gave informed consent to participate in the study (Table 1) which was approved by the local ethics committee. According to the new ICHD-III criteria [3], 19 patients were diagnosed as having chronic migraine (CM) during their first visit. These patients were not affected by medication overuse since the mean monthly tablet intake was 2.7 ± 3.0. Before progressing to CM, all patients had a clear-cut history of episodic migraine without aura (MO, ICHD-II code 1.1). With the exception of 2 patients who had a mild headache (mean VAS = 3), all CM patients underwent the SSEP recordings in a pain-free state. The 2 patients who had a headache had no associated migrainous features. Thirty-four patients were diagnosed as having episodic migraine without aura (ICHD-II code 1.1). Of these, 15 were recorded during the interictal period (MOii), i.e. at least three days before and after an attack, and 19 within a time range of 12 hours before or after the beginning of an attack, then considered as ictal (MOi). Neither chronic nor episodic patients were allowed to take any prophylactic medication in the three months before the recording session. For those patients experiencing a migraine attack, no acute anti-migraine drugs were allowed until the end of the recording session. For comparison, we enrolled 20 healthy volunteers (HV) of comparable age and sex distribution; they had no personal or familial history (1st or 2nd degree relatives) of migraine or any detectable medical conditions. To avoid variability due to hormonal changes, women were recorded outside their pre-menstrual or menstrual periods. All participants received a complete description of the study and granted written informed consent. The project was approved by the ethical review board of the Faculty of Medicine, University of Rome, Italy.

Data acquisition

Somatosensory evoked potentials (SSEPs) were elicited by electrical stimulation applied to the right median nerve at the wrist using a constant current square wave pulse (0.1 ms width, cathode proximal), with a stimulus intensity set at 1.5 times the motor threshold, and a repetition rate of 4.4 Hz. The active electrodes were placed over the contralateral parietal area (C3', 2 cm posterior to C3 in the International 10–20 system) and on the fifth cervical spinous process (Cv5), both referenced to Fz; the ground

Table 1 Demographic data and headache profiles of patients

	HV (n = 20)	MOii (n = 15)	MOi (n = 19)	CM (n = 19)
Women (n)	13	12	13	14
Age (years)	38 ± 10	32 ± 7	33 ± 11	33 ± 14
Duration of history of migraine (years)		18.0 ± 12.7	17.3 ± 13.8	17.3 ± 13.8
Days with headache/month (n)		2.0 ± 1.3	3.7 ± 2.5	25.6 ± 6.2
Severity of headache attacks (0–10)		6.8 ± 0.8	8.0 ± 0.9	7.1 ± 0.9
Duration of the chronic headache (month)				15.2 ± 24.0
Tablet intake/month (n)		1.8 ± 2.1	3.2 ± 2.8	2.5 ± 3.0

Data expressed as mean ± SD. HV healthy volunteers; MOii episodic migraneurs without aura studied interictally; MOi episodic migraneurs without aura studied ictally; CM chronic migraine patients; N number of subjects.

electrode was on the right arm [10]. SSEP signals were amplified with a Digitimer™ D360 pre-amplifier (Digitimer Ltd, UK) (band-pass 0.05-2500 Hz, Gain 1000) and recorded with a CED™ power1401 device (Cambridge Electronic Design Ltd, Cambridge, UK).

Subjects sat relaxed in a comfortable chair in a well-lit room with eyes open. They were asked to fix their attention on the stimulus-induced thumb movement. During continuous median-nerve stimulation at the wrist, we collected 500 sweeps of 50 ms, sampled at 5000 Hz. All recordings were acquired and processed using the Signal™ software package, version 4.10 (CED Ltd). Artefacts were automatically rejected using the Signal™ artefact rejection tool if the signal amplitude exceeded 90% of analog-to-digital converter (ADC) range and controlled by visual inspection. This approach we made sure to exclude all severe artefacts but not to remove any signal systematically because background EEG amplitudes are larger in some

subjects than in others. The EP-signal was corrected off-line for DC-drifts, eye movements and blinks. Five hundred artefact-free evoked responses recorded in each subject were averaged ("grand average").

Low-frequency SSEPs

After digital filtering of the signal between 0–450 Hz, the various SSEP components (N13, N20, P25 and N33) were identified according to their respective latencies. We measured peak-to-peak amplitudes of the cervical N13 component (recorded under the active Cv5 electrode), and the cortical N20-P25 and P25-N33 components (recorded under the active C3′ scalp electrode).

Thereafter, the first 200 evoked responses were partitioned in 2 sequential blocks of 100 responses (Figure 1). Each block was averaged off-line ("block averages") and analyzed for N20-P25 amplitudes. Sensitization was defined as an increased N20-P25 amplitude recorded during

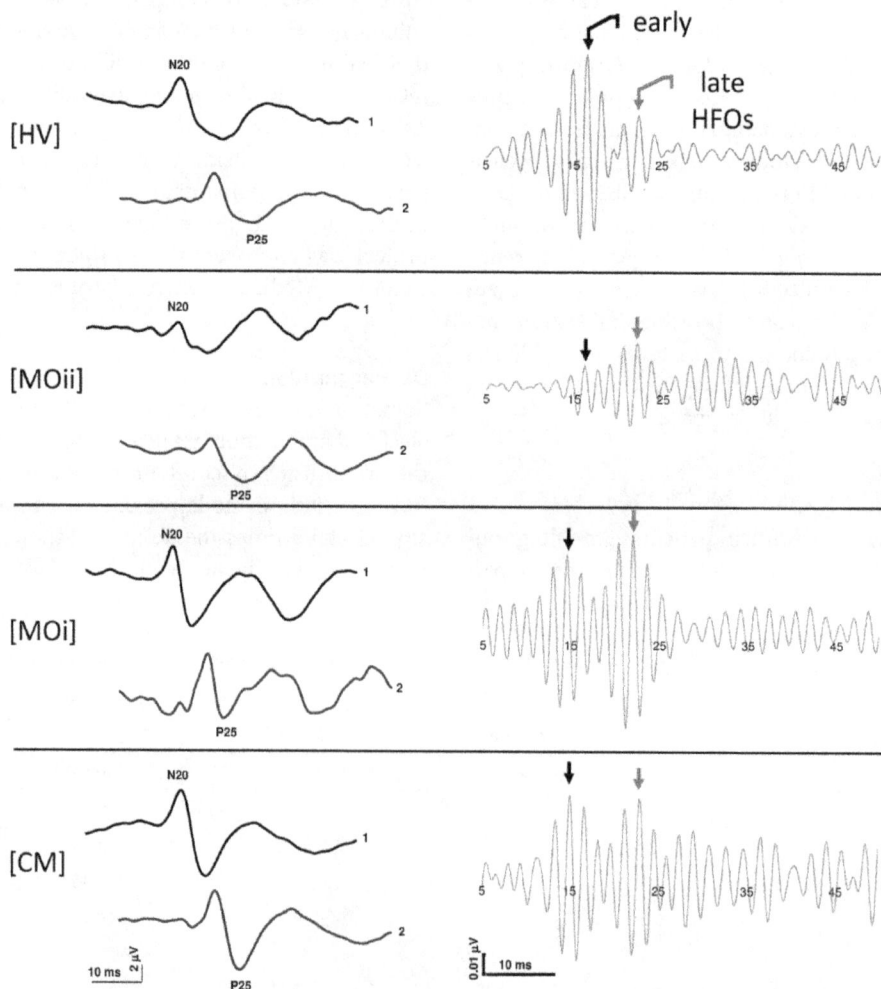

Figure 1 Schematic representation of the changes in somatosensory evoked potentials (SSEPs) N20-P25 amplitude habituation (left panel) and early and late high-frequency oscillations (HFOs) (right panel) in patients in comparison to the responses obtained from a healthy volunteer. (HV, healthy volunteer; MOii, migraine without aura between attacks; MOi, migraine during the attack, CM, chronic migraine).

block 1 (after a low number of 100 stimuli), whereas habituation was expressed as the change in N20-P25 amplitude in block 2 compared to block 1 (over a high number of 200 repetitive stimuli) [10].

High-frequency oscillations (HFOs)

According to the method described elsewhere [6,22], digital zero-phase shift band-pass filtering between 450 and 750 Hz (Barlett-Hanning window, 51 filter coefficients) was applied off-line in order to extract the HFOs embedded in the parietal N20 SSEP component. In the majority of the recorded traces we were able to identify two separate bursts of HFOs: an early burst occurred in the latency interval of the ascending slope of the conventional N20 component and a late burst in the time interval of the descending slope of N20, sometimes extending into the ascending slope of the N33 peak. In general, the frequency of the oscillations was higher in the first than in the second HFO burst and in between the early and late bursts there was a clear frequency and amplitude decrease, which allowed the two bursts to be separated. In recordings in which a clear distinction between the two components was not possible, we considered HFOs occurring before the N20 peak as early burst and those after the N20 peak as late burst.

After eliminating the stimulus artefact, we measured the latency of the negative oscillatory maximum and the maximum peak-to-peak amplitude separately on the two HFO bursts.

Statistical methods

We used the Statistical Package for the Social Sciences (SPSS) for Windows, version 19.0 for all analyses. For grand average SSEPs, component amplitudes were tested in a one-way analysis of variance (ANOVA) with group factor "subjects" (CM patients, MOii and MOi patients, healthy volunteers). To assess changes in SSEP amplitude between blocks 1 and 2, SSEP N20-P25 amplitudes were tested with a repeated-measure ANOVA with group factor "subjects". Tukey's test was used for post hoc analyses. Pearson's correlation coefficient was calculated to test correlations between SSEP amplitudes or habituation and clinical data (disease duration, days with headache, duration of chronic headache). P values of less than 0.05 were considered to indicate statistical significance.

Results

Assessable SSEP recordings were obtained from all patients and controls participating in the study (explicative traces in Figure 1).

Low-frequency (LF-) SSEPs

On grand average SSEP recordings after electrical median nerve stimulation, latencies of N13, N20, P25 and N33 components were not different between groups (for each measure $F_{(3,69)}$, $p > 0.05$).

ANOVA testing SSEP amplitude block averages revealed a main effect for factors group ($F_{(3,69)} = 6.08$, $p < 001$) and a significant interaction of group by block ($F_{(3,69)} = 4.94$, $p = 0.003$). Post hoc analysis showed that the 1st block N20-P25 amplitude was higher in patients with CM ($p = 0.04$) and MOi ($p = 0.02$) and tended to be lower in those with MOii ($p = 0.06$) when compared with HV (Figure 2). Besides, the 1st N20-P25 amplitude block was higher in CM than in MOii patients ($p < 0.001$). In HV, MOi, and CM patients, N20-P25 amplitude decreased from block 1 to block 2, i.e. habituated (slope –0.28 in HV, -0.13 in MOi, -0.39 in CM, $p = 0.594$), while in patients with MOii it increased, i.e. did not habituate (+0.40, $p = 0.002$ vs HV, $p = 0.01$ vs MOi, $p = 0.001$ vs MOii, Figure 2).

Only when patients with episodic and chronic migraine were pooled together, the correlation test revealed that monthly days with headache correlated negatively ($r = –0.366$, $p = 0.01$) with the amplitude slope of LF-SSEP N20-P25, a measure of habituation. The N20-P25 1st amplitude block correlated negatively with the linear regression slope ($r = –549$, $p < 0.001$). The visual analogue scale score did not correlate with any of the neurophysiological parameters.

High-frequency oscillations (HFOs)

Maximum peak-to-peak amplitudes of the early HFO burst differed between groups ($F_{(3,69)} = 3.96$, $p = 0.01$). Post hoc analysis revealed that in MOii patients maximum peak-to-peak amplitudes of the early HFO burst were significantly lower than in HV ($p = 0.03$), MOi ($p = 0.001$), and CM ($p = 0.02$) patients (Figure 3).

Maximum peak-to-peak amplitudes of the late HFO burst differed between groups ($F_{(3,69)} = 3.26$, $p = 0.02$). Post hoc analysis showed that in CM and MOi patients maximum peak-to-peak amplitudes of the late HFO burst were significantly higher than in HV ($p = 0.014$ and $p = 0.013$ respectively) and tended to be higher than in MOii patients (both $p = 0.08$) (Figure 3).

Latency of the negative oscillatory maximum of both early and late HFOs did not differ between groups ($F_{(3,69)} = 2.13$, $p = 0.10$; $F_{(3,69)} = 1.43$, $p = 0.23$ respectively).

When subject groups were considered separately, only in CM and MOi patients was there a positive correlation between early and late HFO maximum peak-to-peak amplitudes ($r = 0.584$, $p = 0.009$; $r = 0.526$, $p = 0.02$ respectively). Nonetheless, this positive correlation was still present when all subject groups (HV, MOii, MOi, CM) were combined ($r = 0.546$, $p < 0.001$), while early and late HFO maximum peak-to-peak amplitudes also positively correlated with the BB-SSEP N20-P25 1st amplitude block ($r = 0.359$, $p = 0.002$ and $r = 0.299$, $p = 0.01$ respectively).

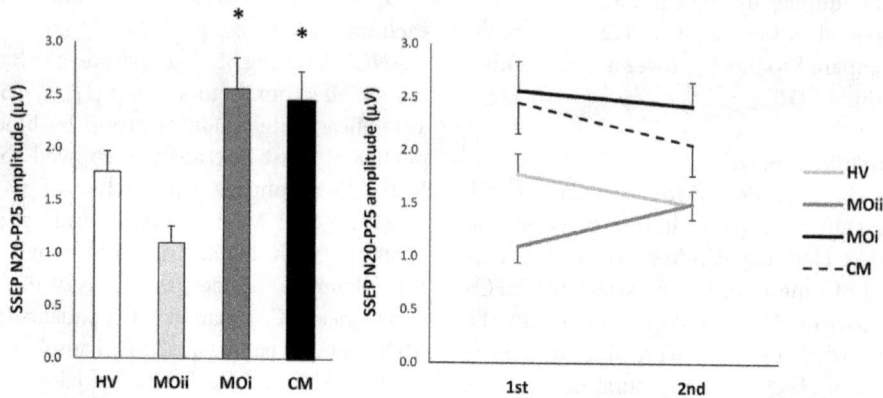

Figure 2 Somatosensory evoked potential (SSEP) 1st amplitude block average (left panel) and habituation (right panel) in each group (data expressed as mean ± SEM). HV, healthy volunteer; MOii, migraine without aura between attacks; MOi, migraine during the attack, CM, chronic migraine. (*P < 0.05 vs. HV).

Discussion

We designed this study to investigate how headache chronification alters subcortico/cortical somatosensory response patterns of episodic migraine patients experiencing progression to chronic migraine without medication overuse.

In our episodic migraineurs between attacks, we have confirmed previous results showing, on the one hand, that the LF-SSEP N20-P25 amplitude lacks habituation during stimulus repetition despite an initially low response amplitude [10,22], and that this comes in parallel to a reduced somatosensory thalamocortical activity [6,23], as reflected by the low amplitude of the early HFO, on the other hand.

Chronic migraine patients have shown a neurophysiological pattern quite similar to that of episodic migraineurs recorded during an attack. In fact, both groups of patients were characterized by higher amplitudes after low numbers of median nerve electrical stimuli (block 1), reflecting sensory cortex sensitization, and by response habituation over sequential block averages. This combination of subcortico/cortical electrophysiological patterns observed in our chronic migraineurs was previously defined as a condition of "never-ending migraine attack" [22]. Moreover, after band-pass filtering, in both CM and MOi patients the interictal episodic amplitude reduction normalized, besides the amplitudes of the primary cortical component consistently increasing with respect to HV and MOii.

In migraine, a strong relationship between clinical and neurophysiological profiles has been demonstrated previously. In episodic migraine, several studies have confirmed between attacks that the amplitude of sensory evoked potentials decreased or tended to be decreased

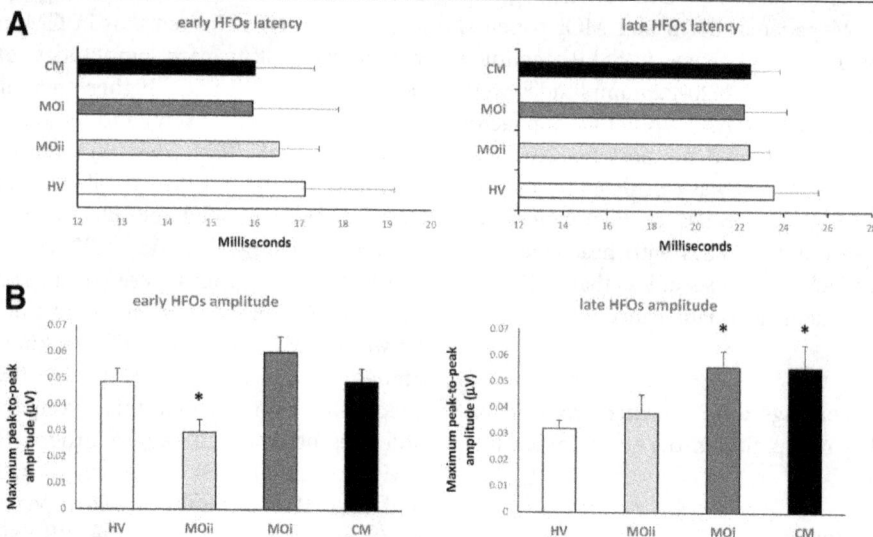

Figure 3 High-frequency oscillations (HFOs) latency of the negative oscillatory maximum (A) and maximum peak-to-peak amplitude (B), separately on the early (left panel) and late (right panel) HFO bursts (data expressed as mean ± SEM). (*P < 0.05 vs. HV).

for low numbers of delivered stimuli and lack of habituation during subsequent block averages [9,10,22]. Contrariwise, close to or during an attack, initial SSEP amplitude increased and deficit of habituation normalized [10,13,16] demonstrating that, on the one hand, the cortical activation state changes between the interictal and ictal periods, and that sensitization disappears between attacks, on the other hand. The electrocortical pattern we found here in our CM patients may thus suggest that the sensory cortex is persistently locked in an "ictal"-like state, associating with both sensitization and habituation. This pattern contrasts with that of episodic migraine where the transition between two electrocortical states (habituation and its lack) alternates following the recurrence of the migraine cycle (ictal and interictal). Similar results were recently observed in a visual EP study [11]. Moreover, this electrophysiological pattern partially differs from that found in chronic headache due to medication overuse (MOH) where, after a similar initial increase in response amplitude, a further increase was observed during stimuli repetitions [10]. Therefore, we considered MOH patients as locked in a "pre-ictal" state, in analogy with the cortical response pattern detected a few days before the beginning of an attack in episodic migraine [15,16]. Nevertheless, further underscoring the clinico-electrophysiological inter-relationship in migraine, this phenomenon in MOH evolved from migraine, was strongly dependent on the drug of overuse, since it was maximal in patients overusing NSAIDs and almost non-existent in those who overuse only triptans [10].

From a behavioural point of view, two distinct and independent processes govern the outcome of repetitive stereotyped sensory stimulation: an increasing one called sensitization, and a reducing one called habituation [24,25]. Sensitization occurs at the beginning of the test session and is responsible for the transitory increase in response amplitude, whereas habituation occurs throughout the test session, and is responsible for the late response decrement [26]. From a physiological point of view, demonstrative of central sensitization are the plastic changes in neural networks devoted to the processing of pain information [27] that results in abnormal neural excitability with decreased nociceptive thresholds and increased responsiveness to noxious and usually innocuous peripheral stimuli, such as, in our case, somatosensory ones [28]. Experimental studies in animals [29] and humans [30] show that SSEP amplitudes increase when transient intense activation of nociceptive afferents induces central sensitization, as happens in clinical pain conditions including chronic headache. Our study shows that sensitization, as reflected by increased initial SSEP amplitudes, is equally present in CM and MOi, although we managed not to record CM patients during a full-blown migraine attack. In CM and episodic migraine attacks central sensitization is associated with increased

excitability both at the trigeminal system [31,32] and the supraspinal levels [33,34]. Interestingly, from our correlation analysis it emerges that the more pronounced the habituation, the more the CM number of headache days and sensory sensitization increase. This further reinforces the evidence for a strong relationship between clinical and neurophysiological features in migraine. A well-recognized clinical expression of central sensitization is cutaneous allodynia, which was shown to be prevalent during episodic migraine attacks at cephalic and extracephalic sites [35,36]. This phenomenon is even more evident in chronic migraine [37-39]. Based on animal models of experimental pain [40,41], some hypothesized that temporary sensitization of third-order thalamic neurons receiving convergent input from the dura, periorbital skin, and skin areas at different body sites explains the spread of cutaneous allodynia beyond the initial pain area during an attack of migraine [36,42]. In a recent study, Burstein and colleagues (2010) studied the effects of sensitizing skin stimuli on the activity of third-order trigeminovascular neurons in the rat thalamus, and on thalamic activation registered by fMRI during migraine in humans. On the one hand, the rat thalamus exhibited long-lasting hyperexcitability to cephalic and extracephalic skin stimuli in response to sensitizing inflammatory soup, and patients undergoing migraine experienced acute thalamic activation during the fMRI in response to extracephalic brush and heat stimuli, on the other hand [42]. The latter data indicate that allodynia is associated with sensitization of third-order thalamic neurons. Taking into account the latter evidence, our finding that the migraine attack modifies a neuronal activity (early HFO) that is generated in the thalamus is not surprising. We observed in both CM and episodic migraineurs recorded ictally an amplitude increase of the usually low thalamo-cortical activation (early HFO) of the interictal episodic migraineurs in parallel with a rise in primary cortical activation (late HFO). These findings may contribute to shed light on the mechanisms of central sensitization, since the elusive mechanisms that are able to ignite the cascade of events that finally lead to an attack facilitate the thalamic activity by reducing latency and augmenting amplitude and, in turn, enhance primary cortical activation at the low (1st SSEP amplitude block) and high frequency bands (late HFOs). This interpretation is supported by the direct correlation we found between the amplitude of the early and that of the late HFO components: in other words, the more the amplitude of the thalamic component increased, the more the cortical activation was enhanced, especially in CM and MOi patients. Furthermore, from the Pearson's analysis it also emerged that the more this sequential thalamic and cortical HF oscillatory activation increased, the more marked the sensitization of the LF-SSEP N20-P25 1st amplitude block.

Only hypotheses can be made about the neural mechanisms by which thalamic neurons become facilitated in CM and in MOi. This process may primarily involve sequential sensitization of first-order or second-order trigeminovascular neurons probably through an evident (aura) or silent (without aura) cortical spreading depression or, more likely, through an indirect activation of pain modulatory structures in the brainstem (raphe magnus, locus coeruleus and other aminergic nuclei) and the forebrain (periaqueductal gray, rostroventral medulla) [43,44]. That the brainstem plays a relevant role in mediating and maintaining central sensitization was recently confirmed by functional neuroimaging studies in healthy humans [45,46]. In Migraine, clear examples of monoaminergic brainstem activation come from both neurophysiology [12,47] and neuroimaging studies where the dorsal rostral brainstem, which contains state-setting aminergic, including serotonergic, nuclei projecting to the thalamus and cortex, was activated immediately before [48] and during an attack of episodic [49,50] and chronic [4,51] migraine.

Conclusions

In conclusion, we show for the first time that not only is the response pattern of the somatosensory cortex in CM patients similar to that found during a migraine attack in episodic migraine patients, in such a way that both habituate normally, as previously observed with visual responses [52], but also that they show an initial response sensitization. Moreover, from the analysis of high-frequency oscillations, it clearly emerges that this sensory sensitization may be explained by the fact that in both groups, the connections between the thalamus and cortex intensify compared to episodic migraine between attacks. Whether this electro-functional behaviour is primary or secondary to daily headache, thus reflecting an electrophysiological fingerprint of the somatosensory system central sensitization process remains to be determined.

Abbreviations
CM: Chronic Migraine; HFOs: High-Frequency Oscillations; HV: Healthy Volunteer; LF: Low-Frequency; MOii: Migraineur without aura recorded interictally; MOi: Migraineur without aura recorded ictally; SSEP: Somatosensory Evoked Potential.

Competing interests
The authors declare that they have no competing interests.

Authors' contributions
GC and EI made substantial contributions to interpretation of data as well as in drafting the manuscript. MS, CDL and FP were implied in the interpretation of data as well as in drafting the manuscript; MB and EI were implied in recording and analyzing data. All authors read and approved the final manuscript.

Author details
[1]G.B. Bietti Foundation IRCCS, Department of Neurophysiology of Vision and Neurophthalmology G.B. Bietti Foundation-IRCCS, Via Livenza 3, Rome 00198, Italy. [2]Department of Medico-Surgical Sciences and Biotechnologies, "Sapienza" University of Rome Polo Pontino, Latina, Italy. [3]Don Carlo Gnocchi Onlus Foundation, Milan, Italy. [4]IRCCS-Neuromed, Pozzilli, IS, Italy.

References
1. Stovner L, Andree C (2010) Prevalence of headache in Europe: a review for the Eurolight project. J Headache Pain 11:289–299
2. Martelletti P, Birbeck G, Katsarava Z, Jensen R, Stovner L, Steiner T, et al. (2013) The Global Burden of Disease survey 2010, Lifting The Burden and thinking outside-the-box on headache disorders. J Headache Pain 14:13
3. Headache Classification Committee of the International Headache Society (IHS) (2013) The International Classification of Headache Disorders, 3rd edition (beta version). Cephalalgia 33:629–808
4. Matharu MS, Bartsch T, Ward N, Frackowiak RSJ, Weiner R, Goadsby PJ, et al. (2004) Central neuromodulation in chronic migraine patients with suboccipital stimulators: a PET study. Brain 127:220–230
5. Sprenger T, Borsook D (2012) Migraine changes the brain: neuroimaging makes its mark. Curr Opin Neurol 25:252–262
6. Coppola G, Vandenheede M, Di Clemente L, Ambrosini A, Fumal A, De Pasqua V, et al. (2005) Somatosensory evoked high-frequency oscillations reflecting thalamo-cortical activity are decreased in migraine patients between attacks. Brain 128:98–103
7. Coppola G, De Pasqua V, Pierelli F, Schoenen J (2012) Effects of repetitive transcranial magnetic stimulation on somatosensory evoked potentials and high frequency oscillations in migraine. Cephalalgia 32:700–709
8. Brighina F, Cosentino G, Vigneri S, Talamanca S, Palermo A, Giglia G, et al. (2011) Abnormal facilitatory mechanisms in motor cortex of migraine with aura. Eur J Pain 15:928–935
9. Coppola G, Pierelli F, Schoenen J (2009) Habituation and migraine. Neurobiol Learn Mem 92:249–259
10. Coppola G, Currà A, Di Lorenzo C, Parisi V, Gorini M, Sava SL, et al. (2010) Abnormal cortical responses to somatosensory stimulation in medication-overuse headache. BMC Neurol 10:126
11. Coppola G, Parisi V, Di Lorenzo C, Serrao M, Magis D, Schoenen J, et al. (2013) Lateral inhibition in visual cortex of migraine patients between attacks. J Headache Pain 14:20
12. Evers S, Quibeldey F, Grotemeyer KH, Suhr B, Husstedt IW (1999) Dynamic changes of cognitive habituation and serotonin metabolism during the migraine interval. Cephalalgia 19:485–491
13. Judit A, Sándor PS, Schoenen J (2000) Habituation of visual and intensity dependence of auditory evoked cortical potentials tends to normalize just before and during the migraine attack. Cephalalgia 20:714–719
14. Kropp P, Gerber WD (1995) Contingent negative variation during migraine attack and interval: evidence for normalization of slow cortical potentials during the attack. Cephalalgia 15:123–8. discussion 78
15. Kropp P, Gerber WD (1998) Prediction of migraine attacks using a slow cortical potential, the contingent negative variation. Neurosci Lett 257:73–76
16. Siniatchkin M, Kropp P, Gerber WD, Stephani U (2000) Migraine in childhood–are periodically occurring migraine attacks related to dynamic changes of cortical information processing? Neurosci Lett 279:1–4
17. Coppola G, Schoenen J (2012) Cortical excitability in chronic migraine. Curr Pain Headache Rep 16:93–100
18. Lorenzo C, Coppola G, Currà A, Grieco G, Santorelli F, Lepre C, et al. (2012) Cortical response to somatosensory stimulation in medication overuse headache patients is influenced by angiotensin converting enzyme (ACE) I/D genetic polymorphism. Cephalalgia 32:1189–1197
19. Gobbelé R, Buchner H, Curio G (1998) High-frequency (600 Hz) SEP activities originating in the subcortical and cortical human somatosensory system. Electroencephalogr Clin Neurophysiol 108:182–189
20. Porcaro C, Coppola G, Di Lorenzo G, Zappasodi F, Siracusano A, Pierelli F, et al. (2009) Hand somatosensory subcortical and cortical sources assessed by functional source separation: an EEG study. Hum Brain Mapp 30:660–674
21. Porcaro C, Coppola G, Pierelli F, Seri S, Di L, Tomasevic L, et al. (2013) Multiple frequency functional connectivity in the hand somatosensory network: an EEG study. Clin Neurophysiol 124:1216–1224
22. Ozkul Y, Uckardes A (2002) Median nerve somatosensory evoked potentials in migraine. Eur J Neurol 9:227–232
23. Schoenen J (2011) Is chronic migraine a never-ending migraine attack? Pain 152:239–240
24. Thompson RF, Spencer WA (1966) Habituation: a model phenomenon for the study of neuronal substrates of behavior. Psychol Rev 73:16–43

25. Groves PM, Thompson RF (1970) Habituation: a dual-process theory. Psychol Rev 77:419–450
26. Rankin CH, Abrams T, Barry RJ, Bhatnagar S, Clayton DF, Colombo J, et al. (2009) Habituation revisited: an updated and revised description of the behavioral characteristics of habituation. Neurobiol Learn Mem 92:135–138
27. Schmidt-Wilcke T, Leinisch E, Straube A, Kämpfe N, Draganski B, Diener HC, et al. (2005) Gray matter decrease in patients with chronic tension type headache. Neurology 65:1483–1486
28. Woolf CJ, Wall PD (1986) Relative effectiveness of C primary afferent fibers of different origins in evoking a prolonged facilitation of the flexor reflex in the rat. J Neurosci 6:1433–1442
29. Lebrun P, Manil J, Colin F (2000) Formalin-induced central sensitization in the rat: somatosensory evoked potential data. Neurosci Lett 283:113–116
30. Baron R, Baron Y, Disbrow E, Roberts TP (2000) Activation of the somatosensory cortex during Abeta-fiber mediated hyperalgesia. A MSI study. Brain Res 871:75–82
31. Kaube H, Katsarava Z, Przywara S, Drepper J, Ellrich J, Diener HC, et al. (2002) Acute migraine headache: possible sensitization of neurons in the spinal trigeminal nucleus? Neurology 58:1234–1238
32. De Marinis M, Pujia A, Colaizzo E, Accornero N (2007) The blink reflex in "chronic migraine". Clin Neurophysiol 118:457–463
33. de Tommaso M, Guido M, Libro G, Losito L, Sciruicchio V, Monetti C, et al. (2002) Abnormal brain processing of cutaneous pain in migraine patients during the attack. Neurosci Lett 333:29–32
34. de Tommaso M, Valeriani M, Guido M, Libro G, Specchio LM, Tonali P, et al. (2003) Abnormal brain processing of cutaneous pain in patients with chronic migraine. Pain 101:25–32
35. Schoenen J, Bottin D, Hardy F, Gerard P (1991) Cephalic and extracephalic pressure pain thresholds in chronic tension-type headache. Pain 47:145–149
36. Burstein R, Cutrer MF, Yarnitsky D (2000) The development of cutaneous allodynia during a migraine attack clinical evidence for the sequential recruitment of spinal and supraspinal nociceptive neurons in migraine. Brain 123(Pt 8):1703–1709
37. Bigal ME, Ashina S, Burstein R, Reed ML, Buse D, Serrano D, et al. (2008) Prevalence and characteristics of allodynia in headache sufferers: a population study. Neurology 70:1525–1533
38. Lovati C, D'Amico D, Bertora P, Rosa S, Suardelli M, Mailland E, et al. (2008) Acute and interictal allodynia in patients with different headache forms: an Italian pilot study. Headache 48:272–277
39. Filatova E, Latysheva N, Kurenkov A (2008) Evidence of persistent central sensitization in chronic headaches: a multi-method study. J Headache Pain 9:295–300
40. Guilbaud G, Kayser V, Benoist J, Gautron M (1986) Modifications in the responsiveness of rat ventrobasal thalamic neurons at different stages of carrageenin-produced inflammation. Brain Res 385:86–98
41. Guilbaud G, Benoist J, Jazat F, Gautron M (1990) Neuronal responsiveness in the ventrobasal thalamic complex of rats with an experimental peripheral mononeuropathy. J Neurophysiol 64:1537–1554
42. Burstein R, Jakubowski M, Garcia-Nicas E, Kainz V, Bajwa Z, Hargreaves R, et al. (2010) Thalamic sensitization transforms localized pain into widespread allodynia. Ann Neurol 68:81–91
43. Lambert G, Truong L, Zagami A (2011) Effect of cortical spreading depression on basal and evoked traffic in the trigeminovascular sensory system. Cephalalgia 31:1439–1451
44. Goadsby P, Akerman S (2012) The trigeminovascular system does not require a peripheral sensory input to be activated–migraine is a central disorder. Focus on 'Effect of cortical spreading depression on basal and evoked traffic in the trigeminovascular sensory system'. Cephalalgia 32:3–5
45. Zambreanu L, Wise R, Brooks J, Iannetti G, Tracey I (2005) A role for the brainstem in central sensitisation in humans. Evidence from functional magnetic resonance imaging. Pain 114:397–407
46. Lee M, Zambreanu L, Menon D, Tracey I (2008) Identifying brain activity specifically related to the maintenance and perceptual consequence of central sensitization in humans. J Neurosci 28:11642–11649
47. Sand T, Zhitniy N, White LR, Stovner LJ (2008) Brainstem auditory-evoked potential habituation and intensity-dependence related to serotonin metabolism in migraine: a longitudinal study. Clin Neurophysiol 119:1190–1200
48. Sakai Y, Dobson C, Diksic M, Aubé M, Hamel E (2008) Sumatriptan normalizes the migraine attack-related increase in brain serotonin synthesis. Neurology 70:431–439
49. Weiller C, May A, Limmroth V, Jüptner M, Kaube H, Schayck RV, et al. (1995) Brain stem activation in spontaneous human migraine attacks. Nat Med 1:658–660
50. Bahra A, Matharu MS, Buchel C, Frackowiak RS, Goadsby PJ (2001) Brainstem activation specific to migraine headache. Lancet 357:1016–1017
51. Aurora S, Barrodale P, Tipton R, Khodavirdi A (2007) Brainstem dysfunction in chronic migraine as evidenced by neurophysiological and positron emission tomography studies. Headache 47:996–1003
52. Chen W, Wang S, Fuh J, Lin C, Ko Y, Lin Y, et al. (2011) Persistent ictal-like visual cortical excitability in chronic migraine. Pain 152:254–258

Permissions

List of Contributors

Sanjay Prakash
Department of Neurology, Medical College, O-19, doctor's quarter, jail road, Baroda, Gujarat 390001, India

Pooja Belani, Ashish Susvirkar and Aditi Trivedi
Department of Medicine, Medical College, Baroda Gujarat, India

Sunil Ahuja and Animesh Patel
Department of Psychiatry, Medical College, Baroda, Gujarat 390001, India

Rongfei Wang, Zhao Dong, Xiaoyan Chen, Mingjie Zhang, Fan Yang, Xiaolan Zhang, Weiquan Jia and Shengyuan Yu
Department of Neurology, Chinese PLA General Hospital, Fuxing Road 28, Haidian District, Beijing 100853, China

Yu-Chen Cheng
Section of Neurology, Department of Internal Medicine, Far Eastern
Memorial Hospital, No. 21, Sec. 2, Nanya S. Rd., Ban-Chiao Dist., New Taipei City 220, Taiwan
Department of Neurology, National Yang-Ming University School of Medicine, Taipei, Taiwan

Kuei-Hong Kuo
Department of Radiology, Far Eastern Memorial Hospital, New Taipei, Taiwan
Department of Neurology, National Yang-Ming University School of Medicine, Taipei, Taiwan

Tzu-Hsien Lai
Department of Neurology, Neurological Institute, Taipei Veterans General Hospital, Taipei, Taiwan
Department of Neurology, National Yang-Ming University School of Medicine, Taipei, Taiwan
Section of Neurology, Department of Internal Medicine, Far Eastern
Memorial Hospital, No. 21, Sec. 2, Nanya S. Rd., Ban-Chiao Dist., New Taipei City 220, Taiwan

Faisal Mohammad Amin, Elisabet Lundholm, Anders Hougaard, Nanna Arngrim, Linda Wiinberg and Messoud Ashina
Danish Headache Center and Department of Neurology, Glostrup Hospital, Faculty of Health and Medical Sciences, University of Copenhagen, Nordre Ringvej 57, DK-2600 Glostrup, Denmark

Patrick JH de Koning
Division of Image Processing, Department of Radiology, Leiden University Medical Center, Leiden, Netherlands

Henrik BW Larsson
Functional Imaging Unit, Diagnostic Department, Glostrup Hospital, Faculty of Health and Medical Sciences, University of Copenhagen, Copenhagen, Denmark

Yassine Zouitina and Mathilde Terrier
Department of Neurology, Amiens University Hospital, 1 Place Victor Pauchet, F-80054 Amiens cedex, France

Marie Hyra
Department of Physical Medicine and Rehabilitation, Amiens University Hospital, Amiens, France

Djohar Seryer
Department of Radiology, Amiens University Hospital, Amiens, France

Jean-Marc Chillon
INSERM U1088, Amiens, France
Department of Clinical Pharmacology, Amiens University Hospital, Amiens, France

Jean-Marc Bugnicourt
Laboratory of Functional Neuroscience and Pathology (EA 4559), Department of Neurology, Amiens University Hospital, Amiens, France
Department of Neurology, Amiens University Hospital, 1 Place Victor Pauchet, F-80054 Amiens cedex, France

Rongfei Wang, Zhao Dong, Xiaoyan Chen, Ruozhuo Liu and Shengyuan Yu
Department of Neurology, Chinese PLA General Hospital, Fuxing Road 28, Haidian District, Beijing 100853, China

Mingjie Zhang
Medical school, Nankai University, Tianjin, China
Department of Neurology, Chinese PLA General

Hospital, Fuxing Road 28, Haidian District, Beijing 100853, China

Jinglong Wu
Biomedical Engineering Laboratory, Graduate School of Natural Science and Technology, Okayama University, 3-1-1 Tsushima-Naka, Okayama 700-8530, Japan

Shih-Pin Chen and Yen-Feng Wang
Faculty of Medicine, School of Medicine, National Yang-Ming University, Taipei, Taiwan
Department of Neurology, Neurological Institute, Taipei Veterans General Hospital, Taipei, Taiwan
Brain Research Center, National Yang-Ming University, Taipei, Taiwan

Jong-Ling Fuh and Shuu-Jiun Wang
Faculty of Medicine, School of Medicine, National Yang-Ming University, Taipei, Taiwan
Department of Neurology, Neurological Institute, Taipei Veterans General Hospital, Taipei, Taiwan
Brain Research Center, National Yang-Ming University, Taipei, Taiwan
Institute of Brain Science, National Yang-Ming University, Taipei, Taiwan

Po-Hsun Huang
Department of Internal Medicine, Division of Cardiology, Taipei Veterans General Hospital, Taipei, Taiwan
Faculty of Medicine, School of Medicine, National Yang-Ming University, Taipei, Taiwan

Chin-Wen Chi
Department and Institute of Pharmacology, School of Medicine, National Yang-Ming University, Taipei, Taiwan
Department of Medical Research & Education, Taipei Veterans General Hospital, Taipei, Taiwan

Aynur Yilmaz Avci, Ulku Sibel Benli and Munire Kilinc
Department of Neurology, Baskent University, Saray Mah, Yunusemre cad, No. 1, Alanya-Antalya 07400 Ankara, Turkey

Hatice Lakadamyali
Department of Radiology, Baskent University, Ankara, Turkey

Serap Arikan
Department of Biochemistry, Baskent University, Ankara, Turkey

Gianluca Coppola, Vincenzo Parisi and Antonio Di Renzo
G.B. Bietti Foundation-IRCCS, Department of Neurophysiology of Vision and Neurophthalmology, Via Livenza 3, 00198 Rome, Italy

Mariano Serrao, Martina Bracaglia and Davide Di Lenola
Department of Medical and Surgical Sciences and Biotechnologies, "Sapienza" University of Rome Polo Pontino, Latina, Italy

Cherubino Di Lorenzo
Fondazione Don Gnocchi, Milan, Italy

Francesco Martelli and Antonello Fadda
Istituto Superiore di Sanità, Dipartimento Tecnologie e Salute, Rome, Italy

Jean Schoenen
Headache Research Unit, Department of Neurology-CHR Citadelle, University of Liège, Liège, Belgium

Francesco Pierelli
IRCCS-Neuromed, Pozzilli, IS, Italy
Department of Medical and Surgical Sciences and Biotechnologies, "Sapienza" University of Rome Polo Pontino, Latina, Italy

Chul-Ho Kim, Min-Uk Jang, Hui-Chul Choi and Jong-Hee Sohn
Department of Neurology, Chuncheon Sacred Heart Hospital, Hallym
University College of Medicine, 153 Gyo-dong, Chuncheon-si, Gangwon-do 200-704, Republic of Korea

Thomas M. Kinfe
Division of Functional Neurosurgery and Neuromodulation, Department of Neurosurgery, Rheinische Friedrich-Wilhelms University, Regina-Pacis-Weg 3, 53113 Bonn, Germany
Department of Neurosurgery, Rheinische Friedrich-Wilhelms University, Regina-Pacis-Weg 3, 53113 Bonn, Germany

Hartmut Vatter, Bogdan Pintea and Sajjad Muhammad
Department of Neurosurgery, Rheinische Friedrich-Wilhelms University, Regina-Pacis-Weg 3, 53113 Bonn, Germany

Sebastian Zaremba
Sleep Medicine, Department of Neurology, Rheinische Friedrich-Wilhelms University, Sigmund-Freud-Str. 25, D-53105 Bonn, Germany
German Centre for Neurodegenerative Diseases (DZNE), Ernst-Robert-Curtius-Str. 12, 53117 Bonn, Germany

Sandra Roeske
German Centre for Neurodegenerative Diseases (DZNE), Ernst-Robert-Curtius-Str. 12, 53117 Bonn, Germany

Bruce J. Simon
electroCore, LLC, 150 Allen Road, Suite 201, Basking Ridge, NJ 07920, USA

Mengqi Liu, Shuangfeng Liu and Lin Ma
Department of Radiology, Chinese PLA General Hospital, Beijing 100853, China

Shengyuan Yu and Xiaoyan Chen
Department of Neurology, Chinese PLA General Hospital, Beijing 100853, China

Zhiye Chen
Department of Neurology, Chinese PLA General Hospital, Beijing 100853, China
Department of Radiology, Chinese PLA General Hospital, Beijing 100853, China

Siyun Shu
Institute of Cognitive Neuroscience, South China Normal University, Guangzhou 510631, China

Gianluca Coppola, Antonio Di Renzo and Vincenzo Parisi
Research Unit of Neurophysiology of Vision and Neurophthalmology, G.B. Bietti Foundation-IRCCS, Via Livenza 3, 00198 Rome, Italy

Marco Scapeccia and Emanuele Tinelli
Department of Neurology and Psychiatry, Neuroradiology Section, "Sapienza" University of Rome, Rome, Italy

Chiara Lepre
Department of Medico-Surgical Sciences and Biotechnologies, Neurology Section, "Sapienza" University of Rome, Rome, Italy

Cherubino Di Lorenzo
Don Carlo Gnocchi Onlus Foundation, Milan, Italy

Giorgio Di Lorenzo
Laboratory of Psychophysiology, Psychiatric Clinic, Department of Systems Medicine, University of Rome "Tor Vergata", Rome, Italy

Mariano Serrao
Department of Medico-Surgical Sciences and Biotechnologies, "Sapienza" University of Rome Polo Pontino, Latina, Italy

Francesco Pierelli
IRCCS Neuromed, Pozzilli, (IS), Italy
Department of Medico-Surgical Sciences and Biotechnologies, "Sapienza" University of Rome Polo Pontino, Latina, Italy

Claudio Colonnese
IRCCS Neuromed, Pozzilli, (IS), Italy
Department of Neurology and Psychiatry, Neuroradiology Section, "Sapienza" University of Rome, Rome, Italy

Jean Schoenen
Headache Research Unit, Department of Neurology-CHR Citadelle, University of Liège, Liège, Belgium

Francesca Cortese, Ilaria Bove and Mariano Serrao
Department of Medico-Surgical Sciences and Biotechnologies, Sapienza
University of Rome Polo Pontino, Corso della Repubblica, 79 – 04100, Latina, Italy

Francesco Pierelli
INM Neuromed IRCCS, Pozzilli (IS), Italy
Department of Medico-Surgical Sciences and Biotechnologies, Sapienza University of Rome Polo Pontino, Corso della Repubblica, 79 – 04100, Latina, Italy

Armando Perrotta
INM Neuromed IRCCS, Pozzilli (IS), Italy

Cherubino Di Lorenzo
Don Carlo Gnocchi, Onlus Foundation, Milan, Italy

Maurizio Evangelista
Università Cattolica del Sacro Cuore/CIC, Istituto di Anestesiologia, Rianimazione e Terapia del Dolore, Rome, Italy

Vincenzo Parisi and Gianluca Coppola
G. B. Bietti Foundation IRCCS, Research Unit of Neurophysiology of Vision and Neuro-Ophthalmology, Rome, Italy

Viviana Lo Buono, Lilla Bonanno, Francesco Corallo, Laura Rosa Pisani, Riccardo Lo Presti, Rosario Grugno, Giuseppe Di Lorenzo and Placido Bramanti
IRCCS Centro Neurolesi "Bonino-Pulejo", S.S. 113 Via Palermo, C.da Casazza, 98124 Messina, Italy

Silvia Marino
Department of Biomedical and Dental Sciences and Morphological and Functional Imaging, University of Messina, Messina, Italy
IRCCS Centro Neurolesi "Bonino-Pulejo", S.S. 113 Via Palermo, C.da Casazza, 98124 Messina, Italy

Shuangfeng Liu and Lin Ma
Department of Radiology, Chinese PLA General Hospital, Fuxing Road 28, Beijing 100853, China

Xiaoyan Chen and Shengyuan Yu
Department of Neurology, Chinese PLA General Hospital, Fuxing Road 28, Beijing 100853, China

Mengqi Liu
Department of Radiology, Hainan Branch of Chinese PLA General Hospital, Sanya 572013, China
Department of Radiology, Chinese PLA General Hospital, Fuxing Road 28, Beijing 100853, China

Zhiye Chen
Department of Radiology, Chinese PLA General Hospital, Fuxing Road 28, Beijing 100853, China
Department of Neurology, Chinese PLA General Hospital, Fuxing Road 28, Beijing 100853, China
Department of Radiology, Hainan Branch of Chinese PLA General Hospital, Sanya 572013, China

Joan Crespi and Erling Tronvik
Department of Neurology, St Olav's University Hospital, Edvards Grieg's gate 8, 7030 Trondheim, Norway
Norwegian Advisory Unit on Headaches, Trondheim, Norway
Department of Neuromedicine and Movement Science, NTNU (University of Science and Technology), Trondheim, Norway

Irina Aschehoug
Department of Neuromedicine and Movement Science, NTNU (University of Science and Technology), Trondheim, Norway

Daniel Bratbak
Department of Neurosurgery, St Olav's University Hospital, Trondheim, Norway

Department of Neuromedicine and Movement Science, NTNU (University of Science and Technology), Trondheim, Norway

David Dodick
Department of Neurology, Mayo Clinic, Phoenix, AZ, USA
Department of Neuromedicine and Movement Science, NTNU (University of Science and Technology), Trondheim, Norway

Manjit Matharu
National Hospital of Neurology and Neurosurgery, London, UK

Kent Are Jamtøy
Department of maxillofacial surgery, St Olav's University Hospital, Trondheim, Norway
Department of Neuromedicine and Movement Science, NTNU (University of Science and Technology), Trondheim, Norway

Samaira Younis, Anders Hougaard, Casper Emil Christensen, Mark and Messoud Ashina
Danish Headache Center, Department of Neurology, Rigshospitalet Glostrup, University of Copenhagen, Copenhagen, Denmark

Henrik Bo Wiberg Larsson and Bitsch Vestergaard
Functional Imaging Unit, Department of Clinical Physiology, Nuclear Medicine and PET, Rigshospitalet Glostrup, University of Copenhagen, Copenhagen, Denmark

Esben Thade Petersen
Danish Research Centre for Magnetic Resonance, Centre for Functional and Diagnostic Imaging and research, Copenhagen University Hospital Hvidovre, Copenhagen, Denmark

Olaf Bjarne Paulson
Neurobiology Research Unit, Department of Neurology, Rigshospitalet, University of Copenhagen, Copenhagen, Denmark

Alessandro Tessitore, Francesca Conte, Daniele Corbo and Manuela De Stefano
Department of Neurology, Second University of Naples, Piazza Miraglia 2 - I-80138, Naples, Italy

Antonio Russo, Alfonso Giordano and Gioacchino Tedeschi
Institute for Diagnosis and Care "Hermitage Capodimonte", Naples, Italy

Sossio Cirillo and Mario Cirillo
Neuroradiology Service, Second University of Naples, Naples, Italy

Fabrizio Esposito
Department of Cognitive Neuroscience, Maastricht University, Maastricht, The Netherlands
Department of Medicine and Surgery, University of Salerno, Salerno, Italy

Ling Zhao, Xilin Dong, Yulin Peng, Fumei Wu and Fanrong Liang
Acupuncture and Tuina School, Chengdu University of Traditional Chinese Medicine, Chengdu, Sichuan 610075, China

Wei Qin, Jinbo Sun, Kai Yuan and Jixin Liu
Life Sciences Research Center, School of Life Sciences and Technology, Xidian University, Xi'an, Shanxi 710071, China

Qiyong Gong
Department of Radiology, The Center for Medical Imaging, Huaxi MR Research Center, West China Hospital of Sichuan University, Chengdu, 610041 Sichuan, China

Todd D Rozen and Jennifer L Beams
Department of Neurology, Geisinger Health System, Geisinger Headache Clinic, MC 37-32, 1000 East Mountain Blvd, Wilkes-Barre, PA 18711, USA

Elisa Candeloro, Isabella Canavero, Maurizia Maurelli, Anna Cavallini and Giuseppe Micieli
Cerebrovascular Diseases and Stroke Unit, Department of Emergency Neurology, IRCCS National Institute of Neurology Foundation Casimiro Mondino, Pavia, Italy

Natascia Ghiotto
Neurosonology Unit, Department of Neuropathophysiology, IRCCS National Institute of Neurology Foundation Casimiro Mondino, Pavia, Italy

Paolo Vitali
Department of Neuroradiology, IRCCS National Institute of Neurology Foundation Casimiro Mondino, Pavia, Italy

Jasem Y Al-Hashel
Department of Neurology, Ibn Sina Hospital, Safat 13115 Kuwait City, Kuwait
Department of Medicine, Faculty of Medicine, Health Sciences Centre, Kuwait University, Kuwait City, Kuwait

Samar Farouk Ahmed
Department of Neurology and Psychiatry, Al-Minia University, Minia, Egypt
Department of Neurology, Ibn Sina Hospital, Safat 13115 Kuwait City, Kuwait

Raed Alroughani
Division of Neurology, Amiri Hospital, Qurtoba 73767 Kuwait City, Kuwait
Division of Neurology, Dasman Diabetes Institute, Dasman 15462 Kuwait City, Kuwait

Peter J Goadsby
Wellcome Trust Clinical Research Facility, Kings College Hospital, London, UK

Gianluca Coppola
G.B. Bietti Foundation IRCCS, Department of Neurophysiology of Vision and Neurophthalmology G.B. Bietti Foundation-IRCCS, Via Livenza 3, Rome 00198, Italy

Elisa Iacovelli, Martina Bracaglia and Mariano Serrao
Department of Medico-Surgical Sciences and Biotechnologies, "Sapienza" University of Rome Polo Pontino, Latina, Italy

Cherubino Di Lorenzo
Don Carlo Gnocchi Onlus Foundation, Milan, Italy

Francesco Pierelli
IRCCS-Neuromed, Pozzilli, IS, Italy

Index